ASSESSMENT

in

Speech-Language Pathology

—■—

A Resource Manual

Second Edition

ASSESSMENT
in
Speech-Language Pathology

■

A Resource Manual

SECOND EDITION

Kenneth G. Shipley, Ph.D.
California State University–Fresno

Julie G. McAfee, M.A.

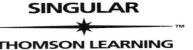

SINGULAR
™
THOMSON LEARNING

Africa • Australia • Canada • Denmark • Japan • Mexico • New Zealand • Philippines
Puerto Rico • Singapore • Spain • United Kingdom • United States

COPYRIGHT © 1998 Delmar. Singular Publishing Group is an imprint of Delmar, a division of Thomson Learning. Thomson Learning™ is a trademark used herein under license.

Printed in Canada
5 6 7 8 9 10 XXX 05 04 03 02 01

For more information, contact Singular Publishing Group, 401 West "A" Street, Suite 325 San Diego, CA 92101-7904; or find us on the World Wide Web at http://www.singpub.com

Library of Congress Cataloging-in-Publication Data:

ISBN: 1-565-93870-4

CONTENTS

Chapter 4 *(continued)*

Chapter 12 *(continued)*

LIST OF TABLES

LIST OF FORMS

LIST OF ILLUSTRATIONS

LIST OF FIGURES

☐ PREFACE ☐

The purpose of the *Assessment in Speech-Language Pathology: A Resource Manual* is to provide students and professionals with a variety of information, materials, and procedures for use in the assessment of communicative disorders. The *Resource Manual* is a practical collection of resource materials applicable to a variety of assessment and diagnostic activities. The items included are practical and easy-to-use. Materials published previously, but unavailable in a single source, as well as materials developed specifically for this work are included.

This second edition features updated and expanded materials included in the first edition, plus the following new materials:

- A separate chapter on the Assessment of Dysphagia, including Assessment of the Tracheostomized Client;
- A new chapter on the Assessment of Three Special Populations: Assessment for Augmentative or Alternative Communication, Assessment of Laryngectomees, and Assessment of Clients with Cleft Lip and/or Palate;
- A new section on the Assessment of Dementia;
- A new section on the Assessment of Right Hemisphere Dysfunction;
- A listing of Standard Medical Abbreviations; and
- Chapter-by-chapter Internet References for pursuing further information.

A valid assessment of an individual's communicative abilities and disabilities is the foundation on which all future clinical activities are based. Clinicians use assessment information to make professional diagnoses and conclusions, identify the need for treatment, determine the focus of treatment, determine the frequency and length of treatment, and identify the need for referral to other professionals. Clinicians also make decisions about the structure of treatment; for example, individual versus group sessions or treatment with or without caregiver involvement. Clearly, all initial clinical decisions are based on information derived from the assessment process.

The following is a general overview of the assessment process:

1. Obtain historical information about the client, the client's family or caregivers, and the nature of the disorder.
2. Interview the client, the client's family or caregivers, or both.
3. Sample and evaluate the client's speech and language use and abilities in the areas of articulation, speech, language, cognition, fluency, voice, and resonance.
4. Evaluate (or screen) the structural and functional integrity of the oral-facial mechanism.
5. Screen the client's hearing or obtain evaluative information about hearing abilities.
6. Evaluate assessment information to determine impressions, diagnosis or conclusions, prognosis, and recommendations.
7. Share clinical findings through an interview with the client or caregiver, formal written records (such as a report), and informal verbal contacts (such as a telephone contact with a physician).

The emphases of an assessment differ depending on the client, the type of disorder, the setting, the client's history, the involvement of the caregiver, and so forth. For example:

- Some disorders will have extensive histories, while others will not.
- Clients will have different primary communicative problems. Some will exhibit problems of articulation, others of voice, still others of fluency, and so forth.
- Some cases will involve extensive interviewing, while others will not.
- Some cases will require detailed written reports, while others will not.

Even though assessment emphases will differ across clients, some consideration of each of the seven general areas just listed will be necessary with most clients.

This resource is divided into two major sections. Part I provides procedures and materials for obtaining assessment information; interpreting assessment findings; and reporting assessment findings to clients, caregivers, and other professionals. It includes case history forms and a wide range of interpretive information; interview questions for various and specific communicative disorders; and materials, instructions, and examples for reporting assessment information.

Part II begins with Chapter 4. This part provides a variety of materials and suggestions for assessing communicative disorders. Chapter 4 includes general assessment procedures, worksheets, and materials that are useful for all speech-language assessments regardless of the specific disorder a client exhibits. Chapters 5 through 10 provide assessment procedures for specific types of communicative disorders. Each of these chapters includes a variety of reference materials, hands-on worksheets, procedural guidelines, and interpretive assessment information that are specifically designed to address the unique characteristics of articulation, fluency, language, voice, resonance, dysphasia, or neurologically based disorders. Chapter 11 presents assessment procedures unique to three special populations—clients who may benefit from augmentative or alternative communication (AAC), laryngectomees, and clients with cleft lip and/or palate. Practical reference materials about the assessment of clients with hearing impairment are provided in Chapter 12.

Appendix A contains information on speech and language differences commonly found with Black, Spanish, and Asian language speakers. Areas to consider when evaluating an assessment instrument, including excerpts from the *Code of Fair Practices in Testing*, are provided in Appendix B. We have attempted to define new or potentially unknown terminology as it was introduced throughout the *Resource Manual*. A Glossary is also included for better understanding of selected terms.

Assessment in Speech-Language Pathology: A Resource Manual can be a valuable resource for beginning or experienced clinicians. To our knowledge, no other manual provides such a comprehensive package of reference materials, explanations of assessment procedures, practical stimulus items, and hands-on worksheets and screening forms. Students and professionals can use these items in a variety of clinical settings. However, the resource is not intended to be a textbook or primary resource for understanding and administering speech-language assessments. We believe that the greatest use of the *Resource Manual* will be as a comprehensive resource for the assessment process. A large and varied collection of materials, guidelines, suggestions, and interpretive information is provided in this single source.

☐ ACKNOWLEDGEMENTS ☐

Our grateful appreciation is extended to our colleagues, friends, and family members who offered support and help with this project. Michelle Austin, Bette J. Baldis, Tracey J. Baldwin, Christine Maul, Deborah Davis, Jeffrey L. Danhauer, Wendy Garabino, M. N. Hegde, Fran Pomaville, Celeste Roseberry-McKibbin, Christine Strike Roussos, and Steven D. Wadsworth reviewed portions or all of the text at various stages of preparation and provided helpful suggestions and comments along the way. We also thank the staff and consultants at Singular Publishing Group, particularly Candice Janco, Marie Linvill, Pam Rider, Randy Stevens, Angie Singh, and Sadanand Singh, for their guidance during the review and production process. Appreciation is also extended to the many publishers and authors who allowed us to include their works in this book. Our families were especially encouraging, supportive, and understanding during the development of this Resource Manual. We extend our love and appreciation to Peggy, Jennifer, Adam, and Mathias.

□ PART I □

Obtaining, Interpreting, and Reporting Assessment Information

□ CHAPTER 1 □

Obtaining Preassessment Information

T horough assessments involve obtaining as much information as possible about your clients and their communicative disorders. We recommend collecting as much information as you can before the actual assessment session is conducted. Primary sources of preassessment information include:

- A written case history;
- An interview with the client, parents, spouse, or other caregivers;
- Information from other professionals.

The preliminary information you gather, combined with your actual assessment results, will enable you to make an accurate diagnosis and develop the most appropriate treatment recommendations possible.

WRITTEN CASE HISTORIES

The written case history is a starting point for understanding clients and their communicative problems. A case history form is typically completed by the client or a caregiver and reviewed by the clinician prior to the initial meeting. This enables the clinician to anticipate those areas that will require assessment, identify topics requiring further clarification, and preselect appropriate evaluation materials and procedures for use during the evaluation session. Be aware, though, that sometimes the value of a case history form as a preassessment tool can be limited because of such possible reliability problems as:

1. *The respondent may not have understood all the terminology on the form.* As a result, inaccurate and/or incomplete information may be provided.

2. *Insufficient time may have been provided to complete the entire form.* Realize that it can take considerable time to collect certain requested information, such as dates of illnesses or developmental history.

3. *The respondent may not have known, or may have only vaguely recalled, certain information.* Naturally, the amount and accuracy of information provided is related to the length and depth of the relationship between the client and the person completing the form. The client's parent, grandparent, spouse, sibling, social worker, teacher, or others will not all have equal knowledge of the client's history and communicative handicap.

4. *Significant time may have elapsed between the onset of the problem and the speech-language assessment.* Respondents will usually have a greater recollection of recent events than events that occurred months or even years ago.

5. *Other life events or circumstances may have hindered the respondent's ability to recall certain information.* For example, the parent of an only child will probably remember developmental milestones more clearly than the parent who has several children. Or, the parent of a child with multiple medical, communicative, and academic problems will likely be less focused on specific speech and language development than the parent of a child who has only a communication disorder.

6. *Cultural differences may have interfered with accurate provision of information.* The respondent may not understand cultural innuendos reflected in the case history's queries or by their own responses.

Clearly, there are potential dangers to overrelying on the information obtained in a case history. However, when viewed cautiously, case histories provide an excellent starting point for understanding clients, the problems they have experienced, and the difficulties they are facing.

In the field of communicative disorders, a standard case history form used by all professionals does not exist (Peterson & Marquardt, 1994; Shipley, 1992). Practitioners in different settings typically develop or adapt forms that reflect the information they feel is needed. Appendix 1–A is a case history form for use with children and Appendix 1–B is designed for use with adults. These are basic forms that can be adapted for your particular practice or setting.

INFORMATION-GETTING INTERVIEWS

Professionals in communicative disorders generally conduct three types of interviews. These are information-getting, information-giving, and counseling interviews (Shipley, 1992). The information-getting interview, sometimes called an intake interview, consists of three phases—the opening, the body, and the closing. The basic content of each phase includes:

Opening Phase

Introduce yourself.

Describe the purpose of the meeting.

Indicate approximately how much time the session will take.

For example: "I am Mrs. Smith, the speech pathologist who will be evaluating Vicki's speech today. I'd like to begin by asking you some questions about her speech. Then I'll spend some time with Vicki by herself and get together with you again when we are finished. This should take about 90 minutes."

Body of the Interview

Discuss the client's history and current status in depth. This discussion will focus on communicative development, abilities, and problems, along with such other pertinent information as the client's medical, developmental, familial, social and/or educational histories. If a written case history has already been completed, the clinician can clarify and confirm relevant information during this portion of the interview.

Closing Phase

Summarize the major points from the body of the interview.

Express your appreciation for the interviewee's help.

Indicate the steps that will be taken next.

<u>For example:</u> "Thank you for all of the helpful information. Now I'd like to spend some time with Vicki and evaluate her speech. In about an hour we will get together again, and I'll share my findings with you."

The opening and closing phases are generally brief and succinct. A majority of the interview occurs in the second phase—the body of the interview—during which the major content areas are discussed. The content and length of this phase are directly influenced by the amount and type of information provided on the written case history, the concerns of the client and/or the caregiver, and the needs of the clinician to best understand the client and the problems he or she is experiencing.

Questions Common to Various Communicative Disorders

During an interview, both open-ended questions (e.g., *How would you describe your speech?*) and closed-ended questions (e.g., *Which sounds are difficult?*) are asked. Closed-ended questions typically elicit short, direct responses. Open-ended questions are less confining, allowing the respondent to provide more general and elaborate answers. It is usually best to begin an interview with open-ended questions. This will help you identify primary concerns that often require further clarification and follow-up through closed-ended questions.

The following questions are often asked about most communicative disorders during the body of the interview. You may use some or all of these questions with your clients, their caregivers, or both. Select those that are appropriate and integrate them into the interview. Answers to these questions, when combined with information from the case history, provide insight into your client's communicative handicap and become a springboard for asking questions that are more specific to the presenting disorder.

- ☐ Please describe the problem.
- ☐ When did the problem begin?
- ☐ How did it begin? Gradually? Suddenly?
- ☐ Has the problem changed since it was first noticed? Gotten better? Gotten worse?
- ☐ Is the problem consistent or does it vary? Are there certain circumstances that create fluctuations or variations?
- ☐ How do you react or respond to the problem? Does it bother you? What do you do?
- ☐ Where else have you been seen for the problem? What did they suggest? Did it help?
- ☐ How have you tried to help the problem? How have others tried to help?
- ☐ What other specialists (physician, teachers, hearing aid dispensers, etc.) have you seen?
- ☐ Why did you decide to come in for an evaluation? What do you hope will result? (Shipley, 1992)

Questions Common to Specific Communicative Disorders

Once you have asked the general questions, you will be ready to ask more specific questions related to the presenting disorder. Questions that are common to the disorders of articulation, language, fluency, or voice are listed below. Be aware that asking every question is not necessary or even appropriate with all clients. Do not use the questions as an interviewing checklist; rather, select appropriate questions and adapt as needed to help you gain a more complete understanding of your client's problems. When questioning a parent or caregiver about a child, substitute the words *your child* or the child's name for *you* or *your*.

Articulation

- ☐ Describe your concerns about your speech.
- ☐ What is your native language? What language do you speak most often?
- ☐ What language is spoken most often at home? At school? At work?
- ☐ How long have you been concerned about your speech? Who first noticed the problem?
- ☐ Describe your speech when the problem was first noticed. Has it improved over time?
- ☐ What do you think is the cause of your speech problem?
- ☐ What sounds are most difficult for you?
- ☐ Is it difficult for you to repeat what other people have said?
- ☐ Are there times when your speech is better than others?
- ☐ How well does your family understand you? Do they ask you to repeat yourself?
- ☐ How well do your friends and acquaintances understand you? Do they ask you to repeat yourself?
- ☐ Does your speech affect your interactions with other people? How does it affect your work? Your social activities? Your school activities?
- ☐ What have you done to try to improve your speech?
- ☐ Have you had speech therapy before? When? Where? With whom? What were the results?
- ☐ During the time you have been with me, has your speech been typical? Is it better or worse than usual?

Language (Child)

Use the child's name rather than "your child" whenever possible.

- ☐ Describe your concerns about your child's language.
- ☐ What is your child's native language? What language does your child speak most often?
- ☐ What language is spoken most often at home? At school? At work?

☐ Who does your child interact with most often? What kinds of activities do they do together?

☐ Does your child seem to understand you? Others?

☐ How well do you understand your child?

☐ Does your child maintain eye contact?

☐ How does your child get your attention (through gestures, verbalizations, etc.)?

☐ How does your child express needs and wants?

☐ Approximately how many words does your child understand?

☐ Approximately how many words does your child use?

☐ Provide an estimate of your child's average sentence length. Approximately how many words does your child use in his or her longest sentences?

☐ Does your child follow:
    Simple commands (e.g., put that away)?
    Two-part commands (e.g., get your shoes and brush your hair)?
    Three-part commands (e.g., pick up your toys, brush your teeth, and get in bed)?

☐ Does your child ask questions?

☐ Does your child use:
    Nouns (e.g., boy, car)?
    Verbs (e.g., jump, eat)?
    Adjectives (e.g., big, funny)?
    Adverbs (e.g., quickly, slowly)?
    Pronouns (e.g., he, they)?
    Conjunctions (e.g., and, but)?
    -ing endings (e.g., going, jumping)?
    Past-tense word forms (e.g., went, jumped)?
    Plurals (e.g., dogs, toys)?
    Possessives (e.g., my mom's, the dog's)?
    Comparatives (e.g., slower, bigger)?

☐ Does your child appear to understand cause-and-effect relationships? The function of objects?

☐ Is your child able to imitate immediately? Following a short lapse of time? How accurate is the imitation?

☐ Can your child narrate or talk about experiences?

☐ Does your child know how to take turns in conversation?

☐ Is your child's speech usually appropriate to the situation?

☐ Does your child participate in symbolic play (e.g., use of a stick to represent a microphone)?

Language (Adult)

☐ What is your native language? What language do you speak most often?

☐ Do you have a problem in your native language *and* in English?

☐ How long have you been concerned about your language? Who first noticed the problem?

☐ Describe your language abilities when the problem was first noticed. Has it improved over time?

☐ Do you read? How often? What kinds of books do you read?

☐ Describe your education. Did you have any problems learning?

☐ What do you think is the cause of your language problem?

☐ What does your family think about the problem?

☐ Does your language affect your interaction with other people? How does it affect your work? Your social activities?

☐ Have you had any accidents or illnesses that have affected your language?

☐ What have you done to try to improve your language skills?

☐ Have you had language therapy before? When? Where? With whom? What were the results?

Stuttering

☐ Describe your concerns about your speech.

☐ When did you first begin to stutter? Who noticed it? In what type of speaking situations did you first notice it?

☐ Describe your stuttering when it was first noticed. How has it changed over time?

☐ Did anyone else in the family stutter (parents, brothers, sisters, grandparents, uncles, aunts, cousins, etc.)? Do they still stutter? Did they have therapy? If so, did it help?

☐ Why do you think you stutter?

☐ Does the stuttering bother you? How?

☐ How does your family react to the problem?

☐ How do your friends and acquaintances react to the problem?

☐ What do you do when you stutter?

☐ When you stutter, what do you do to try to stop it? Does your strategy work? If yes, why do you think it works? If no, why not?

☐ In what situations do you stutter the most (over the telephone; speaking to a large group; speaking to your spouse, boss, or someone in a position of authority; etc.)?

☐ In what situations do you stutter the least (speaking to a child, speaking to your spouse, etc.)?

☐ Do you avoid certain speaking situations? Describe these.

☐ Do you avoid certain sounds or words? Describe these.

☐ Does your stuttering problem vary from day to day? How does it vary? Why do you think it varies?

☐ What have you done to try to eliminate the stuttering (previous therapy, self-help books, etc.)? What were the results?

☐ Have you had speech therapy before? When? Where? With whom? What were the results?

☐ Does your stuttering give you difficulties at work, at school, or at home? Are there other places that it gives you trouble?

☐ Have you had any illnesses or accidents that seemed to affect your speech? Describe these.

☐ During the time you have been with me, has your speech been typical? Are you stuttering more or less than usual?

Voice

☐ Describe your concerns about your voice?

☐ How long have you had the voice problem? Who first noticed it?

☐ Describe your voice when the problem was first noticed. How has it changed over time?

☐ What do you think is the cause of your voice problem?

☐ Do you speak a lot at work? At home? On the telephone? At social events or in large groups?

☐ What types of activities are you involved in?

☐ Do you ever run out of breath when you talk? Describe those situations.

☐ In what speaking situations is your voice the worst?

☐ In what situations is your voice the best?

☐ Is your voice better or worse at different times of the day?

☐ How does your family react to your voice problem?

☐ How do your friends and acquaintances react to your voice?

☐ How does your voice affect your interactions with other people? How does it affect your work? Your social activities? School?

☐ What have you done to try to resolve the problem?

☐ Have you seen an ear, nose, and throat specialist? What were the results?

☐ Have you had speech therapy before? When? Where? With whom? What were the results?

☐ Have you had any illnesses or accidents that seemed to affect your voice? Describe these.

☐ During the time you have been with me, has your voice been typical? Is it better or worse than usual?

INFORMATION FROM OTHER PROFESSIONALS

Information is sometimes available from other professionals who have seen the client. Occasionally, such information is necessary before commencing treatment (as in the case of an otolaryngologic evaluation before the initiation of voice therapy), and this information is often helpful for understanding the disorder more thoroughly before making a diagnosis. There are many sources for such preassessment information, including: other speech-language pathologists or audiologists, physicians (general or family practitioners, pediatricians, otolaryngologists, neurologists, psychiatrists, etc.), dentists or orthodontists, regular and special educators (classroom teachers, reading specialists, etc.), school nurses, clinical or educational psychologists, occupational or physical therapists, and rehabilitation or vocational counselors. Of course, this list is not all-inclusive. Professionals from other fields may also be involved with a client.

The information obtained from other professionals often ranges in its importance and potential use. It may be minimally useful, somewhat helpful, very helpful, or even vitally important. In some cases the value of such information will not be known until it has been received and reviewed by the clinician. Such information may help identify:

- The history or etiology of a disorder.
- Associated or concomitant medical, social, educational, and familial problems.
- Treatment histories, including the effects of treatment.
- Prognostic implications.
- Treatment options and alternatives.

Be aware that information from other professionals can potentially lead to a biased view of your client's condition. It is important to maintain an objective position throughout the assessment, relying primarily on your direct observation and evaluation results.

Other professionals or agencies should never be contacted for information, either by telephone or in writing, without the client's or caregiver's permission. A written permission is sometimes required, and it is always advisable. Licensure requirements in many states, ethical practice principles, and common sense dictate that students should never contact an outside professional or agency without the full knowledge and permission of their clinical supervisor.

Permissions that are granted by telephone should be followed-up by a written document, including a notation in the patient's records. Virtually all speech and hearing clinics have specific procedures and protocols for contacting outside agencies. These are available by contacting your clinic supervisor, the office staff, or the clinic director.

Another word of caution is needed about information from outside sources. Such information is confidential and should be used only for the specific purpose for which it was requested. Even though you may file such information with the client's other records, it is not appropriate for you to share it with other individuals or agencies. For example, if another professional or agency requests information about a given client, you should only provide reports generated by you or within your facility. Even if additional information is available in the client's file, the professional requesting the additional information should obtain that information only from the original source—not from you.

CONCLUDING COMMENTS

Three primary sources of obtaining information about a client were discussed in this chapter. These were written case histories, information-getting interviews, and information from other professionals. It is best to obtain as much information as possible to aid in diagnosing the communicative disorder, designing a treatment program, assessing prognosis, and preparing recommendations. Important information may include various histories of the disorder, current levels of functioning, and previous and current reports of evaluations or treatment. The amount, quality, and clinical applicability of the information you collect will vary. Some information will be immensely helpful, while other information will be of less use. The degree of applicability is, of course, related to the information itself and to the clinician's ability to use it. Information can sometimes be like a computer—a dust collector to one person and an indispensable tool to another. Information and its use is, indeed, in the hands of the holder.

SOURCES OF ADDITIONAL INFORMATION

Case Histories

Emerick, L. L., & Haynes, W. O. (1986). *Diagnosis and evaluation in speech pathology* (3rd ed.). Englewood Cliffs, NJ: Prentice-Hall.

Haynes, W. O., Pindzola, R. H., & Emerick, L. L. (1992). *Diagnosis and evaluation in speech pathology* (4th ed.). Englewood Cliffs, NJ: Prentice-Hall.

Meitus, I. J., & Weinberg, B. (Eds.). (1983a). *Diagnosis in speech-language pathology.* Austin, TX: PRO-ED.

Peterson, H. A., & Marquardt, T. P. (1994). *Appraisal and diagnosis of speech and language disorders* (3rd ed.). Englewood Cliffs, NJ: Prentice-Hall.

Shipley, K. G. (1996). *Interviewing and counseling in communicative disorders: Principles and procedures* (2nd ed.). Needham Heights, MA: Allyn & Bacon.

Interviews

Emerick, L. (1969). *The parent interview.* Danville, IL: Interstate Press.

Emerick, L. L., & Haynes, W. O. (1986). *Diagnosis and evaluation in speech pathology* (3rd ed.). Englewood Cliffs, NJ: Prentice-Hall.

Haynes, W. O., Pindzola, R. H., & Emerick, L. L. (1992). *Diagnosis and evaluation in speech pathology* (4th ed.). Englewood Cliffs, NJ: Prentice-Hall.

Hutchinson, B. B., Hanson, M. L., & Mecham, M. J. (Eds.). (1979). *Diagnostic handbook of speech pathology.* Baltimore: Williams & Wilkins.

Schulman, E. D. (1991). *Intervention in human services: A guide to skills and knowledge* (4th ed.). New York: Merrill.

Shipley, K. G. (1992). *Interviewing and counseling in communicative disorders: Principles and procedures.* New York: Merrill/Macmillan.

Stewart, C. J., & Cash, W. B. (1991). *Interviewing: Principles and practices* (6th ed.). Dubuque, IA: William C. Brown.

Articulation

Bernthal, J. E., & Bankson, N. W. (1993). *Articulation and phonological disorders* (3rd ed.). Englewood Cliffs, NJ: Prentice-Hall.

Creaghead, N. A., Newman, P. W., & Secord, W. (1989). *Assessment and remediation of articulatory and phonological disorders* (2nd ed.). Columbus, OH: Merrill.

Hegde, M. N. (1995). *Introduction to communicative disorders* (2nd ed.). Austin, TX: PRO-ED.

Language

Lahey, M. (1988). *Language disorders and language development.* New York: Macmillan.

McCormick, L., & Schiefelbusch, R. L. (1990). *Early language intervention* (2nd ed.). Columbus, OH: Merrill.

Owens, R. E. (1995). *Language disorders: A functional approach to assessment and intervention* (2nd ed.). Needham Heights, MA: Allyn & Bacon.

Reed, V. A. (1994). *An introduction to children with language disorders* (2nd ed.). New York: Macmillan.

Wiig, E. H., & Semel, E. (1984). *Language assessment and intervention for the learning disabled* (2nd ed.). Columbus, OH: Merrill.

Stuttering

Conture, E. G. (1990). *Stuttering* (2nd ed.). Englewood Cliffs, NJ: Prentice-Hall.

Ham, R. (1986). *Techniques of stuttering therapy.* Englewood Cliffs, NJ: Prentice-Hall.

Peters, T. J., & Guitar, B. (1991). *Stuttering: An integrated approach to its nature and treatment.* Baltimore: Williams & Wilkins.

Van Riper, C. (1973). *The treatment of stuttering.* Englewood Cliffs, NJ: Prentice-Hall.

Wells, G. B. (1987). *Stuttering treatment: A comprehensive clinical guide.* Englewood Cliffs, NJ: Prentice-Hall.

Voice

Aronson, A. E. (1990). *Clinical voice disorders: An interdisciplinary approach* (3rd ed.). New York: Thieme.

Boone, D. R., & McFarlane, S. C. (1994). *The voice and voice therapy* (5th ed.). Englewood Cliffs, NJ: Prentice-Hall.

Case, J. L. (1991). *Clinical management of voice disorders* (2nd ed.). Austin, TX: PRO-ED.

Colton, R. H., & Casper, J. K (1996). *Understanding voice problems: A physiological perspective for diagnosis and treatment* (2nd ed.). Baltimore: Williams & Wilkins.

Wilson, D. K (1987). *Voice problems of children* (3rd ed.). Baltimore: Williams & Wilkins.

Internet Sources

American Speech-Language-Hearing Association
http://www.asha.org
Listservers of Interest to Communication Disorders Folks
http://www.shc.uiowa.edu/wjshc/iiscdl.html

APPENDIX 1–A

Child Case History Form

General Information

Child's Name: _____ Date of Birth: _____

Address: _____ Phone: _____

City: _____ Zip: _____

Does the child live with both parents? _____

Mother's Name: _____ Age: _____

Mother's Occupation: _____ Business Phone: _____

Father's Name:_____ Age: _____

Father's Occupation: _____ Business Phone: _____

Referred By:_____ Phone: _____

Address: _____

Pediatrician: _____ Phone: _____

Address: _____

Family Doctor:_____ Phone: _____

Address: _____

Brothers and Sisters (include names and ages):

_____

_____

_____

_____

What languages does the child speak? What is the child's primary language?

What languages are spoken in the home? What is the primary language spoken?

With whom does the child spend most of his or her time?

Describe the child's speech-language problem.

How does the child usually communicate (gestures, single words, short phrases, sentences)?

When was the problem first noticed? By whom?

What do you think may have caused the problem?

Has the problem changed since it was first noticed?

Is the child aware of the problem? If yes, how does he or she feel about it?

Have any other speech-language specialists seen the child? Who and when? What were their conclusions or suggestions?

Have any other specialists (physicians, psychologists, special education teachers, etc.) seen the child? If yes, indicate the type of specialist, when the child was seen, and the specialist's conclusions or suggestions.

Are there any other speech, language, or hearing problems in your family? If yes, please describe.

Prenatal and Birth History

Mother's general health during pregnancy (illnesses, accidents, medications, etc.).

Length of pregnancy: _____   Length of labor: _____

General condition: _____   Birth weight:_____

Circle type of delivery: head first   feet first   breech   Caesarian

Were there any unusual conditions that may have affected the pregnancy or birth?

Medical History

Provide the approximate ages at which the child suffered the following illnesses and conditions:

Allergies_____	Asthma _____	Chicken Pox_____
Colds _____	Convulsions _____	Croup _____
Dizziness _____	Draining Ear _____	Ear Infections _____
Encephalitis _____	German Measles _____	Headaches _____
High Fever_____	Influenza _____	Mastoiditis _____
Measles _____	Meningitis _____	Mumps _____
Pneumonia_____	Seizures _____	Sinusitis _____
Tinnitus _____	Tonsillitis _____	Other _____

Has the child had any surgeries? If yes, what type and when (e.g., tonsillectomy, tube placement, etc.)?

Describe any major accidents or hospitalizations.

Is the child taking any medications? If yes, identify.

Have there been any negative reactions to medications? If yes, identify.

Developmental History

Provide the approximate age at which the child began to do the following activities:

Crawl _____ Sit _____ Stand _____

Walk _____ Feed self_____ Dress self _____

Use toilet _____

Use single words (e.g., no, mom, doggie, etc.): _____

Combine words (e.g., me go, daddy shoe, etc.): _____

Name simple objects (e.g., dog, car, tree, etc.): _____

Use simple questions (e.g., Where's doggie? etc.): _____

Engage in a conversation: _____

Does the child have difficulty walking, running, or participating in other activities which require small or large muscle coordination?

Are there or have there ever been any feeding problems (e.g., problems with sucking, swallowing, drooling, chewing, etc.)? If yes, describe.

Describe the child's response to sound (e.g., responds to all sounds, responds to loud sounds only, inconsistently responds to sounds, etc.).

Educational History

School:_____Grade: _____

Teacher(s): _____

How is the child doing academically (or preacademically)?

Does the child receive special services? If yes, describe.

How does the child interact with others (e.g., shy, aggressive, uncooperative, etc.)?

If enrolled for special education services, has an Individualized Educational Plan (IEP) been developed? If yes, describe the most important goals.

Provide any additional information that might be helpful in the evaluation or remediation of the child's problem.

Person completing form: _____

Relationship to child: _____

Signed: _____ Date: _____

APPENDIX 1–B
Adult Case History Form

General Information

Name: _____ Date of Birth: _____

Address: _____ Phone: _____

City: _____ Zip: _____

Occupation: _____ Business Phone: _____

Employer:_____

Referred By:_____ Phone: _____

Address: _____

Family Physician:_____ Phone: _____

Address: _____

Single _____ Widowed _____ Divorced _____ Spouse's Name _____

Children (include names, gender, and ages):

_____

_____

_____

_____

Who lives in the home?

What languages do you speak? If more than one, which one is your primary language?

What was the highest grade, diploma, or degree earned?

Describe your speech-language problem.

What do you think may have caused the problem?

Has the problem changed since it was first noticed?

Have you seen any other speech-language specialists? Who and when? What were their conclusions or suggestions?

Have you seen any other specialists (physicians, psychologists, neurologists, etc.)? If yes, indicate the type of specialist, when you were seen, and the specialist's conclusions or suggestions.

Are there any other speech, language, learning, or hearing problems in your family? If yes, please describe.

Medical History

Provide the approximate ages at which you suffered the following illnesses and conditions:

Adenoidectomy _____	Allergies _____	Asthma _____
Chicken Pox _____	Colds _____	Convulsions _____
Croup _____	Dizziness_____	Draining Ear_____
Ear Infections _____	Encephalitis _____	German Measles _____
Headaches_____	Hearing Loss _____	High Fever _____
Influenza _____	Mastoiditis _____	Measles_____
Meningitis_____	Mumps _____	Noise Exposure _____
Otosclerosis _____	Pneumonia _____	Seizures _____
Sinusitis _____	Tinnitus _____	Tonsillectomy _____
Tonsillitis _____	Other _____	

Do you have any eating or swallowing difficulties? If yes, describe.

List all medications you are taking.

Are you having any negative reactions to these medications? If yes, describe.

Describe any major surgeries, operations, or hospitalizations (include dates).

Describe any major accidents.

Provide any additional information that might be helpful in the evaluation or remediation process.

Person completing form: _____

Relationship to child: _____

Signed: _____ Date: _____

APPENDIX 1–C

Sample Request for Information

ABC Clinic
123 Main Street
Anytown, CA 99999
209-555-1529

September 12, 1997

Timothy Aspinwall, M.A.
321 Main Street
Anytown, CA 99999

Re: Audiological records for Laura Tolle

Dear Mr. Aspinwall:

Please send a copy of your most recent audiological findings and other appropriate information about Laura's hearing to the ABC Clinic. The information will be used in the evaluation of Laura's speech.

Permission is hereby granted to release and forward this information by:

_____   _____
Name   Signature

_____   _____
Relationship to Client   Date

_____   _____
Address   Phone

_____   _____
Witness   Date

Thank you.

_____
Name of Professional Requesting Information
Title

APPENDIX 1–D

Sample Referral for Medical Evaluation[1]

This example was designed for referring a person for a medical evaluation of the larynx. The model is adaptable for various uses.

Date:_____

Name: _____

Address: _____

Re: _____ Date of Birth: _____

Dear Dr. _____:

_____ was seen for a voice evaluation on _____.

The presenting problem was:

My primary findings were:

Prior to initiating voice therapy, a medical evaluation of the laryngeal area appears to be necessary. Following your evaluation, I would appreciate it if you would complete the second page of this form and return it to me.

Thank you very much.

_____

Speech-Language Pathologist

_____   _____

Address   Telephone

_____

[1]From K G. Shipley, *Systematic Assessment of Voice* (pp. 61–62). Oceanside, CA: Academic Communication Associates. Copyright © 1990 and used by permission.

Voice Client:_____

Results of Laryngeal Evaluation

Was evidence of vocal pathology found?   Yes _____   No _____

If so, please summarize the medical diagnosis below:

Describe the pathology in terms of
size and show location on the vocal folds.
Please indicate the size and location
on the illustration.

Is voice therapy recommended from your point of view?   Yes _____   No _____

Comments:

_____

Physician

_____   _____

Address   Telephone

□ CHAPTER 2 □

Evaluating Preassessment Information

- Speech, Language, and Motor Development
- Medical Conditions Associated With Communicative Disorders
- Syndromes Associated With Communicative Disorders
- Standard Medical Abbreviations
- Concluding Comments
- Sources of Additional Information

Several methods of gathering information for a complete diagnostic evaluation were described in Chapter 1, including information-getting interviews, written case histories, and information from other professionals. Occasionally, clinicians obtain valuable information from one or more of these sources without really understanding the potential clinical implications. The materials in this chapter are provided to help you interpret preassessment information.

Use care when interpreting the information given in this chapter and applying it to individual cases. Normal development, disorder severity, and clinical manifestations of medical conditions and syndromes vary tremendously. For example, some normal children begin talking at 9 months while others may be almost 2 years of age before beginning to talk. Also, retardation is frequently seen in Prader-Willi syndrome but some children with the disorder have above-normal intelligence. Just because something is listed on a case history or mentioned during an interview does not necessarily mean it is contributing to a specific communicative disorder.

SPEECH, LANGUAGE, AND MOTOR DEVELOPMENT

The outline below provides a general summary of the developmental sequence of speech, language, and motor skills in normal children. Because children develop at different rates, avoid strictly applying the age approximations. The time intervals are provided only as a general guideline for age appropriateness. This information was compiled from a variety of sources, which included the American Speech-Language-Hearing Association (1983); Boone and Plante (1993); Gard, Gilman, and Gorman (1980); Hegde (1995b); Kunz and Finkel (1987); Lane and Molyneaux (1992); and Lenneberg (1969).

0–6 Months

Speech and Language Skills

☐ Repeats the same sounds;
☐ Frequently coos, gurgles, and makes pleasure sounds;
☐ Uses a different cry to express different needs;
☐ Smiles when spoken to;
☐ Recognizes voices;
☐ Localizes sound by turning head;
☐ Listens to speech;
☐ Uses the phonemes /b/, /p/, and /m/ in babbling;
☐ Uses sounds or gestures to indicate wants.

Motor Skills

☐ Smiles;
☐ Rolls over from front to back and back to front;
☐ Raises head and shoulder from a face-down position;
☐ Sits while using hands for support;

☐ Reaches for objects with one hand but often misses;
☐ Blows bubbles on lips;
☐ Visually tracks people and objects;
☐ Watches own hands.

7–12 Months

Speech and Language Skills

☐ Understands *no* and *hot*;
☐ Responds to simple requests;
☐ Understands and responds to own name;
☐ Listens to and imitates some sounds;
☐ Recognizes words for common items (e.g., cup, shoe, juice);
☐ Babbles using long and short groups of sounds;
☐ Uses a song-like intonation pattern when babbling;
☐ Uses a large variety of sounds in babbling;
☐ Imitates some adult speech sounds and intonation patterns;
☐ Uses speech sounds rather than only crying to get attention;
☐ Listens when spoken to;
☐ Uses sound approximations;
☐ Begins to change babbling to jargon;
☐ Uses speech intentionally for the first time;
☐ Uses nouns almost exclusively;
☐ Has an expressive vocabulary of 1 to 3 words;
☐ Understands simple commands.

Motor Skills

☐ Crawls on stomach;
☐ Stands or walks with assistance;
☐ Attempts to feed self with a spoon;
☐ Rises to a sitting position;
☐ Attempts to imitate gestures;
☐ Uses smooth and continuous reaches to grasp objects;
☐ Sits unsupported;
☐ Drinks from a cup;
☐ Pulls self up to stand by furniture;
☐ Holds own bottle;
☐ Plays ball with a partner;
☐ Has poor aim and timing of release when throwing;
☐ Enjoys games like peek-a-boo and pat-a-cake;
☐ Uses a primitive grasp for writing, bangs crayon rather than writes;
☐ Cooperates with dressing, puts foot out for shoe, and places arms through sleeves.

13–18 Months

Speech and Language Skills

- ☐ Uses adult-like intonation patterns;
- ☐ Uses echolalia and jargon;
- ☐ Uses jargon to fill gaps in fluency;
- ☐ Omits some initial consonants and almost all final consonants;
- ☐ Produces mostly unintelligible speech;
- ☐ Follows simple commands;
- ☐ Receptively identifies 1 to 3 body parts;
- ☐ Has an expressive vocabulary of 3 to 20 or more words (mostly nouns);
- ☐ Combines gestures and vocalization;
- ☐ Makes requests for more of desired items.

Motor Skills

- ☐ Points to recognized objects;
- ☐ Runs but falls frequently;
- ☐ Imitates gestures;
- ☐ Removes some clothing items (e.g., socks, hat);
- ☐ Attempts to pull zippers up and down.

19–24 Months

Speech and Language Skills

- ☐ Uses words more frequently than jargon;
- ☐ Has an expressive vocabulary of 50 to 100 or more words;
- ☐ Has a receptive vocabulary of 300 or more words;
- ☐ Starts to combine nouns and verbs;
- ☐ Begins to use pronouns;
- ☐ Maintains unstable voice control;
- ☐ Uses appropriate intonation for questions;
- ☐ Is approximately 25–50% intelligible to strangers;
- ☐ Answers "what's that?" questions;
- ☐ Enjoys listening to stories;
- ☐ Knows 5 body parts;
- ☐ Accurately names a few familiar objects.

Motor Skills

- ☐ Walks without assistance;
- ☐ Walks sideways and backwards;
- ☐ Uses pull toys;
- ☐ Strings beads;
- ☐ Enjoys playing with clay;

- ☐ Picks up objects from the floor without falling;
- ☐ Stands with heels together;
- ☐ Walks up and down stairs with help;
- ☐ Jumps down a distance of 12 inches;
- ☐ Climbs and stands on chair;
- ☐ Rotates head while walking;
- ☐ Reaches automatically with primary concern on manipulation of object;
- ☐ Inserts key into lock;
- ☐ Stands on one foot with help;
- ☐ Seats self in a child's chair;
- ☐ Makes a tower 3 cubes high.

2–3 Years

Speech and Language Skills

- ☐ Speech is 50–75% intelligible;
- ☐ Understands *one* and *all*;
- ☐ Verbalizes toilet needs (before, during, or after act);
- ☐ Requests items by name;
- ☐ Points to pictures in a book when named;
- ☐ Identifies several body parts;
- ☐ Follows simple commands and answers simple questions;
- ☐ Enjoys listening to short stories, songs, and rhymes;
- ☐ Asks 1- to 2-word questions;
- ☐ Uses 3- to 4-word phrases;
- ☐ Uses some prepositions, articles, present progressive verbs, regular plurals, contractions, and irregular past tense forms;
- ☐ Uses words that are general in context;
- ☐ Continues use of echolalia when difficulties in speech are encountered;
- ☐ Has a receptive vocabulary of 500–900 or more words;
- ☐ Has an expressive vocabulary of 50–250 or more words (rapid growth during this period);
- ☐ Exhibits multiple grammatical errors;
- ☐ Understands most things said to him or her;
- ☐ Frequently exhibits repetitions — especially starters, "I," and first syllables;
- ☐ Speaks with a loud voice;
- ☐ Increases range of pitch;
- ☐ Uses vowels correctly;
- ☐ Consistently uses initial consonants (although some are misarticulated);
- ☐ Frequently omits medial consonants;
- ☐ Frequently omits or substitutes final consonants;
- ☐ Uses approximately 27 phonemes;
- ☐ Uses auxiliary *is* including the contracted form;
- ☐ Uses some regular past tense verbs' possessive morphemes, pronouns, and imperatives.

Motor Skills

- ☐ Walks with characteristic toddling movements;
- ☐ Begins developing rhythm;
- ☐ Walks up and down stairs alone;
- ☐ Jumps off floor with both feet;
- ☐ Balances on one foot for one second;
- ☐ Walks on tip-toes;
- ☐ Turns pages one by one, or two to three at a time;
- ☐ Folds paper roughly in half on imitation;
- ☐ Builds a tower of 6 cubes;
- ☐ Scribbles;
- ☐ Uses a palmer grip with writing tools;
- ☐ Paints with whole arm movements;
- ☐ Steps and rotates body when throwing;
- ☐ Drinks from a full glass with one hand;
- ☐ Chews food;
- ☐ Undresses self.

3–4 Years

Speech and Language Skills

- ☐ Understands object functions;
- ☐ Understands differences in meanings (stop–go, in–on, big–little);
- ☐ Follows 2- and 3-part commands;
- ☐ Asks and answers simple questions (who, what, where, why);
- ☐ Frequently asks questions and often demands detail in responses;
- ☐ Produces simple verbal analogies;
- ☐ Uses language to express emotion;
- ☐ Uses 4 to 5 words in sentences;
- ☐ Repeats 6- to 13-syllable sentences accurately;
- ☐ Identifies objects by name;
- ☐ Manipulates adults and peers;
- ☐ May continue to use echolalia;
- ☐ Uses up to 6 words in a sentence;
- ☐ Uses nouns and verbs most frequently;
- ☐ Is conscious of past and future;
- ☐ Has a 1,200–2,000 or more word receptive vocabulary;
- ☐ Has an 800–1,500 or more word expressive vocabulary;
- ☐ May repeat self often, exhibiting blocks, disturbed breathing, and facial grimaces during speech;
- ☐ Increases speech rate;
- ☐ Whispers;
- ☐ Masters 50% of consonants and blends;
- ☐ Speech is 80% intelligible;
- ☐ Sentence grammar improves, although some errors still persist;

☐ Appropriately uses *is, are*, and *am* in sentences;
☐ Tells two events in chronological order;
☐ Engages in long conversations;
☐ Uses some contractions, irregular plurals, future tense verbs, and conjunctions;
☐ Consistently uses regular plurals, possessives, and simple past tense verbs.

Motor Skills

☐ Kicks ball forward;
☐ Turns pages one at a time;
☐ Learns to use blunt scissors;
☐ Runs and plays active games with abandonment;
☐ Rises from squatting position;
☐ Balances and walks on toes;
☐ Unbuttons but cannot button;
☐ Holds crayon with thumb and fingers, not fist;
☐ Uses one hand consistently for most activities;
☐ Traces a square, copies a circle, and imitates horizontal strokes;
☐ Puts on own shoes, but not necessarily on the correct foot;
☐ Rides a tricycle;
☐ Builds a tower of 9 cubes;
☐ Alternates feet while walking up and down stairs;
☐ Jumps in place with both feet together;
☐ Uses a spoon without spilling;
☐ Opens doors by turning the handle.

4–5 Years

Speech and Language Skills

☐ Understands concept of numbers up to 3;
☐ Continues understanding of spatial concepts;
☐ Recognizes 1 to 3 colors;
☐ Has a receptive vocabulary of 2,800 or more words;
☐ Counts to 10 by rote;
☐ Listens to short, simple stories;
☐ Answers questions about function;
☐ Uses grammatically correct sentences;
☐ Has an expressive vocabulary of 900 to 2,000 or more words;
☐ Uses sentences of 4 to 8 words;
☐ Answers complex 2-part questions;
☐ Asks for word definitions;
☐ Speaks at a rate of approximately 186 words per minute;
☐ Reduces total number of repetitions;
☐ Enjoys rhymes, rhythms, and nonsense syllables;
☐ Produces consonants with 90% accuracy;

☐ Significantly reduces number of persistent sound omissions and substitutions;
☐ Frequently omits medial consonants;
☐ Speech is usually intelligible to strangers;
☐ Talks about experiences at school, at friends' homes, etc.;
☐ Accurately relays a long story;
☐ Pays attention to a story and answers simple questions about it;
☐ Uses some irregular plurals, possessive pronouns, future tense, reflexive pronouns, and comparative morphemes in sentences.

Motor Skills

☐ Runs around obstacles;
☐ Pushes, pulls, and steers wheeled toys;
☐ Jumps over 6-inch-high object and lands on both feet together;
☐ Throws ball with direction;
☐ Balances on one foot for 5 seconds;
☐ Pours from a pitcher;
☐ Spreads substances with a knife;
☐ Uses toilet independently;
☐ Skips to music;
☐ Hops on one foot;
☐ Walks on a line;
☐ Uses legs with good strength, ease, and facility;
☐ Grasps with thumb and medial finger;
☐ Releases objects with precision;
☐ Holds paper with hand when writing;
☐ Draws circles, crosses, and diamonds;
☐ Descends stairs without assistance;
☐ Carries a cup of water without spilling;
☐ Enjoys cutting and pasting.

5–6 Years

Speech and Language Skills

☐ Names 6 basic colors and 3 basic shapes;
☐ Follows instructions given to a group;
☐ Follows 3-part commands;
☐ Asks *how* questions;
☐ Answers verbally to *hi* and *how are you*?;
☐ Uses past tense and future tense appropriately;
☐ Uses conjunctions;
☐ Has a receptive vocabulary of approximately 13,000 words;
☐ Names opposites;
☐ Sequentially names days of the week;
☐ Counts to 30 by rote;

☐ Continues to drastically increase vocabulary;
☐ Reduces sentence length to 4 to 6 words;
☐ Reverses sounds occasionally;
☐ Exchanges information and asks questions;
☐ Uses sentences with details;
☐ Accurately relays a story;
☐ Sings entire songs and recites nursery rhymes;
☐ Communicates easily with adults and other children;
☐ Uses appropriate grammar in most cases.

Motor Skills

☐ Walks backward heel-to-toe;
☐ Does somersaults;
☐ Cuts on a line with scissors;
☐ Prints a few capital letters;
☐ Cuts food with a knife;
☐ Ties own shoes;
☐ Builds complex structures with blocks;
☐ Gracefully roller skates, skips, jumps rope, and rides a bicycle;
☐ Competently uses miniature tools;
☐ Buttons clothes, washes face, and puts toys away;
☐ Reaches and grasps in one continuous movement;
☐ Catches a ball with hands;
☐ Makes precise marks with crayon, confining marks to a small area.

6–7 Years

Speech and Language Skills

☐ Names some letters, numbers, and currencies;
☐ Sequences numbers;
☐ Understands *left* and *right*;
☐ Uses increasingly more complex descriptions;
☐ Engages in conversations;
☐ Has a receptive vocabulary of approximately 20,000 words;
☐ Uses a sentence length of approximately 6 words;
☐ Understands most concepts of time;
☐ Recites the alphabet;
☐ Counts to 100 by rote;
☐ Uses most morphologic markers appropriately;
☐ Uses passive voice appropriately.

Motor Skills

☐ Enjoys strenuous activities like running, jumping, racing, gymnastics, playing chase, and tag games;

☐ Shows reduced interest in writing and drawing;
☐ Draws a recognizable *man*, *tree*, and *house*;
☐ Uses adult-like writing, but it is slow and labored;
☐ Draws pictures that are not proportional;
☐ Runs lightly on toes;
☐ Walks on a balance beam;
☐ Cuts out simple shapes;
☐ Colors within lines;
☐ Indicates well-established right- or left-handedness;
☐ Dresses self completely;
☐ Brushes teeth without assistance;
☐ Follows advanced rhythms.

MEDICAL CONDITIONS ASSOCIATED WITH COMMUNICATIVE DISORDERS

The following medical conditions may be listed on a typical case history form. It is important to know what each condition is and how it can affect a patient's communicative abilities. Keep in mind that most illnesses or conditions have potential implications for the development of a speech and language disorder. For example, the person who is prone to frequent illnesses, whether or not the illnesses are serious, is also more prone to a communicative disorder. This is especially true for children who have had multiple hearing losses during the crucial period of speech-language acquisition, or those who have frequently missed school and now lag behind their peers in communicative, social, and educational development.

A disease condition acquired by a pregnant woman may also influence the normal growth of her unborn child. Specific disruptions' in fetal development are related to the time during gestation that the illness was acquired. First trimester illnesses impose the greatest developmental risks on the growing baby. Many congenital disorders have associated speech and language impairments. Descsriptions of the following medical conditions are based on the works of Brace and Pacanowski (1985), Gerber (1990), Kunz and Finkel (1987), Reese and Douglas (1983), and Sparks (1984). The term *complication* as used in the following section refers to additional problems often associated with the specific illness. These complications may or may not be directly attributable to the primary illness.

Acquired Immune Deficiency Syndrome (AIDS)

Description

AIDS is a disease in which some of the body's white blood cells are destroyed, resulting in an impaired natural defense mechanism. It is caused by the human T-cell lymphotropic virus III (HTL VIII). AIDS symptoms in adults include fever, weight loss, swollen glands, general weakness, headaches, drowsiness, confusion, and infections of the mouth, skin, or chest. Children who have AIDS exhibit symptoms such as low birth weight, developmental delay, upper respiratory infections, pneumonia, ear diseases, and sensorineural hearing loss. A person infected with HTL VIII may appear healthy for several years or a lifetime before developing AIDS. The virus is transmitted through infected semen or blood. An unborn baby will acquire the virus if its mother is a carrier.

Complications

AIDS is a fatal disease. A person with AIDS is at great risk for multiple infections (especially pneumonia, swollen lymph glands, fever, and encephalitis), various types of cancer (particularly skin cancer), progressive weight loss, generalized weakness, and eventual death. Children who have AIDS are prone to more severe infections than adults, simply because their immune systems are not mature. Infected children are especially at risk for cancer of the external ear, cancer of the oral cavity, and cortical atrophy.

Adenoidectomy

Description

An adenoidectomy is a partial or complete surgical removal of the adenoids. This procedure is usually performed when a child's adenoids enlarge and block the nasopharynx or eustachian tubes on a recurrent basis. The blockage often results in breathing difficulties or frequent bouts of otitis media. A successful adenoidectomy alleviates complications resulting from middle ear infections.

Complications

In most cases, there are no negative complications associated with an adenoidectomy. Velopharyngeal incompetence resulting in hypernasality occurs in rare cases.

Allergies

Description

Allergies are physical disorders caused by hypersensitivity to substances that are eaten, inhaled, injected, or brought into contact with the skin. Symptoms of an allergy attack often include headache, shock, excessive mucus production, constriction of bronchioles, and such skin conditions as redness, swelling, and itching. These allergic reactions are caused by a breakdown in the body's natural immune system, particularly an excessive release of the body chemical histamine. Allergies are fairly common and are often associated with asthma, allergic rhinitis (hay fever), eczema, dermatitis, hives, farmer's lung, celiac disease (a disease of the small intestine), allergic bronchitis, and some forms of conjunctivitis (inflammation of the eyelid lining).

Complications

Allergies are typically not complicated. A potential complication is otitis media resulting from fluid build-up in the middle ear.

Asthma

Description

Asthma is a disorder characterized by periodic attacks of wheezing, tightness in the chest, and breathing difficulties. Such attacks occur when muscles of the bronchial walls contract, obstructing the air passages to and from the lungs. Asthma is most often triggered by allergies, emotional stress, or infection. Other contributing factors may be drug use, inhalation of irritants, vigorous exercise, or a psychosomatic disorder. Asthma is relatively common among school-age children and there is a tendency to outgrow the condition over time. Asthma attacks vary in frequency and severity, lasting from a few minutes to several days.

Complications

Asthma attacks are usually not complicated and can be kept under control with medical assistance. In rare cases, people who suffer successive and severe attacks may acquire a permanent disability or even die because of the reduced oxygen supply to the body.

Chicken Pox
(also called Varicella)

Description

Chicken pox is a mild, infectious disease caused by a herpes virus. The primary symptom is a rash that appears mostly on the skin and the lining of the mouth and throat. Within a few days, the characteristic small, fluid-filled spots burst or dry out and develop crusts. The crusts eventually fall off, leaving pink marks that disappear entirely over time. The primary irritation is itching of the spots. Some children also experience a slight fever. Adults with chicken pox may have flu-like symptoms 2–3 days before the rash appears. Chicken pox primarily affects children between the ages of 5 and 9. It is rare in adults. The disease is highly contagious, with symptoms appearing after an incubation of from 7–21 days. In children, recovery is fast (7–10 days); adults are more prone to complications and a slower recovery period.

Complications

Chicken pox is usually a mild illness with no complications. Reye's syndrome occurs in rare cases. If the chicken pox occurs in the ears, there may be a toxic effect that results in bilateral hearing loss.

Colds

Description

The common cold is usually caused by a viral infection of the nose and throat, although the larynx and lungs may also be involved. Symptoms include nasal congestion, runny nose, sneezing, mild sore throat, watery eyes, hoarseness, abdominal pain, and coughing. A temporary conductive hearing loss may also be present. A normal head cold typically lasts for about 7 days. Colds usually occur in winter months, and children are most prone to acquiring them. Immunity to cold viruses increases as a child grows older; therefore, the frequency of infection and severity are reduced over time. Symptoms appear following an incubation period of 2–4 days.

Complications

Colds are not serious in most cases, although infections can spread to the middle ears, sinuses, larynx, trachea, or lungs. This can result in secondary bacterial infections with complications such as laryngitis, bronchitis, otitis media, and sinusitis.

Convulsions
(also called Seizures)

Description

Convulsions are uncontrollable muscle contractions caused by abnormal nerve cell activity in the brain. They vary considerably in severity. During a grand mal convulsion, the person loses consciousness and exhibits jerking movements of the whole body. The seizure may last several minutes before the person regains consciousness and then falls into a deep sleep. Most febrile convulsions (those associated with a fever) are of this type.

Petit mal convulsions are much less severe. The person may exhibit a blank stare and appear to be daydreaming for several seconds. After the convulsion is over, he or she does not remember that it has happened. This type of convulsion can occur many times in one day.

A psychomotor convulsion, also called a temporal lobe attack, occurs when a person exhibits violent behavior, laughs, or cries for no apparent reason. The seizure lasts for a few minutes. Afterward, he or she is not aware that it occurred.

Infantile spasms are sudden episodes in which a baby or toddler drops its head to its chest and doubles up at the waist. Afterward the child may fall asleep. These convulsions last only a second to a few seconds and can occur several times a day.

Convulsions occur most often in children and are often outgrown by adulthood. People prone to convulsions usually have idiopathic epilepsy or a minor fever-causing infection. Other causes include meningitis, encephalitis, hypoglycemia, brain damage, cerebral palsy, or a brain tumor.

Complications

A majority of convulsions are not harmful. One primary risk is that the person will hit his or her head during the convulsion and incur a brain injury. However, this rarely occurs. The most serious of the convulsions is the grand mal—as multiple, prolonged episodes may lead to injury during the seizures.

Croup

Description

Croup is a viral disorder characterized by a barking-like cough, hoarseness, respiratory distress, and inhalatory stridor resulting from swelling of the larynx and trachea. In most cases, it is a complication of influenza or a cold. Croup is a childhood disorder, primarily affecting children between the ages of 3 months and 3 years (although it can affect children up to 7 years of age). Attacks usually occur at night and subside after a few hours, and the condition may continue for several days. It is most common in the fall and winter months.

Complications

Croup is not usually complicated. In rare cases, an emergency tracheotomy is necessary to supply oxygen to the body. Severe croup is an indication of epiglottidis, which can be fatal.

Dizziness

Description

Dizziness is a sensation of spinning, either within the person or in the person's environment. It is not a disease or condition; rather, it is a symptom of several types of neurological or aural disturbances. The person with dizziness may also feel nauseated, vomit, and have reduced control of balance. The term vertigo is often used interchangeably with dizziness, but they are not the same. Vertigo is dizziness experienced secondary to middle or inner ear pathology such as Ménière's disease, otitis media, labyrinthitis, or ototoxicity.

Dizziness can occur as a result of a severe blow to the head. It may also be an indication of a stroke, transient ischemic attack, subdural hemorrhage or hematoma, or brain tumor.

Complications

Most cases of dizziness are temporary and uncomplicated. Because dizziness is a symptom rather than a disease, complications must be viewed in terms of specific etiologies. However, dizziness itself does have some inherent risks. Because dizziness is associated with balance problems, a person may fall down and suffer a head injury.

Draining Ear

Description

Draining ear is not a disease condition, but is a common symptom of certain disorders. A greenish-yellow discharge from the ear canal may be an indication of otitis externa, otitis media, or mastoiditis. The infected person may also experience pain in the ear during head movement.

Complications

Complications associated with draining ear must be evaluated according to the etiology of the condition. When the drainage obstructs the outer ear canal, a temporary hearing loss often occurs.

Encephalitis

Description

Encephalitis is an inflammation of the brain cells. The condition may have noninfectious origins, although it is caused by a viral infection (such as mumps, measles, or infectious mononucleosis) in most cases. Symptoms of mild encephalitis are similar to those of most viral infections, including fever, headache, and a loss of energy and appetite. In severe cases, the person has obvious brain dysfunction. Symptoms may include irritability, restlessness, drowsiness (which may deepen into a coma in the most severe cases), loss of muscular power in the arms or legs, double vision, and impairment of speech and hearing.

Complications

Mild cases of encephalitis are rather common and uncomplicated, but severe cases can be extremely serious. Permanent brain damage or even death may result. Babies and the elderly are at the highest risk for such complications. Recovery from a severe episode of encephalitis may be very slow, requiring long-term rehabilitation.

German Measles
(also called Rubella)

Description

German measles is a contagious viral disease that begins with a low fever, sore throat, body aches, and swollen glands behind the ears and on the neck. Within 2–3 days a rash of small, flat, reddish-pink spots appears on the face and neck. It then spreads to the trunk and limbs. The rash does not itch and it fades away within 1–2 days. The total course of the disease lasts only 4–5 days. German measles is most common among children. Symptoms appear following an incubation of 14–21 days. Immunization is available for people over the age of 12 months.

Complications

People who have contracted German measles are, themselves, at little risk for serious complications. However, the developing fetuses of pregnant women who have contracted the disease or received a vaccine within the 3 months preceding conception are at great risk for serious birth defects. These defects can include premature birth, congenital pneumonia, malformation, cataracts, jaundice, cardiac defects, mental retardation, microcephaly, hydrocephaly, meningoencephalitis, and deafness. The behaviors the child may exhibit include hyperactivity, impulsivity, poor attention span, sleep disturbances, and delayed speech and language development.

Headaches

Description

Headaches occur because of increased strain on muscles of the face, neck, and scalp (called tension headaches), or because of increased swelling of the blood vessels in the head (called vascular headaches). The resulting pain is located in the meninges, not the brain tissues themselves. Many factors can lead to headaches, including stress, alcohol consumption, overeating, exposure to noise, eyestrain, poor body posture, and head injury. Headaches are common and usually last only a few hours. They can be a symptom of another medical condition, such as a viral infection or a hemorrhage. Common headaches should be differentiated from migraine headaches, which are more intense and incapacitating.

Complications

In most cases, headaches are not complicated. However, if they occur frequently or last for over 24 hours, the person may have a central nervous system disorder or a depressive illness.

High Fever

Description

A high fever is a rise in body temperature above 100°F. The sufferer may also be irritable, flushed, and sleepy. In children, high fever can be a symptom of influenza, a cold, an acute infection of the middle ear, a respiratory tract infection, measles, mumps, or meningitis. A high fever in adults can be a symptom of pneumonia, acute bronchitis, influenza, meningitis, gastroenteritis (inflammation of the digestive tract), pharyngitis (inflammation of the pharynx), tonsillitis, a kidney infection, or cystitis (a urinary tract infection).

Complications

Although most high fevers are not harmful, there can be serious complications in some cases. The fever can generate damaging toxins, resulting in a permanent injury such as a hearing loss. In children, especially those under the age of 5, a high fever can lead to febrile convulsions. If the fever is very high (up to or above 107°F), permanent brain damage can result.

Influenza
(also called Flu)

Description

Influenza is a viral disease that is characterized by chills, high fever, muscular pains, headache, sore throat, and sneezing. These symptoms are followed by a dry, hacking cough, possible chest pains, and runny nose. Complete recovery typically occurs within 1–2 weeks. The disease is highly contagious and usually occurs in epidemics, especially in the winter and spring months. Symptoms appear following a 1–2 day incubation.

Complications

In most cases influenza is not complicated. The primary risk is the spread of a bacterial infection to the lungs, causing bronchitis or bacterial pneumonia. A viral pneumonia can occur in rare cases. Other complications include otitis media, fever convulsions, skin rash, Reye's syndrome, and Guillain-Barré syndrome.

Mastoiditis

Description

Mastoiditis is an inflammation of all or part of the mastoid process. It occurs most commonly when a middle ear infection spreads to the mastoid. Symptoms include intense pain behind the ear, fever, a rapid pulse rate, discharge from the affected ear, swelling behind the affected ear, and a pronounced hearing loss.

Complications

If the mastoiditis does not respond to antibiotics, a mastoidectomy (partial or complete removal of the mastoid) may be necessary. Another potential complication of mastoiditis is meningitis.

Measles
(also called Rubeola)

Description

Measles is a viral disease that primarily affects the skin and the respiratory tract. The 7–10 day course of the disease begins with a fever, runny nose, watery eyes, dry cough, and possibly diarrhea. Within a few days, the fever is reduced and small white spots appear in the mouth. Next, the fever rises again and a red rash develops, beginning on the head and spreading to the rest of the body. In a short time, the rash and all other symptoms fade away. Measles is a highly contagious and dangerous disease. It often occurs in epidemics but, because immunization is available for children over 15 months old, it is not common. Symptoms appear following an incubation of about 7–14 days. A person who has acquired measles is immune from future occurrences. It should not be confused with German measles (rubella) which is much less serious, except during pregnancy.

Complications

Measles is a potentially serious disorder that can lead to severe complications such as hearing loss, otitis media, bronchitis, bronchopneumonia, learning disabilities, encephalitis, meningitis, permanent brain damage, mental retardation, ulceration of the cornea, vision problems, seizures, and even death. A pregnant woman who contracts measles is at risk for premature labor or spontaneous abortion. Her newborn baby may have a low birth weight and, if the disease was contracted during the first trimester of fetal development, congenital malformation.

Meningitis

Description

Meningitis is an inflammation of the meninges (the membranous coverings of the brain and spinal cord). Bacteria or viruses can spread to these membranes through the bloodstream or cavities and bones of the skull, or from a skull fracture. Symptoms include fever, headache, chills, nausea, vomiting, irritability, a stiff neck, and photophobia (inability to tolerate bright light). A deep red or purplish skin rash occurs in some cases.

Complications

The viral form of meningitis usually imposes no associated complications. Meningitis stemming from a bacterial infection, however, is a very serious condition requiring aggressive medical treatment. Complications associated with bacterial meningitis include convulsions, coma, permanent deafness, permanent blindness, mental deterioration, or death. Babies and the elderly are especially prone to these serious complications.

Mumps

Description

Mumps is a viral infection of the salivary glands, particularly of the parotid glands located just anterior to the ears. Swelling of these glands occurs initially on one side of the face and then on the other side within a couple of days. The infected person may also experience difficulty opening the mouth, dryness of the mouth, pain during swallowing, fever, diarrhea, vomiting, and/or general feelings of illness. Mumps can occur at any age, but it is most common in children between the ages of 5 and 15. It rarely occurs more than once in a lifetime. It is a contagious disease usually spread through the breath of an infected person. Symptoms appear after a 14–28 day incubation. Immunization is available for people over the age of 12 months.

Complications

Most cases of mumps are relatively mild and uncomplicated. Inflammation of the testicles or ovaries is the most common complication. Other risks include meningitis, encephalitis, pancreatitis, febrile (fever) convulsions, respiratory tract infections, and ear infections. In rare conditions, a mild-to-severe hearing loss can occur. The hearing loss is typically (but not exclusively) unilateral.

Otitis Media

Description

Otitis media is an infection of the middle ear. The infection may be viral or bacterial, and it usually spreads from the nose and throat to the ear through the eustachian tube. The infection can also enter the middle ear through a ruptured eardrum. The symptoms of acute otitis media include a feeling of fullness in the affected ear that is followed by pain, fever, and hearing loss. If untreated, the acute condition may lead to chronic otitis media, which is much more serious and permanently damaging. Otitis media is very common among children, particularly those under 6 years of age.

Complications

Otitis media is nearly always associated with a temporary hearing loss. This can directly influence speech and language development as repeated infections are common among children, primarily during the critical years of speech and language acquisition. Viral acute otitis media is usually less complicated and serious than the bacterial type. If untreated, bacterial otitis media may lead to such intense middle ear pressure from pus buildup that the eardrum bursts. Acute otitis media can also lead to mastoiditis or chronic otitis media. If the chronic form of otitis media continues untreated, the person is at risk for much more permanent and serious damage including damaged or destroyed ossicles, a ruptured eardrum, cholesteatoma (an enlarged collection of skin tissue near the eardrum), a mastoidectomy, and permanent hearing impairment.

Parkinson's Disease

Description

Parkinson's disease is a degenerative condition caused by gradual deterioration of nerve centers in the brain. This deterioration disrupts the brain's normal balance of dopamine and acetylcholine, resulting in progressive loss of control of movement. One of the first symptoms of Parkinsonism is rhythmic tremors of the hands and/or head, often accompanied by involuntary rubbing together of the thumb and forefinger. As the condition progresses, automatic physical movements associated with walking, writing, and speaking also become impaired. Other symptoms include excessive salivation, abdominal cramps, and, in the latest stages of the disease, deterioration of memory and thought processes. It most often affects people who are late middle age and older.

Complications

Parkinson's disease can result in mild-to-profound communication and/or swallowing impairments, depending on the individual and the stage of progression of the disease. Dysphagia and hypokinetic dysarthria are characteristic. As deterioration increases, cognitive function may also be impaired. Parkinson's disease is sometimes medically controlled with L-Dopa, which can significantly reduce the severity of the condition.

Pneumonia
(also called Pneumonitis)

Description

Pneumonia is a general term for inflammation of the lungs. The several types of pneumonia are differentiated by their origins and severity. Most cases are viral or bacterial in origin although fungi, inhalation of food, vomit, or pus, or inhalation of poisonous gas can also cause pneumonia. Symptoms vary according to the type of pneumonia. Most types are characterized by nasal congestion, cough, fever, chills, shortness of breath, and bluish skin. Additional symptoms often include chest pain, sweating, blood in the phlegm, or possible mental confusion.

Complications

Severity varies considerably from mild and uncomplicated to extremely dangerous and life-threatening. Viral pneumonias, which do not respond to antibiotics, pose the greatest danger. People who already have health problems and whose natural defense mechanisms are reduced usually have the most threatening complications. The most serious risk is death. Other complications include pleurisy (inflammation of the lining around the lungs and inner side of the ribs) and empyema (an accumulation of pus in the lining around the lungs).

Sinusitis

Description

Sinusitis is an inflammation of the mucuous membranes of the frontal and/or maxillary sinuses. It is usually spread through the nose after a common cold (viral infection) and may be complicated by a bacterial infection. Symptoms include coughing, a greenish discharge through the nose, increased nasal congestion, and a general feeling of illness. When the frontal sinuses are affected, the person may experience headaches, increased pain when first waking up or bending the head forward, and tenderness just above the eyes. When the maxillary sinuses are affected, the person may experience pain in one or both cheeks and in one or more upper teeth. Sinusitis is fairly common. Some people have repeated attacks nearly every time they have a cold. The condition can also be acquired through damage to the nasal bones, nasal obstruction by a foreign object, or a nasal deformity.

Complications

Sinusitis is rarely complicated. If untreated, however, the infection can spread to the bones or into the brain.

Stroke

Description

A cerebral vascular accident (CVA), commonly known as a *stroke*, occurs when part of the brain is damaged because its blood supply is disrupted. There are three etiologies of a stroke.

A cerebral hemorrhage occurs when an artery bursts or leaks and blood seeps into the brain tissue. A cerebral thrombosis occurs when a clot forms in an artery and eventually grows until it partially or completely blocks the flow of blood at that point. A cerebral embolism occurs when foreign material is carried through the bloodstream and becomes caught, obstructing the flow of blood to the brain. The result of a stroke is dependent on the area of the brain affected and the severity of the damage. Symptoms of a stroke include headache, blurred or double vision, confusion, dizziness, slurred speech or an inability to talk, weakness or numbness on only one side of the body, difficulty swallowing, and/or loss of consciousness. These symptoms persist for a period of at least 24 hours, and usually significantly longer (unlike a transient ischemic attack).

Complications

Depending on the severity of the stroke, the consequent deficits can be mild to profound. Speech, language, swallowing, and/or cognition can be affected, resulting in dysarthria, aphasia, apraxia, dysphagia, and/or cognitive-linguistic impairments.

Tinnitus

Description

Tinnitus is an unwanted ringing noise in the ear that varies in quality and pitch among people with the condition. Various descriptions of tinnitus have included a buzzing sound, a high-pitched whistle, a grinding noise, or a low-pitched roar. Some people experience the condition continuously, while others report intermittent attacks of tinnitus. Tinnitus is usually associated with an impairment of the hearing mechanism. It is often an initial indication that something is wrong in the auditory system. The condition can be triggered by a large number of factors including stress, a virus, exposure to loud noise, diet, thyroid problems, hypertension, head trauma, drug intake, and dental problems.

Complications

Since tinnitus typically is associated with an auditory impairment, it should not be ignored as a medical condition. It can be an early symptom of progressive hearing loss, meningitis, encephalitis, ototoxicity (loss of hearing from medications), or an acoustic neurinoma (a tumor in the ear).

Tonsillitis

Description

Tonsillitis is an inflammation of the tonsils caused by a bacterial or viral infection. In adults, the symptoms include sore throat, headache, chills, fever, and red, inflamed tonsils. Glandular swelling around the infected area is also common. Children who acquire tonsillitis may have difficulty swallowing, sore throat, fever, vomiting, coughing, stomach pains, swollen glands on the neck, and, in some cases, febrile (fever) convulsions. The disease is common among children, especially those between 2 and 6 years of age. Tonsillitis is highly infectious and is often accompanied by an infection of the adenoids.

Complications

Tonsillitis is rarely complicated. Complications include otitis media and sinusitis. If the condition occurs frequently or is especially severe, a tonsillectomy may be recommended.

Transient Ischemic Attack

Description

A transient ischemic attack (TIA) occurs when there is an interference of normal blood flow to the brain. Typically, a foreign material flowing through the bloodstream becomes caught and disrupts the brain's blood supply, much like a cerebral embolism (see *Stroke*). The symptoms are very similar to a stroke and include headache, dizziness, blurred or double vision, confusion, slurred speech, swallowing difficulty, and weakness or numbness on one side of the body. These symptoms, however, are short lived (less than 24 hours) as the foreign material is eventually dislodged or broken up and blood circulation to the brain is restored.

Complications

A transient ischemic attack is usually not complicated, as the resulting impairments are temporary, although it is often a warning of an impending stroke.

SYNDROMES ASSOCIATED WITH COMMUNICATIVE DISORDERS

A syndrome is a distinct collection of symptoms that have a common cause. The etiology may be viral, bacterial, genetic, chromosomal, teratogenic (a foreign agent causing embryonic or fetal structural abnormalities), or traumatic. Many syndromes have been named and described, yet many more remain unidentified by medical experts. Some of the major syndromes that affect communicative abilities, and therefore may be seen by clinicians for speech, language, or hearing services, are described in this section. Use caution when using this information and consider these factors:

1. *Syndrome severity varies tremendously.* A child diagnosed with a given syndrome may exhibit barely detectable symptoms, or may be a "textbook example."
2. *Individual symptoms vary.* For example, a child with mental retardation may be severely impaired intellectually, or may be nearly normal.
3. *All symptoms associated with a syndrome need not be present.* Syndromes are a collection of many symptoms which appear in varying degrees; some symptoms may not appear at all.

4. *Symptoms that are not described in this section may also be present.* We have highlighted only the major characteristics of each syndrome. Other less common symptoms may also be observed.

5. *These descriptions are presented only as a starting point of inquiry about syndromes associated with communicative disorders.* The information in this section is based primarily on Gerber's (1990) *Prevention: The Etiology of Communicative Disorders* and Jung's (1989) *Genetic Syndromes in Communication Disorders.* Both of these excellent resources will help you further explore these and other syndromes.

Acquired Immune Deficiency Syndrome (AIDS)

See **Acquired Immune Deficiency Syndrome (AIDS)** (pp. 40–41) under **Medical Conditions Associated with Communicative Disorders**.

Alport Syndrome

This hereditary syndrome is characterized by nephritis (inflammation of the kidneys) and deafness. These symptoms tend to be more serious and progress faster in males. The associated hearing loss is typically bilateral, sensorineural, and progressive. Research has shown that approximately 1% of all genetically based hearing losses are attributed to Alport syndrome. Speech and language problems associated with hearing loss have also been reported.

Apert Syndrome

Craniosynostosis (premature fusion of the cranial sutures) resulting in a tall head shape, midfacial hypoplasia (underdevelopment), and strabismus are characteristic of Apert syndrome. Hand or toe syndactyly (webbing) or synostosis (joining of two bones) is also common, typically affecting the second through fourth digits. Conductive hearing loss, cleft palate, hyponasality, mouth breathing, and/or a forward posturing of the tongue are common symptoms associated with communicative disorders. Articulation problems related to structural abnormalities and/or hearing loss and language difficulties associated with mental retardation may be present.

Brachman–de Lange Syndrome

See **Cornelia de Lange Syndrom**e.

Cornelia de Lange Syndrome

This syndrome is also called the *de Lange* or *Brachman–de Lange Syndrome*. It is characterized by a short stature, infantile posture, microcephaly, synophrys (abundant eyebrows joined at the midline), a small and dysmorphic (abnormal) nose, a thin and downturned upper lip, small extremities, and contracted elbows. Congenital heart failure often allows for early medical diagnosis of the syndrome. Failure to thrive may also occur. Symptoms associated with communication disorders include cleft palate, micrognathia (underdeveloped mandible), severe speech and language problems, hearing loss, and/or severe mental retardation.

Cri du Chat Syndrome

This chromosomal syndrome results from a deletion of the short arm of the fifth chromosome. The most outstanding symptom is the infant's characteristic cry, which resembles a crying cat (thus the French name *Cri du Chat*, or "cry of the cat"). A narrow oral cavity, low set ears, and/or mental impairment are also common symptoms.

Crouzon Syndrome

Craniosynostosis (premature fusion of the cranial sutures), midfacial and maxillary hypoplasia (underdevelopment), a "beak-shaped" or "parrot-like" nose, strabismus, hypertelorism (increased distance between the eyes), and brachydactyly (shortness of fingers) are characteristic of Crouzon syndrome. A malocclusion, typically Class III, may be present. The head has an irregular shape with a short front-to-back distance and a tall forehead. Ptosis (drooping of the eyelids) is also common. Hearing loss (usually conductive but occasionally sensorineural) and structural problems in the oral cavity often contribute to speech and language disorders.

de Lange Syndrome

See **Cornelia de Lange Syndrome**.

Down Syndrome (Trisomy 21)

Down syndrome is the most common and well-known disorder resulting from a chromosome abnormality. Its name *Trisomy 21* refers to a triplicate (rather than the normal duplicate) of chromosome 21, which results in a total of 47 rather than the usual 46 chromosomes. This chromosomal distinction is present in about 95% of all patients with Down syndrome. Its major characteristics include general hypotonia, open-mouth posture with tongue protrusion, a flat facial profile, brachycephaly (shortened anterior to posterior diameter of the skull), mental retardation or developmental delay, abnormal auricles, and cardiac malformations (in about 40% of patients).

Approximately 75% of all children with Down syndrome have unilateral or bilateral hearing loss, most commonly a mild-moderate conductive impairment. Associated hearing loss is also common among adults, with an increase in the number of sensorineural losses when compared to the normal population. Speech development is typically delayed and complicated by oral-facial abnormalities. A language delay or disorder is common. Abnormal voice and resonance features may also be present.

Ectrodactyly-Ectodermal Dysplasia-Clefting Syndrome (EEC Syndrome)

This syndrome is characterized by ectrodactyly (absence of one or more fingers or toes) or syndactyly (webbing between digits), sparse hair, cleft lip and palate, dental abnormalities, and maxillary hypoplasia (underdevelopment). Chronic serous otitis media in early childhood often results in conductive hearing loss. Various speech problems associated with cleft lip, cleft palate, velopharyngeal incompetence, and dental/ maxillary abnormalities may be present. Intellectual capabilities are typically within normal expectations and mental retardation is not characteristic.

EEC Syndrome

See **Ectrodactyly-Ectodermal Dysplasia-Clefting Syndrome**.

Facio-Auriculo-Vertebral Syndrome

See **Goldenhar Syndrome**.

Fetal Alcohol Syndrome (FAS)

Fetal alcohol syndrome, caused by maternal consumption of alcohol, is the leading cause of birth defects and the third leading cause of mental retardation in the United States. The syndrome may result even if the mother is a light, "social" drinker. Characteristics vary depending, at least in part, on the amount of alcohol consumed and the developmental stage of the fetus. Common features include prenatal and postnatal growth deficiencies in which the child does not "catch up," short palpebral fissures (slits of the eyes), a short and upturned nose, maxillary hypoplasia (underdevelopment), micrognathia (underdeveloped mandible), microcephaly, hypotonia, congenital heart abnormalities, renal (kidney) anomalies, and poor motor coordination. Irritability during infancy and hyperactivity during childhood are also common. Abnormalities of the outer ear may be present, but hearing is generally normal. Children with this syndrome often have impaired mental functioning, language-learning disabilities, hyperactivity, speech impairments, voice problems, and/or fluency disorders. There is a higher incidence of cleft palate among children with this syndrome than in the general population.

First and Second Branchial Arch Syndrome

See **Goldenhar Syndrome**.

Fragile X Syndrome

This syndrome is the second most common cause of genetically based mental retardation (second to Down syndrome). It occurs when there is a fragile spot on the long arm of the X chromosome (technically, Xq27). Characteristics include a large head, prominent forehead, a long and narrow chin, and large ears. The child with this syndrome may exhibit autism or autistic-like behaviors, shyness, or friendliness. Delayed speech and motor development are common. Also, these children exhibit a higher than normal incidence of psychiatric and behavioral problems.

Goldenhar Syndrome

This syndrome has also been referred to as *Hemifacial Microsomia, Facio-AuriculoVertebral Malformation Sequence, Ocular-Auriculo-Vertebral Dysplasia,* and *First and Second Branchial Arch Syndrome.* It is characterized by hypoplasia (underdevelopment) of the face resulting in facial asymmetry (usually unilateral but it may be bilateral), mandibular hypoplasia, facial palsy, microtia (underdeveloped ears), atresia, and/or hemifacial microsomia (portions or all of the head are small). Hearing loss (usually conductive but occasionally sensorineural) may be present. Cleft palate, velar asymmetry, velar paresis, or other oral structure malformations contribute to articulation and resonance disorders in some cases. Retardation is rarely associated with this syndrome.

Hemifacial Microsomia

See **Goldenhar Syndrome**.

Hurler Syndrome

See **Mucopolysaccharidosis Syndromes**.

Hunter Syndrome

See **Mucopolysaccharidosis Syndromes**.

Maroteaux-Lamy Syndrome

See **Mucopolysaccharidosis Syndromes**.

Moebius Syndrome

Characteristics of this syndrome include facial diplegia (bilateral paralysis) resulting in an expressionless, mask-like facial appearance, and unilateral or bilateral loss of abductor muscles. Although not seen in all clients, there is a higher than normal incidence of retardation, cleft palate, hypoplasic (underdeveloped) mandible, and hypoplasic limbs. Hearing loss (usually conductive) may be present. Involvement of the facial nerve (CN VII) and hypoglossal nerve (CN VI) often cause symptoms such as bilabial paresis (partial paralysis or weakness) and difficulties lateralizing, elevating, depressing, or protruding the tongue. Articulatory movements may be limited in strength, range, and speed of movement. Some language development problems are reported, presumably associated with early hospitalizations for aspiration, lack of early growth due to feeding problems, and/or reduced parental expectations for development.

Morquio Syndrome

See **Mucopolysaccharidosis Syndromes**.

Mucopolysaccharidosis Syndromes (including Hurler, Scheie, Hunter, Sanfilippo, Morquio, Morateaux-Lamy, and Sly Syndromes)

The Mucopolysaccharidosis syndromes (MPS) are a group of rare disorders (perhaps 100–700 occurrences per year in the United States). The common characteristic is the excessive storage of complex carbohydrates (mucopolysaccharidosis) in the body. The disorders are progressive and result in mental and physical deterioration, including the possibility of premature death. The most common MPS are Hurler and Hunter syndromes. The differential diagnosis of Hunter syndrome is essential because it is a recessively inherited syndrome which carries a 25% chance of subsequent recurrence. Symptoms of each MPS vary considerably. Speech, language, and hearing problems occur in all of the MPS disorders, but there is limited documentation about specific communication impairments associated with each syndrome.

Noonan Syndrome

This syndrome is characterized by congenital heart disease, narrow chest, short stature, and/or webbing of the neck. Facial features include hypertelorism (increased distance between the eyes) and ptosis (drooping of the eyelids). The ears may also be abnormally shaped, have prominent pinnae, and be set low with a slight posterior rotation. Mental retardation may or may not be present. Oral-facial defects such as lingual and oral malformations and hearing loss (conductive or sensorineural) are often reported. Noonan syndrome has been called the "Turner-like syndrome" since many of the outward manifestations are similar to Turner syndrome (a chromosomally based syndrome).

Oculo-Auriculo-Vertebral Dysplasia

See **Goldenhar Syndrome**.

Oro-Facial-Digital Syndromes
(including Mohr Syndrome)

There are six or seven Oro-Facial-Digital syndromes. The most common is Oro-Facial-Digital syndrome Type II, or Mohr syndrome. This syndrome is characterized by cleft lip, cleft lip and palate, short labial frenulum, absent central incisors, hypoplasic (underdeveloped) mandible, micrognathia (underdeveloped or recessed lower jaw), and tongue malformations such as partial clefting or nodules. The person with this syndrome often has a short stature and digital abnormalities, such as short digits and/ or polydactyly (extra fingers and toes). There may also be an early medical diagnosis of failure to thrive. Conductive hearing loss is common, usually resulting from atresia, ossicular chain malformation, or chronic otitis media (particularly subsequent to cleft palate). Speech impairments may be caused by oral-facial abnormalities, retardation, and/or hearing loss. Intellectual abilities vary considerably from extreme mental retardation to normal intelligence. Naturally, the child's language-learning abilities are related to his or her intellectual capabilities.

Oto-Palatal-Digital Syndrome (OPD)

This syndrome is also known as *Taybi Syndrome*. It is characterized by bone dysplasia (abnormal tissue development), which may result in short and broad finger or toe tips and limited ability to bend the elbows, micrognathia (small or recessed chin), upper airway obstruction, small stature and/or a short torso, and mild hypertelorism (increased distance between the eyes). Cleft palate, missing teeth, and bilateral conductive hearing loss are common with this syndrome; these problems often cause speech and language delays, articulation disorders, and palatopharyngeal difficulties. Mental retardation and associated learning disabilities are reported frequently. Some children with this syndrome also exhibit early chewing, sucking, and swallowing difficulties.

Parkinson's Disease

See **Parkinson's Disease** (p. 49) under **Medical Conditions Associated With Communicative Disorders**.

Pendred Syndrome

This syndrome is a recessively inherited genetic disorder characterized by congenital hearing loss, defective thyroid metabolism, and/or goiter. A profound hearing loss is most characteristic, although mild-moderate losses occur occasionally. Conductive, sensorineural, or mixed hearing losses have been reported and may be progressive in some cases. Speech and language skills can be influenced by the severity and type of hearing impairment. Mental retardation is typically not associated with this syndrome.

Pierre-Robin Sequence
(or Syndrome)

Pierre-Robin sequence is not a true syndrome since it is a combination of several clinical findings caused by one or many etiologies. It may also be called *Pierre-Robin Syndrome*, *Robin Sequence*, or *Robin Deformation Sequence*. Characteristics include mandibular hypoplasia (underdevelopment), glossoptosis (downward displacement of the tongue), and cleft palate (usually the soft palate). The cleft is typically U-shaped (rather than the more common V-shape) or in the form of a bifid uvula (which is most clearly seen during phonation of "ah"). Respiratory problems resulting from the medical diagnosis of failure to thrive and hypoxic (lack of oxygen) brain damage are reported in some cases. Low-set ears, deformed pinnae, an unusual angle of the ear canal, and ossicular defects may also be present. Hearing loss (usually conductive but occasionally sensorineural), speech disorders, language delays, and resonance problems associated with the ear abnormalities and/or the clefting are common. Post-hypoxic brain damage may also cause language problems, learning disabilities, or mental retardation.

Prader-Willi Syndrome

This disorder is sometimes referred to as *Prader-Labhart-Willi Syndrome*. Symptoms include small stature, hypotonia, obesity (especially after the second year of life), and hypogonadism. Excessive appetite and weight gain are long-term problems that must be managed. The frequency of hearing loss is similar to, or only slightly higher than, the general population. Delayed language development is typical. Delayed speech, dysarthria, and/or apraxia may also be present in some cases. Intelligence may be normal, although some degree of retardation (ranging from mild to severe) is more common.

Refsum Syndrome

Symptoms of this syndrome include chronic polyneuritis (inflammation of the nerves), cerebellar ataxia,, and retinitis pigmentosa (a deteriorating condition involving inflammation and pigment infiltration in the retina). Approximately 50% of all patients with this syndrome have a progressive sensorineural hearing loss, often beginning in the 20s or 30s. Associated speech disorders may result from the hearing loss. Ataxic dysarthria, with its characteristic errors of articulation, voice, rate, and prosody, may also be present.

Robin Sequence (or Syndrome)

See **Pierre-Robin Sequence**.

Rubella

See **German Measles** (pp. 45–46) under **Medical Conditions Associated with Communicative Disorders**.

Sanfilippo Syndrome

See **Mucopolysaccharidosis Syndromes**.

Scheie Syndrome

See **Mucopolysaccharidosis Syndromes**.

Sly Syndrome

See **Mucopolysaccharidosis Syndromes**.

Stickler Syndrome

Characteristics of this syndrome include mild midfacial hypoplasia (underdevelopment); micrognathia (underdeveloped chin); severe myopia; and long, thin extremities often with prominent ankle, knee, or wrist joints. Conductive and/or sensorineural hearing loss, and chronic serous otitis media are common. Language and learning abilities can be affected by the hearing loss. Submucosal or overt cleft palate with its associated palatopharyngeal valving problems, early chewing, sucking, and swallowing problems, and articulation and resonance disorders may also be found. Intelligence is usually normal.

Taybi Syndrome

See **Oto-Palatal-Digital Syndrome.**

Treacher Collins Syndrome

Facial abnormalities occur frequently, including mandibular and/or maxillary hyperplasia (underdevelopment), overt or submucosal cleft palate, short or immobile palate, downward slanting palpebral fissures, coloboma (clefting defect) of the eyelids, dental malocclusion, hyperplasia (underdevelopment) of the teeth, beak-shaped nose, and an open bite. Upper respiratory problems that affect breathing may also be present. Atresia, malformations of the pinnae, and/or middle ear structural abnormalities are very common. Inner ear malformations (such as enlarged cochlear aqueducts or absent horizontal canals) occur in severe cases. Language-learning problems associated with hearing loss are typical. Early problems with chewing, sucking, and swallowing, as well as various speech problems, are often seen in the presence of oral-facial abnormalities. Intelligence is usually normal.

Turner Syndrome

This syndrome, also called *XO Syndrome*, is a chromosomal disorder that affects only females. It is characterized by a short stature, reduced angle of the elbow, excessive skin or webbing of the neck, sexual infantilism, amenorrhea (absence of the menstrual cycle), and infertility. A narrow maxilla and palate and micrognathia (underdeveloped chin) may also be present. Auricular deformities and hearing loss (usually mild-moderate sensorineural) are common. Some authorities report that the hearing loss is congenital, while others suggest that it is degenerative. Middle ear pathology is common before age 10. Mental retardation and language problems occur in almost all cases. Speech problems resulting from hearing loss and/or structural abnormalities of the face are also characteristic.

Usher Syndrome

Congenital hearing loss and progressive blindness due to retinitis pigmentosa are the distinguishing characteristics of this syndrome. Usher syndrome is the leading cause of deafness/blindness in the United States. The hearing loss is typically sensorineural, associated with incomplete development or atrophy at the basal end of the organ of Corti in the cochlea. High frequencies are usually more affected than low frequencies, which is consistent with cochlear involvement. Vestibular problems are also very common. Speech and language problems are often associated with the severe-profound hearing loss.

Van der Woude Syndrome

The most common symptom of this syndrome is the presence of congenital pits (fistulae) or mounds on the lower lip. They are typically bilateral and directly inferior to the nares. Cleft lip or palate may also be seen. The upper lip may have a wide cupid's bow or "gull-wing" appearance. Velopharyngeal incompetence is common, especially if there is a deep pharynx and/or submucosal or overt clefting. Chewing, sucking, and swallowing problems are common in early childhood. Hearing loss (usually conductive but occasionally sensorineural or mixed) may be associated with cleft palate or deficient palatal function. The lip pits do not normally cause speech problems since bilabial closure is not affected. However, speech and resonance problems associated with clefting, palatal-pharyngeal inadequacy, and hearing loss may be present. Intelligence is typically normal.

Waardenburg Syndrome

Symptoms of this syndrome include pigment abnormalities such as heterochromia irides (different colors of the iris), vitiligo (unpigmented, pale patches of skin), and the most noticeable feature — a white forelock in the hair (which may be masked if the entire scalp turns white prematurely). Short palpebral fissures, cleft lip or palate, and/ or a prognathic (markedly projected) mandible may also be present. There are two types of Waardenburg syndrome, and both are associated with profound sensorineural hearing loss. The loss may be unilateral or bilateral. Articulation and resonance problems may be associated with clefting, palatal insufficiency, a prognathic mandible, and/or hearing loss. Intelligence is typically normal.

XO Syndrome

See **Turner Syndrome**.

STANDARD MEDICAL ABBREVIATIONS

Some of the preassessment information you gather might be written documents from other health care professionals, such as physician reports or nurses notes. Professionals in the medical industry often use abbreviations when documenting information about a client. Until you are experienced in reading medical notes, understanding the content of such documentation can be a challenge. Below is a list of many of the most commonly used medical abbreviations.

$\bar{a}$	before
Ⓐ	assisted
ADL	activity of daily living
bid	twice per day
$\bar{c}$	with
ca	cancer
c/o	complains of
CVA	cerebral vascular accident
dc	discontinue
dx	diagnosis
fld	fluid
gi	gastrointestinal
H & P	history and physical
hx	history

Ⓘ	independent
iv	intravenous
Ⓛ	left
liq	liquid
med	medical or medication
npo	nothing by mouth
OT	occupational therapy or therapist
p̄	after
per	by or through
PH	past history
PLF	prior level of function
PMH	past medical history
po	by mouth
prn	whenever necessary
PT	physical therapy or therapist
pt	patient
q	every
qd	every day
qid	four times a day
Ⓡ	right
RT	respiratory therapy or therapist
Rx	prescription
s̄	without
sig	marked or significant
SOAP	subjective, objective, assessment, plan
ST	speech therapy or therapist
tid	three times a day
tx	treatment
wt	weight
WFL	within functional limits
WNL	within normal limits
x	times (e.g., 2x = twice)
y/o	years old
Δ	change
2°	secondary to
~	approximately

CONCLUDING COMMENTS

The materials in this chapter are provided to help you understand preassessment information received from a case history. The materials are somewhat general and introductory in nature. Further investigation into additional resources will be necessary in many cases. The "Sources of Additional Information" section lists several sources that may be helpful for more in-depth inquiry into specific areas.

SOURCES OF ADDITIONAL INFORMATION

Speech, Language, and Motor Development

American Speech-Language-Hearing Association. (1983). *How does your child hear and talk?* Rockville,MD: National Association for Hearing and Speech Action.

Boone, D. R., & Plante, E. (1993). *Human communication and its disorders* (2nd ed.). Englewood Cliffs, NJ: Prentice-Hall.

Gard, A., Gilman, L., & Gorman, J. (1980). *Speech and language development chart.* Salt Lake City, UT: Word Making Productions.

Gleason, J. Berko. (Ed.). (1993). *The development of language* (3rd ed.), New York: Macmillan.

Hegde, M. N. (1995). *Introduction to communicative disorders* (2nd ed.). Austin, TX: PRO-ED.

James, S. (1990). *Normal language acquisition.* Boston: Little, Brown.

Kunz, J. R. M., & Finkel, A., J. (Eds.). (1987). *The American Medical Association family medical guide.* New York: Random House.

Lane, V. W., & Molyneaux, D. (1992). *The dynamics of communicative development.* Englewood Cliffs, NJ: Prentice-Hall.

Lenneberg, E. (1969). On explaining language. *Science, 164,* 636.

Owens, R. E. (1996). *Language development: An introduction* (4th ed.). Needham Heights, MA: Allyn & Bacon.

Reich, P. A., (1986). *Language development.* Englewood Cliffs, NJ: Prentice-Hall.

Medical Conditions and Syndromes

Brace, E. R., & Pacanowski, J. P. (1985). *Childhood symptoms.* New York: Harper & Row.

Hamann, B. (1994). *Disease: Identification, prevention, and control.* St. Louis: Mosby.

Gerber, S. E. (1990). *Prevention: The etiology of communicative disorders in children.* Englewood Cliffs, NJ: Prentice-Hall.

Jung, J. H. (1989). *Genetic syndromes in communicative disorders.* Boston: Little, Brown.

Kunz, J. R. M., & Finkel, A. J. (Eds.). *The American Medical Association family medical guide.* New York: Random House.

Larson, D. E. (Ed.). (1990). *Mayo Clinic family health book.* New York: William Morrow.

Reese, R. E., & Douglas, R. G. (Eds.). *A practical approach to infectious diseases.* Boston: Little, Brown.

Rothenberg, M. A., & Chapman, C. F. (1989). *Dictionary of medical terms for the nonmedical person* (2nd ed.). New York: Barron's Educational Series.

Sparks, S. N. (1984). *Birth defects and speech-language disorders.* San Diego, CA: College-Hill Press.

Thomas, C. L. (Ed.). (1989). *Taber's cyclopedic medical dictionary* (16th ed.). Philadelphia: F. A. Davis.

Internet Sources

Interactive Guide to Learning Disabilities for Parents, Teachers, and Children. (Search under *LD in Depth* for information related to Speech-Language Pathology.)
   http://www.ldonline.org

☐ CHAPTER 3 ☐

Reporting Assessment Findings

There are two primary methods for conveying clinical findings, conclusions, and recommendations: information-giving interviews and written reports. In some cases the telephone may be used to convey information. For example, you may wish to call the client's physician to report findings to expedite insurance coverage. Information conveyed by telephone is typically a brief, summarized oral report of clinical findings and often followed up by written correspondence.

INFORMATION-GIVING INTERVIEWS

Information-giving interviews are conducted with the client and/or the client's caregivers. They are typically completed in person, but can be conducted over the telephone in some cases. Information-giving interviews usually consist of three phases: an opening, the body, and a closing (Shipley, 1992). The basic information in each phase includes:

Opening Phase

>Introduce the purpose of the meeting.
>Indicate approximately how much time the session will take.
>Report whether adequate information was obtained during the assessment.
>If reporting to caregivers, describe the client's behavior during the assessment.

>For example: "Vicki was very cooperative and I enjoyed working with her. I was able to get all of the information I needed. I'd like to spend the next 10–15 minutes sharing my results and recommendations with you. Here's what I found . . ."

Body of the Interview

>Discuss the major findings and conclusions from the assessment.
>Keep your language easy to understand and jargon-free.
>Emphasize the major points so that the listener will be able to understand and retain the information you present.

Closing Phase

>Summarize the major findings, conclusions, and recommendations.
>Ask if the listener has any further questions.
>Thank the person for his or her help and interest.
>Describe the next steps that will need to be taken (e.g., seeing the client again, making an appointment with a physician, beginning treatment, etc.).

>For example: "Thank you for bringing Vicki in today. Do you have any more questions before we finish? Once again, (restate major points) . . . That's why I think the next thing we should do is . . ."

ILLUSTRATIONS TO USE WHEN CONVEYING INFORMATION

Many disorders, such as aphasia, hearing loss, certain articulation problems, and some voice or resonance disorders, result from physiological damage or dysfunction. In these cases, visual illustrations of the anatomic areas affected are often useful for helping clients and caregivers understand the information you provide during the information-giving interview. To help you with this information-giving process, illustrations of the brain, ear, oral cavity, vocal folds, and vocal tract are provided in this section.

A chart of the phonetic symbols of the English language is included on page 72 (Table 3–1). This is useful for conveying information to clients or caregivers who are more familiar with the 26 letters in the English alphabet than with the sounds of the language. Several additional items for conveying information about hearing impairment are presented in Chapter 12. These items include an acoustic-phonetic audiogram (p. 420), a chart of environmental noise (dB) levels (p. 421), and a guide to troubleshooting hearing aid problems (pp. 423). The acoustic-phonetic audiogram and chart of environmental noise levels will help you describe how different hearing losses affect a person's ability to hear speech sounds and environmental noises. The troubleshooting guide can help you and your clients identify hearing aid problems that may interfere with communication.

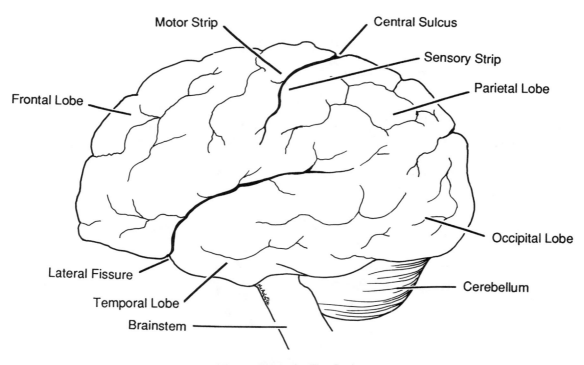

Illustration 3–1. The Brain.

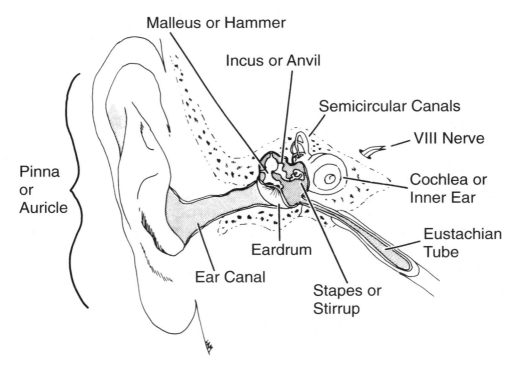

Illustration 3–2. The Ear.

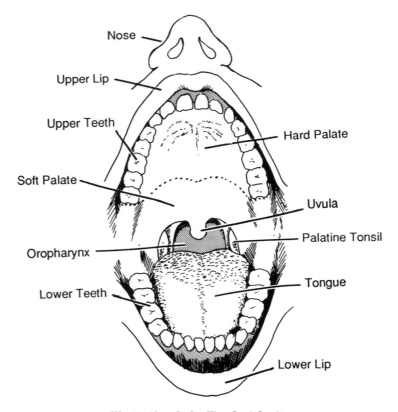

Illustration 3–3. The Oral Cavity.

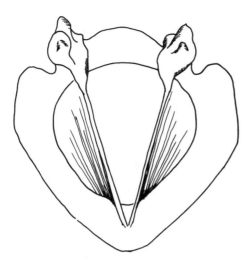

Illustration 3–4. The Vocal Folds—Open.

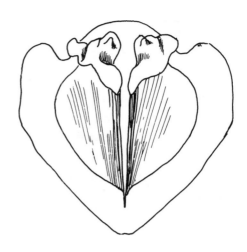

Illustration 3–5. The Vocal Folds—Closed.

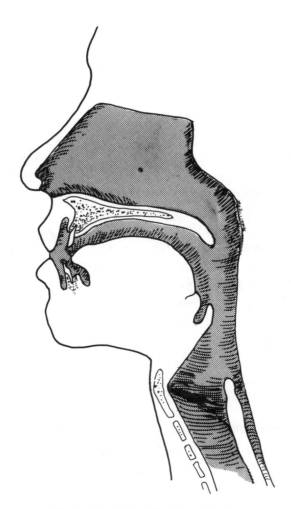

Illustration 3–6. The Vocal Tract.

Table 3–1. Phonetic Symbols of the English Language

Consonants				Vowels					
Voiced		**Unvoiced**						**Blends**		**Diphthongs**	
/b/	as in *b*ig	/p/	as in *p*in	/i/	as in m*ee*t	/ʒ /	as in s*u*re	/aɪ/	as in b*ye*
/d/	as in *d*og	/t/	as in *t*ie	/ɪ/	as in *i*t		(stressed)	/eɪ/	as in cr*ay*on
/g/	as in *g*o	/k/	as in *c*at	/e/	as in *eigh*t	/ɚ/	as in moth*er*	/ɑʊ/	as in *ou*t
/v/	as in *v*ase	/f/	as in *f*ar	/ɛ/	as in m*e*t		(unstressed)	/ɔɪ/	as in b*oy*
/z/	as in *z*oo	/s/	as in *s*it	/æ/	as in *a*sk	/oʊ/	as in m*o*de		
/ð/	as in *th*is	/θ/	as in *th*ink	/ə/	as in c*o*ntrol				
/ʒ/	as in mea*s*ure	/ʃ/	as in *sh*ake		(unstressed)				
/dʒ/	as in *j*ump	/tʃ/	as in *ch*ip	/ʌ/	as in c*ou*ntry				
/m/	as in *m*op	/h/	as in *h*i		(stressed)				
/n/	as in *n*o			/u/	as in t*oo*				
/ŋ/	as in si*ng*			/ʊ/	as in b*oo*k				
/l/	as in *l*ight			/o/	as in g*o*				
/r/	as in *r*ake			/ɔ/	as in d*o*g				
/j/	as in *y*es			/ɑ/	as in s*aw*				
/w/	as in *w*et								

WRITING ASSESSMENT REPORTS

The precise format, style, scope, length, and degree of detail needed for a diagnostic report varies across settings, university programs, and even different supervisors in the same setting. To find any two supervisors who agree on precisely what constitutes a fully acceptable, good report seems to be unusual. Such varying expectations frequently frustrate students during clinical education, particularly as they must "perfect" one style one term and then another style the next term. Perhaps the consolation for students is that, when you graduate and practice professionally, you will be able to "pick and choose" aspects you like from those different models, so you can develop your own unique style of writing assessment reports. Despite individual variations, most assessment or diagnostic reports have a similar format and generally present the same basic information, which includes:

Identifying Information

> Name
> Date of birth/Age
> School/Teacher/Grade (if appropriate)
> Address
> Phone numbers
> Physician(s)
> Billing party (if appropriate)

Overview/Background/Presenting Complaint

> Referral source
> Dates and locations of previous evaluations
> Presenting complaint (unintelligible speech, dysfluency, voice problem, etc.)
> Previous treatment

Histories

> Speech, language, and hearing
> Medical
> Educational
> Psychological/Emotional
> Developmental/Motor
> Familial
> Social
> Occupational (adult)

Assessment Information

> Articulation
>> Conversational speech (sound errors, intelligibility)
>> Identification and analysis of sound errors
>> Consistency of sound errors Patterns of sound errors (errors types, severity of errors, phonological processes)
>> Stimulability of errors (i.e., whether correct sounds can be made)
>> Rate, prosody, intonation, inflection, and so on

> Language
>> Receptive language, including information from formal and informal evaluations, primarily of semantics and syntax
>> Expressive language, including information from formal and informal language samples of semantics, syntax, morphologic features, and pragmatics
>> Cognition (if appropriate)

> Fluency
>> Types and frequencies of dysfluencies
>> Associated motor behaviors (hand movements, eyeblinking, etc.)
>> Avoidance of sounds, words, or situations; anticipation of stuttering
>> Speech rates with and without dysfluencies
>> Stimulability of fluent speech

> Voice
>> Quality (hoarse, aphonic, etc.)
>> Pitch (too high, too low, variable)

Resonance (nasal, denasal, mixed)
Breath support; type of breathing used (diaphragmatic, thoracic, clavicular)
Muscular tension
Stimulability of improved voice

Oral-facial Examination

Structures and functions that affect speech production
Peripheral areas (if appropriate). For example, hand and arm movements that indicate alternative communication potential

Hearing

Hearing screening or more sophisticated auditory assessment

Summary

Statement of diagnosis
Concise statement of most significant findings
Prognosis

Recommendations

Treatment, no treatment, recheck at a later time
Referral to other professionals
Suggestions to the client and/or caregivers

The specific format of the report, including which headings to use, is dependent on the acceptable expectations within your setting. Examples of assessment reports with slightly different formats and styles are found in Haynes, Pindzola, and Emerick (1992); Hegde, 1994; Hegde and Davis (1995); Meitus (1983a); Nation and Aram (1991); Peterson and Marquardt (1994); and Sanders (1979). Two sample reports are also included in Appendix 3–A. We do recommend that you consult with your supervisor to secure specific report formats and styles in your clinical setting.

Some time ago, Haynes and Hartmann (1975) wrote that while report styles do vary, most supervisors have "remarkably similar criteria for what should not be presented in a report and what is considered to be an error" (p. 10). The following guidelines are based, in part, on their article. Consider these suggestions when reviewing your own reports.

11. Does it contain all of the major information needed?

12. Is the information appropriately categorized? For example, is the historical information presented under a *history* heading or subheading? Is the information from language testing under *language*?

13. Is there redundancy of words, phrases, or topics?

14. Is it too wordy? Are any sentences too long?

5. Is all terminology used correctly? Are professional words used appropriately? Should professional terminology be used instead of lay terms?

6. Is the report written objectively?

7. Are the "facts" truly based on fact? Or are there facts that are actually interpretations or presumptions?

8. Is the focus on the major points? Are there any major points that have been omitted or underemphasized? Are secondary points overemphasized?

9. Does the report contain ambiguities that could be misinterpreted? Is it specific?

10. Is it written in a logical progression? Do introductory sections lead to assessment findings, which then lead to conclusions and recommendations?

11. Are the mechanics appropriate (spelling, punctuation, grammar, etc.)?

Instructors often recommend that students ask peers or family members to read their class-related papers for basic readability, organization, spelling, and grammar. Keep in mind that this is inappropriate for most clinical reports, as it would violate the client's confidentiality—whether the outside reader knows the client or not.

CLINICAL CORRESPONDENCE

Letters to other professionals are common in clinical practice. Recipients of clinical information may include physicians, social workers, mental health professionals, insurance companies or other third-party payors (such as an employer), departments of vocational rehabilitation, or others. The written correspondence will vary in length and scope depending on the client, the findings, and the recipient. Many professionals, particularly physicians, prefer a short letter that simply "gets to the point" without excessive background or verbiage. Three sample letters, varying in length and scope, are presented in Appendix 3–B.

CONCLUDING COMMENTS

Once you have gathered your assessment information and completed the diagnostic evaluation, you are ready to begin the process of sharing your results with the client, caregivers, and/or other professionals. Results and suggestions are typically conveyed through an information-giving interview, a clinical assessment report, and/or specific correspondence to other professionals. In all cases, the effectiveness of the information you convey depends on adequate assessment data, knowledgeable interpretations of the data, and the use of good oral or written reporting skills. Acceptable, useful presentation and dissemination of clinical findings is extremely important. Remember that the best assessment in the world may have little effect unless the information is presented effectively to others.

SOURCES OF ADDITIONAL INFORMATION

Information-giving Interviews

Meitus, I. J. (1983b). Talking with patients and their families. In I. J. Meitus & B. Weinberg (Eds.), *Diagnosis in speech-language pathology* (pp. 311–337). Austin, TX: PRO-ED.

Shipley, K. G. (1992). *Interviewing and counseling in communicative disorders: Principles and procedures*. New York: Merrill/Macmillan.

Stewart, C. J., & Cash, W. B. (1991). *Interviewing: Principles and practices* (6th ed.). Dubuque, IA: William C. Brown.

Written Reports

Emerick, L. L., & Haynes, W. O. (1986). *Diagnosis and evaluation in speech pathology* (3rd ed.). Englewood Cliffs, NJ: Prentice-Hall.

Haynes, W. O., & Hartmann, D. E. (1975). The agony of report writing: A new look at an old problem. *Journal of the National Student Speech and Hearing Association, 3*, 7–15.

Haynes, W. O., Pindzola, R H., & Emerick, L. L. (1992). *Diagnosis and evaluation in speech pathology* (4th ed.). Englewood Cliffs, NJ: Prentice-Hall.

Hegde, M. N. (1997). *A coursebook on scientific and professional writing in speech-language pathology*. San Diego, CA: Singular Publishing Group.

Hegde, M. N., & Davis, D. (1995). *Clinical methods and practicum in speech-language pathology*. (2nd ed.). San Diego, CA: Singular Publishing Group.

Knepfler, K. (1976). *Report writing*. Danville, IL: Interstate Printers & Publishers.

Meitus, I. J. (1983a). Clinical report and letter writing. In I. J. Meitus & B. Weinberg (Eds.), *Diagnosis in speech-language pathology* (pp. 287–309). Austin, TX: PRO-ED.

Peterson, H. A., & Marquardt, T. P. (1994). *Appraisal and diagnosis of speech and language disorders* (3rd ed.). Englewood Cliffs, NJ: Prentice-Hall.

Sanders, L.J. (1979). *Procedure guides for evaluation of speech and hearing disorders in children* (4th ed.). Danville, IL: Interstate Printers & Publishers.

Internet Sources

Interactive Guide to Learning Disabilities for Parents, Teachers, and Children. (Search under *LD in Depth* for information related to Speech-Language Pathology.)
http://www.ldonline.org

APPENDIX 3–A
Sample Clinical Reports

Sample Report I

University Clinic
123 Main Street
Anytown, CA 99999
209-555-1529

Diagnostic Evaluation

Name: Adam McCune

Birthdate: 4-2-90

Age: 7 years, 5 months

Address: 4574 E. 1st St.

           Anytown, CA 99999

School Status: 2nd grade, Holt Elementary

Date: September 14, 1997

Clinic File No.: 12345

Diagnosis: Fluency Disorder

Phone: 555-8942

History and Presenting Complaint

Adam, a 7-year 5-month-old male, was seen for a speech-language evaluation at the University Clinic on September 14, 1997. He was accompanied by his mother.

Adam attended Holt Elementary School and received speech therapy two times per week for remediation of dysfluent speech. Mrs. McCune reported that Adam began stuttering at approximately 3 years of age. She also stated that his stuttering fluctuated and increased during stressful situations. Mrs. McCune stated that her father also stuttered.

Adam's medical history was unremarkable.

Assessment Findings

Speech: The *Goldman-Fristoe Test of Articulation* was administered to assess Adam's production of consonants in fixed positions at the word level. Adam lateralized /s/ and /z/ in all positions. He substituted /nk/ for /n/ in the medial and final positions. Adam was stimulable for /s/ and /z/ at the word level.

A 384-word conversational speech sample revealed similar errors. He also omitted /d/ and /t/ in the final position during connected speech. Adam was 100% intelligible during this sample.

Oral-facial Examination: An oral-facial examination was administered to assess the structural and functional integrity of the oral mechanism. Facial features were symmetrical.

Labial and lingual strength and range of motion were normal during speech and nonspeech tasks. Lingual size and shape were normal. Mandibular movement revealed a slight crossbite, and a lateral view of the central incisors indicated a slight overjet Appropriate velar movement was observed during productions of /a/.

Diadochokinetic syllable tasks were administered to assess rapid movements of the speech musculature. Adam repeated /pʌtəkə/ at a rate of 4.04 repetitions per second. This was within normal limits for a child his age.

Language: The *Peabody Picture Vocabulary Test* (Form L) was administered to assess receptive vocabulary. A raw score of 92 and a standard score of 108 were obtained. Age equivalency was 8:0 and percentile rank was 70. The results indicated average to above-average receptive vocabulary skills.

Analysis of the conversational speech-language sample revealed appropriate expressive language skills. Syntactic, morphologic, and semantic structures of the language were appropriate. Adam's average length of utterance was 10.9 words.

Voice: Adam exhibited a normal vocal quality. An s/z ratio of 1.0 was obtained.

Fluency: A 384-word spontaneous sample was elicited to assess Adam's fluency rate, and he was 82% fluent on a word-by-word basis. Dysfluencies averaged 2 seconds in duration with a range of .8 seconds to 4 seconds. Dysfluencies included:

	# Dysfluencies	Percentage
Sound Interjections	28	17.3%
Word Interjections	11	10.3%
Sound Repetitions	19	15.0%
Word Repetitions	18	12.1%
Phrase Repetitions	18	12.1%
Revisions	13	10.8%
Prolongations	12	10.5%
Total	**69**	**18.1%**

Adam was stimulable for fluent speech at the 3-syllable phrase level when he was required to use an easy onset and syllable stretching.

Hearing: A hearing screen was administered at 20 dB HTL for the frequencies of 250, 500, 1000, 2000, 4000, and 6000 Hz. Adam responded to all sounds bilaterally.

Summary and Recommendations

Adam exhibited moderate dysfluency characterized by sound interjections and sound, word, and phrase repetitions. He was stimulable for fluent speech, which suggests a good prognosis for improvement with therapy. Adam also exhibited mild articulatory errors of substitutions and additions. He was stimulable for all phonemes. Expressive and receptive language abilities were age appropriate.

It was recommended that Adam receive speech therapy to train fluent speech and correct his articulation errors.

Stephen D. Marshall, M.A., CCC/SIP
Speech-Language Pathologist

Sample Report 2

University Clinic
123 Main Street
Anytown, CA 99999
209-555-1529

Diagnostic Evaluation

Name: Lisa Breckenridge

Birthdate: 12-12-61

Age: 35

Address: 4574 Cedar Ave.

Anytown, CA 99999

Occupation: High School Mathematics Instructor

Date: 6-2-97

Clinic file No.: 98765

Diagnosis: Voice Disorder

Phone: 555-0809

History and Presenting Complaint

Mrs. Breckenridge, a 35-year-old female, was referred to the University Clinic by Stuart Goehring, M.D., subsequent to the development of bilateral vocal nodules. The patient complained of a hoarse voice. She reported that the problem started about five months ago and had become especially problematic during the last two months.

At the time of the evaluation, Mrs. Breckenridge reported that she taught four periods of high school mathematics per day at San Joaquin High School. There were approximately 35 students per class. She stated that she needed to project her voice during that time.

Mrs. Breckenridge stated that she liked to sing, but did so rarely because it aggravated her voice problem. She reported that she did not smoke, and consumed a minimal amount of alcohol (e.g., a glass of wine once in a while). She also stated that she did not yell excessively, use inhalants, talk in noisy environments (other than the classroom), or cough excessively. She did not report a history of allergies, asthma, or frequent colds. Caffeine intake included, at most, one or two iced teas per day.

Assessment Findings

Mrs. Breckenridge exhibited the symptoms of vocal nodules. Her voice was characterized by hoarseness, intermittent breathiness, pitch breaks, and intermittent glottal fry. The symptoms were exacerbated when she was asked to increase her vocal intensity. Attempts to increase her loudness levels were accompanied by increased feelings of discomfort in the laryngeal region.

Mrs. Breckenridge's fundamental frequency was approximately 220 Hz when sustaining "ah" for 15+ seconds. An increase in breathiness and the occurrence of pitch breaks were noted during the last 5+ seconds of these vocalizations.

She exhibited a low vertical focus in the use of her voice. This created a lower pitch and poor vocal projection. In an attempt to increase her projection, she increased her vocal effort. This type of vocal abuse is typically associated with the development of vocal nodules

With instruction and modeling, Mrs. Breckenridge was able to raise her vertical focus and produce clearer, louder, nonhoarse, and nonbreathy vocal productions. During these stimulability tasks, Mrs. Breckenridge reported that she was not feeling the vocal tension and aggravation that typically accompanied her speech and voice use. This indicated a good prognosis for improved voice quality with therapy.

Diagnosis and Recommendations

Mrs. Breckenridge was diagnosed as having bilateral vocal nodules by her referring physician, Dr. Goehring. Vocal symptoms of this diagnosis were apparent during the assessment. She exhibited a hoarse and breathy vocal quality. She appeared to be an excellent candidate for voice therapy.

Sixteen 30-minute sessions of voice therapy (i.e., twice per week for two months) were recommended. Additional steps that may be needed will be reconsidered at that time.

———————————————

Autumn Noel, M.A., CCC/SLP
Speech-Language Pathologist

APPENDIX 3–B

Sample Clinical Correspondence

A Brief Example

ABC Clinic
123 Main Street
Anytown, CA 99999
209-555-1529

January 13, 1997

Curtis Clay, M.D.
4242 W. Oak Street
Anytown, CA 99999

Re: Peggy Kiskaddon (DOB: 4-2-1992)

Dear Dr. Clay:

Peggy was seen for an evaluation on January 12, 1997. She has difficulty producing several speech sounds—specifically *r*, *l*, *th*, and most consonant blends (such as *br*, *pl*, and *thr*).

I was able to stimulate several sounds during the session, and she could produce these new sounds in several words and short phrases. Peggy will be enrolled for therapy to improve her misarticulations beginning in two weeks. Her prognosis for improvement with therapy is good.

I will forward a complete report of my findings if it would be helpful to you. Please let me know if you would like a copy. Thank you very much.

Sincerely,

———————————————

Linda J. Rees, M.A., CCC/SLP
Speech-Language Pathologist

cc: Mr. and Mrs. Kiskaddon

A More Detailed Example

ABC Clinic
123 Main Street
Anytown, CA 99999
209-555-1529

January 19, 1997

Mark Lapsley, M.D.
7772 1st Street, Suite 12
Anytown, CA 99999

Re: Eric Armstrong (DOB: 10-13-92)

Dear Dr. Lapsley:

Thank you for referring Eric to our clinic. His speech was evaluated on January 17, 1997. He was cooperative throughout the 75-minute evaluative session and a good sample of his speech was obtained.

Eric exhibited a severe stuttering disorder. His speech was approximately 40% dysfluent and included five different types of dysfluencies. Eric and his mother confirmed that his stuttering was bothersome to both of them, that he avoids certain speaking situations, and that the stuttering patterns have become more prominent during the last six months.

Several techniques (particularly an easier onset of speech and a slower rate) resulted in fluent speech in the clinic. Eric's and his mother's levels of concern, their motivation, and the child's ability to produce fluent speech were considered good signs for teaching him a more fluent speech pattern with therapy. He will be enrolled for 40-minute sessions three times per week beginning this June.

Other areas of communication (articulation, hearing, language, and voice) were normal or above-normal. Thus, I will focus only on his ability to produce fluent speech.

A report of my findings has been written. Please contact me if this is of interest to you. I will send you periodic reports of Eric's progress in treatment.

Again, thank you for referring Eric to us.

Sincerely,

Darlene Blackwood, M.A., CCC/SLP
Speech-Language Pathologist

cc: Mr. and Mrs. Armstrong

A Detailed Example[1]

Purdue University Speech and Hearing Clinic
West Lafayette, IN 47907

July 17, 1982

Robert J. Black, M.D.
2901 Reading Road
Lafayette, IN 47905

Re: JONES, David M.
DOB: 10-23-70
PUSHC #: 82-999

Dear Doctor Black:

This is a summary report on David M. Jones, an 11-year, 9-month-old boy you referred to our clinic because "his voice did not sound normal." David was examined on July 15, 1982. He was accompanied by his mother who felt that David's primary problem was "huskiness" of the voice.

Significant historical information included Mrs. Jones' report that David's voice disturbance began "about 1 year ago." David received no prior examination or treatment for this problem. His development has been unremarkable and his health history is excellent. David's school progress has been outstanding. Mrs. Jones reported that their family is a "close-knit group," is "highly verbal," and is "very affectionate." There is a negative familial history of speech or voice disturbance.

During the course of the direct interview with David, he acknowledged that he has a voice problem. He correctly indicated that his voice problem is mild and that it does not have a significant negative influence on his school achievement or his social relationships. He was unaware of why his voice problem exists. Both David and his mother agreed that there are times when his voice sounds "better" (e.g., when rested, when not in school, when not participating in sports, and in the morning). They agreed that David often engages in "shouting" and that he speaks excessively.

David cooperated fully in all phases of the examination. He appeared to us to be a capable 11-year-old who freely expresses his feelings. The results of our examination of David's speech and hearing mechanism were unremarkable. A comprehensive examination of various aspects of David's voice production was completed. His voice had a consistent breathy component. Vocal pitch and loudness characteristics were perceptually unremarkable, and no pitch breaks or interruptions of the voice were noted during the examination. Significant changes in David's voice were not apparent during the examination. He was not able to modify the breathy component to his voice in response to several facilitative techniques we attempted.

Various types of respiratory testing were also completed. The results of these forms of testing revealed that: 1) airflow rate through David's larynx (0.25–0.35 LPS) was higher than normal; 2) laryngeal airway resistance (about 34 cm H_2O LPS) was well within normal limits; 3) he was able to supply adequate pressure to the larynx during voice production; and 4) his chest wall movements and air volume characteristics associated with voice production were unremarkable.

---

[1]From I.J. Meitus and B. Weinberg, *Diagnosis in Speech-Language Pathology* (pp. 306–307). Austin, TX: PRO-ED. Copyright © 1983 and used by permission of Allyn and Bacon, current copyright holder.

With one exception, David's speech and language function was judged to be normal. The exception was that he consistently distorted the /s/ sound, but was able to produce acceptable /s/ sounds with limited instruction.

Our impression is that David has a mild voice disorder characterized by the consistent presence of breathy voice quality. Statements about the etiology of this problem and plans to initiate voice therapy must await laryngological examination. The etiology of David's isolated speech sound error is also unknown and has not been of concern to David and his family. David's ability to modify this isolated error was an indication that speech therapy would be productive.

The following recommendations were made and accepted by David and his mother:

1. A laryngological examination was scheduled (July 23, 1982) with George B. Wilson, M.D.
2. A return visit was scheduled with us for August 15, 1982. During this visit we expect to discuss that laryngological finding and possible voice remediation, and initiate a therapy program for the /s/ sound.

We appreciate your referral of the Jones family and urge you to contact us if further information concerning David is needed.

Sincerely yours,

John D. Williams, CCC/SP
Speech Pathologist

□   PART II   □

Resources for Assessing Communicative Disorders

□ CHAPTER 4 □

Assessment Procedures Common to Most Communicative Disorders

This chapter contains eight basic methods for assessing most speech and language disorders—particularly articulation, language, voice, and fluency. You will not need every procedure for each client, although a majority of your assessments will include several, if not most, of the procedures described here.

ORAL-FACIAL EXAMINATION

The oral-facial evaluation is an important component of a complete speech assessment (Form 4–1). Its purpose is to identify or rule out structural or functional factors that relate to a communicative disorder. Minimally, you will need a small flashlight and a tongue depressor. For some clients, you may also need a bite block (to disassociate tongue and jaw movements), cotton gauze (to hold the tongue in place), an applicator stick (to assess velopharyngeal movement), and/or a mirror. When evaluating young children, especially those who are reluctant to participate, foods such as peanut butter or applesauce can be strategically placed in the oral cavity to help you assess lip and tongue movements.

A complete oral examination includes an assessment of diadochokinetic rates, which measures a client's ability to produce rapidly alternating articulatory movements. The "Assessing Diadochokinetic Syllable Rates" worksheet presented later in this chapter is provided to help you assess these abilities.

Interpreting the Oral-facial Examination

Valid interpretation of findings from an oral-facial examination requires an understanding of the anatomic, physiologic, and neurologic bases of the oral-facial structures and their functions, combined with experience in performing oral-facial examinations and assessing the relationship between oral-facial integrity and communicative function. Sophistication in administering these examinations takes time and a good deal of experience to develop.

Several common observations from an oral-facial examination and possible clinical implications are described below. Recognize that this is not an all-inclusive list, nor does it exhaust the potential implications of each finding. Beginning clinicians will need to rely on class notes and anatomy, physiology, and neurology textbooks, as well as the chapters on oral examinations in diagnostic textbooks (e.g., Haynes, et al., 1992; Meitus & Weinberg, 1983b; Nation & Aram, 1991; Peterson & Marquardt, 1994). Additional sources are listed in the "Sources of Additional Information" section at the end of this chapter. Resources for motor speech disorders (e.g., Darley, Aronson, & Brown, 1975; Dworkin, 1991; Johns, 1985; Love, 1992; Yorkston, Beukelman, & Bell, 1988) are also useful.

☐ *Abnormal color of the tongue, palate, or pharynx:* There are several abnormal colors you may observe. A grayish color is normally associated with muscular paresis or paralysis. A bluish tint may result from excessive vascularity or bleeding. A whitish color present along the border of the hard and soft palate is a symptom of a submucosal cleft. An abnormally dark or a translucent color on the hard palate may be an indication of a palatal fistula or a cleft. Dark spots may indicate oral cancer.

☐ *Abnormal height or width of the palatal arch:* The shape of the palatal arch may vary considerably from client to client. If the arch is especially wide or high, the client may experience difficulties with palatal-lingual sounds. An abnormally low or narrow arch in the presence of a large tongue may result in consonant distortions.

☐ *Asymmetry of the face or palate:* This is often associated with neurological impairment or muscle weakness.

☐ *Deviation of the tongue and/or uvula to the left or right:* This may indicate neurological involvement. If so, the tongue may deviate to the weaker side because the weaker half of the tongue is unable to match the extension of the stronger half. On phonation, the uvula may deviate to the stronger side as the palatal muscles on that strong side pull the uvula farther toward the velopharyngeal opening. Facial asymmetry is also likely to be present. The client may exhibit concomitant aphasia and/or dysarthria.

☐ *Enlarged tonsils:* Many children have large tonsils with no adverse affect on speech production. In some cases, however, enlarged tonsils interfere with general health, normal resonance, and/or hearing acuity (if the eustachian tubes are blocked). A forward carriage of the tongue may also persist, resulting in abnormal articulation.

☐ *Missing teeth:* Depending on which teeth are missing, articulation may be impaired. It is important to determine whether the missing teeth are the primary cause of, or a contributor to, the communicative disorder. In most cases, especially in children, missing teeth do not seriously affect articulation.

☐ *Mouth breathing:* The client may have a restricted passageway to the nasal cavity. If this is a persistent problem and the client also exhibits hyponasal (denasal) speech, a referral to a physician is warranted. Mouth breathing may also be associated with anterior posturing of the tongue at rest.

☐ *Poor intraoral pressure:* Poor maintenance of air in the cheeks is a sign of labial weakness and/or velopharyngeal inadequacy—more specifically, velopharyngeal insufficiency (a structural problem) or velopharyngeal incompetence (a functional problem). Check for nasal emission or air escaping from the lips. This client may also have dysarthria and/or hypernasality.

☐ *Prominent rugae:* This may indicate an abnormally narrow and/or low palate, or abnormally large tongue in relation to the palatal areas. Pronounced rugae is also associated with tongue thrust.

☐ *Short lingual frenum:* This may result in an articulation disorder. If the client is unable to place the tongue against the alveolar ridge or the teeth to produce sounds such as /t/, /d/, /n/, /l/, /tʃ/, and /dʒ/, the frenum may need to be clipped by a physician.

☐ *Weak or absent gag reflex:* This often indicates muscular weakness in the velopharyngeal area. Neurological impairment may be present. A warning though—do not make this conclusion without considering other factors. Some clients have a very high tolerance for gagging and will not gag even if muscular integrity is normal.

☐ *Weakness of the lips, tongue, and/or jaw:* This is common among clients with neurological impairments. Aphasia and/or dysarthria may be present.

Form 4–1. Oral-facial Examination Form

Name: _____ Age:_____ Date:_____

Examiner: _____

Instructions: Check and circle each item noted. Include descriptive comments in the right-hand margin.

Evaluation of Face   **Comments**

_____   symmetry: normal/droops on right/droops on left _____

_____   abnormal movements: none/grimaces/spasms _____

_____   mouth breathing: yes/no _____

_____   other:_____

Evaluation of Jaw and Teeth

Tell client to open and close mouth.

_____   range of motion: normal/reduced _____

_____   symmetry: normal/deviates to right/deviates to left _____

_____   movement: normal/jerky/groping/slow/asymmetrical _____

_____   TMJ noises: absent/grinding/popping _____

_____   other:_____

Observe dentition:

_____   occlusion (molar relationship): normal/neutroclusion (Class I)/distoclusion (Class II)/mesioclusion (Class III)/_____

_____   occlusion (incisor relationship): normal/overbite/underbite/crossbite _____

_____   teeth: all present/dentures/teeth missing (specify) _____

_____   arrangement of teeth: normal/jumbled/spaces/misaligned _____

_____   hygiene: _____

_____   other:_____

Evaluation of Lips

Tell client to pucker.

_____   range of motion: normal/reduced_____

(continued)

Form 4–1 *(continued)*

Comments

_____   symmetry: norma/droops bilaterally/droops right/droops left _____

_____   strength (press tongue blade against lips): normal/weak _____

_____   other: _____

Tell client to smile.

_____   range of motion: normal/reduced _____

_____   symmetry: normal/droops bilaterally/droops right/droops left _____

_____   other: _____

Tell client to puff cheeks and hold air.

_____   lip strength: normal/reduced _____

_____   nasal emission: absent/present _____

_____   other: _____

Evaluation of Tongue

_____   surface color: normal/abnormal (specify) _____

_____   abnormal movements: absent/jerky/spasms/writhing/fasciculations _____

_____   size: normal/small/large _____

_____   frenum: normal/short _____

_____   other: _____

Tell client to protrude the tongue.

_____   excursion: normal/deviates to right/deviates to left _____

_____   range of motion: normal/reduced _____

_____   speed of motion: normal/reduced _____

_____   strength (apply opposing pressure with tongue blade): normal/reduced _____

_____   other: _____

Tell client to retract tongue.

_____   excursion: normal/deviates to right/deviates to left _____

_____   range of motion: normal/reduced _____

(continued)

Comments

_____ speed of motion: normal/reduced _____

_____ other: _____

Tell client to move tongue tip to the right.

_____ excursion: normal/incomplete/groping _____

_____ range of motion: normal/reduced _____

_____ strength (apply opposing pressure with tongue blade): normal/reduced:_____

_____ other: _____

Tell client to move the tongue tip to the left.

_____ excursion: normal/incomplete/groping _____

_____ range of motion: normal/reduced _____

_____ strength (apply opposing pressure with tongue blade): normal/reduced:_____

_____ other: _____

Tell client to move the tongue tip up.

_____ movement: normal/groping: _____

_____ range of motion: normal/reduced _____

_____ other: _____

Tell client to move the tongue tip down.

_____ movement: normal/groping: _____

_____ range of motion: normal/reduced _____

_____ other: _____

Observe rapid side-to-side movements.

_____ rate: normal/reduced/slows down progressively _____

_____ range of motion: normal/reduced on left/reduced on right _____

_____ other: _____

Evaluation of Pharynx:

_____ color: normal/abnormal _____

_____ tonsils: absent/normal/enlarged _____

_____ other: _____

(continued)

Form 4–1 *(continued)*

Comments

Evaluation of Hard and Soft Palates:

_____ color: normal/abnormal _____

_____ rugae: normal/very prominent _____

_____ arch height: normal/high/low _____

_____ arch width: normal/narrow/wide _____

_____ growths: absent/present (describe) _____

_____ fistula: absent/present (describe) _____

_____ clefting: absent/present (describe) _____

_____ symmetry at rest: normal/lower on right/lower on left_____

_____ gag reflex: normal/absent/hyperactive/hypoactive _____

_____ other:_____

Tell client to phonate using /a/.

_____ symmetry of movement: normal/deviates right/deviates left _____

_____ posterior movement: present/absent/reduced _____

_____ lateral movement: present/absent/reduced _____

_____ uvula: normal/bifid/deviates right/deviates left _____

_____ nasality: absent/hypernasal _____

_____ other:_____

Summary of Findings:

ASSESSING DIADOCHOKINETIC SYLLABLE RATES

Diadochokinetic syllable rates are used to evaluate a client's ability to make rapidly alternating speech movements. There are two primary ways to obtain these measures. The first is by counting the number of syllable repetitions a client produces within a predetermined number of seconds. For example, how many repetitions of /pʌ/ can the client produce in 15 seconds? The second method is timing how many seconds it takes the client to repeat a predetermined number of syllables. For example, how many seconds does it take to produce 20 repetitions of /pʌ/

The diadochokinetic worksheet, Form 4–2, is based on the works of Fletcher (1972, 1978). The norms are based on the second method described above—the total seconds taken to repeat a specific number of syllables. A total of 384 children from 6 to 13 years of age, including 24 boys and 24 girls from each age group, participated in the norming sample (see Fletcher, 1972).

Before obtaining diadochokinetic syllable rates, provide adequate instructions for the tasks, model the target behaviors, and allow the client to practice the tasks. Then, using a stopwatch to keep accurate time, say the word "go." Count the number of syllables (e.g., /pʌ/ the client produces. When the predetermined number of seconds has elapsed, say "stop." Redo the task if the client stops or slows down intentionally before the allotted time is expired. After each syllable has been assessed individually, evaluate the client's production of the /pʌtəkə/ sequence. Use the "Diadochokinetic Syllable Rates Worksheet," Form 4–2, to record the results of your evaluation.

With practice, most clinicians are able to accurately count the number of syllables produced during the time interval tested. If you are inexperienced or feel unsure of your accuracy, count the productions with a hand-held counter or tape record the test for review at a later time. If you are involved in research and need more information about the normative data, or if you desire to evaluate additional diadochokinetic tasks (i.e., /fʌ/, /lʌ/, /pʌtə/, /pʌkə/, and /tʌkə/), consult Fletcher's (1972, 1978) works.

Form 4–2. Diadochokinetic Syllable Rates Worksheet[1]

Name:_____ Age:_____ Date:_____

Examiner: _____

Instructions: Time the number of seconds it takes your client to complete each task the prescribed number of times. The average number of seconds for children from 6 to 13 years of age is reported in the right-hand side of the table.

The standard deviation (SD) from the norm (mean or average) is also found in the table. Subtract the SD from the norm to determine each SD interval. For example, using the /pʌ/ norm with a 6-year-old, 3.8 (4.8–1.0) is one SD, 2.8 (4.8–2.0) is two SDs, 2.3 (4.8–2.5) is two-and-a-half SDs, etc. Therefore, a 6year-old child who needed 2.6 seconds to complete the /pʌ/ sequence would be two SDs below the mean.

| | | | *Norms in seconds for diadochokinetic syllable rates* | | | | | | | |
| | | | Age: | | | | | | | |
Task	Repetitions	Seconds	16	17	8	9	10	11	12	13
pʌ	20	_____	14.8	14.8	4.2	4.0	3.7	3.6	3.4	3.3
tʌ	20	_____	14.9	14.9	4.4	4.1	3.8	3.6	3.5	3.3
kʌ	20	_____	15.5	15.3	4.8	4.6	4.3	4.0	3.9	3.7
	Standard Deviation:		11.0	11.0	0.7	0.7	0.6	0.6	0.6	0.6
pʌtəkə	10	_____	10.3	10.0	8.3	7.7	7.1	6.5	6.4	5.7
	Standard Deviation:		12.8	12.8	2.0	2.0	1.5	1.5	1.5	1.5

Comments: _____

_____

_____

_____

_____

_____

[1]Norms are from S. G. Fletcher (1972), "Time-by-Count Measurement of Diadochokinetic Syllable Rate." *Journal of Speech and Hearing Disorders, 15*, 763–770; and S. G. Fletcher (1978), *Time-by-Count Test Measurement of Diadochokinetic Syllable Rate*. Austin, TX: PRO-ED. Used by permission.

SPEECH AND LANGUAGE SAMPLING

Speech-language samples are invaluable in the assessment of a client's communicative abilities and disorders (Bailey & Wolery, 1989; Haynes et al., 1992; Lahey, 1988; Owens, 1995; Peterson & Marquardt, 1994). They can be the basis for determining whether a problem exists and, if so, identifying the client's specific deficiencies and needs. A speech-language sample should be long enough to obtain a true, representative sample of the client's speech and language. A minimum of 50–100 distinct utterances is needed for a language sample (Bloom & Lahey, 1978; James, 1993), and we emphasize the word *minimum*. Collecting 50–100 utterances does not guarantee that you have an adequate sample; rather, 200 or more different utterances provide a better data base, although a sample of this length may not always be possible (Lahey, 1988).

To help you obtain a reliable and valid speech-language sample, we offer the following recommendations:

- Strive for a long sample.
- Vary the subject matter of the sample.
- Seek out multiple environments (e.g., clinic, playground, home, work place, etc.).
- Alter the contexts (e.g., conversation, narratives, responses to pictures, etc.).
- Request other people to record samples for you (e.g., spouse, parent, teacher, etc.).

Owens (1995) offers several other suggestions for collecting samples, including:

- Establish a positive relationship before collecting a sample.
- Assume more of a "conversational equal" role rather than an "authority" role.
- Be as unobtrusive as possible. Minimize your interruptions and distractions; try to "fade into the woodwork."
- Keep your talking to a minimum; don't be afraid to "wait out" the child.
- Avoid using yes/no questions or other stimuli that elicit short answers.
- Preselect materials and topics that will be interesting to the client, and follow the client's lead in elaborating or changing topics.
- Model topics or responses if necessary. This is particularly helpful if the client responds in a repetitive or stereotypic manner (adapted from pp. 144–45).

We suggest using "tell me about . . ." and "tell me more about . . ." stimuli rather than "what is . . ." or "what are . . ." questions. For example, consider some typical responses to "what is/are . . ." questions:

- What are they doing. *I don't know*
- What is that? *a car*
- What color is it? *green*
- What were you doing in class? *nothing*

These examples illustrate why it is better to use declarative, open-ended stimuli such as "tell me about . . ." to elicit an adequate speech-language sample.

Conversation Starters for Eliciting a Speech-language Sample

Obtaining an adequate speech-language sample from an adult client is usually an uncomplicated task. If the client is verbal and the clinician uses open-ended stimuli (e.g., "tell me about . . .") to elicit responses, an adequate sample may be collected during the information-getting interview. If this does not occur, however, you can ask specific questions about the client's interests (e.g., hobbies, occupation, sports, family, current events, etc.) to encourage more speech.

Obtaining a representative speech-language sample is usually a bigger challenge with children, particularly if they are quiet by nature or are reticent about the situation. We have provided sample stimulus questions and statements to help you elicit a speech-language sample. These suggestions are extracted from our own clinical experiences and from Peterson's (1981) *Conversation Starters for Speech-Language Pathology*. Adapt them as needed with different clients to obtain the best speech-language sample possible.

- ☐ Tell me about your favorite movie (or TV show).
- ☐ What is your favorite video game? Tell me how to play it.
- ☐ Tell me about your favorite book.
- ☐ Tell me what you and your friends play (or talk about) together.
- ☐ Tell me what you did last weekend (or this morning, yesterday, last night, etc.).
- ☐ Tell me what you are going to do after you leave here today.
- ☐ Tell me about your favorite family vacation.
- ☐ Tell me what you would do if you won a million dollars.
- ☐ Tell me about your favorite babysitter. What do you like about her/him?
- ☐ Pretend I've never had pizza before. Describe it to me.
- ☐ Pretend I've never used a telephone before. Tell me how to use one.
- ☐ Pretend I've never used a library before. Tell me how to use one.
- ☐ What do people mean when they say, "It's raining cats and dogs?"
- ☐ Tell me the difference between a mouse and a fish.
- ☐ Tell me the difference between a dentist and a teacher.
- ☐ How do you make a hamburger (or taco, spaghetti, or other food)?
- ☐ Tell me the story of the "Three Little Pigs" (or another children's story).
- ☐ What is the Super Bowl? Tell me about it.
- ☐ Tell me what your bedroom looks like.
- ☐ Tell me what you would do if you were the President.
- ☐ When was the last time you were really mad. Why were you mad?
- ☐ What do you like the best about being in the _____ grade?
- ☐ What do you like the least about being in the _____ grade?
- ☐ If you could have three wishes, what would you wish for? Why?

☐ What would you get at the grocery store if you were going to make dinner for your family?

☐ Tell me how to make popcorn (or cookies, a cake, or another treat).

With younger children, introduce different activities, objects, or toys into the environment to elicit speech or vocalizations. For example, play *pat-a-cake* or *peek-a-boo*; present animals, cars, planes, dolls, or other toys; play matching games; use a puppet to name common objects, body parts; and so forth.

Pictures

The pictures on the next four pages (Figures 4–1 through 4–4) are provided to help you elicit a speech-language sample. For some clients, additional pictures may be needed to collect an adequate sample. It is important to use pictures that illustrate a variety of activities. Pictures that show little action, depict few things to describe, or elicit naming-only responses are of little use.

Narratives With Pictures

Another method of obtaining a speech-language sample is to tell a story and then have the child repeat it back to you. We have provided two narratives with pictures to help you complete that task (Figures 4–5 and 4–6 on pages 104–111). After you read the story, encourage your client to retell it with as much detail as possible. Other sources of narratives include commercially available sequencing cards and the *Goldman-Fristoe Test of Articulation* (Goldman & Fristoe, 1986), which has two narrative stories.

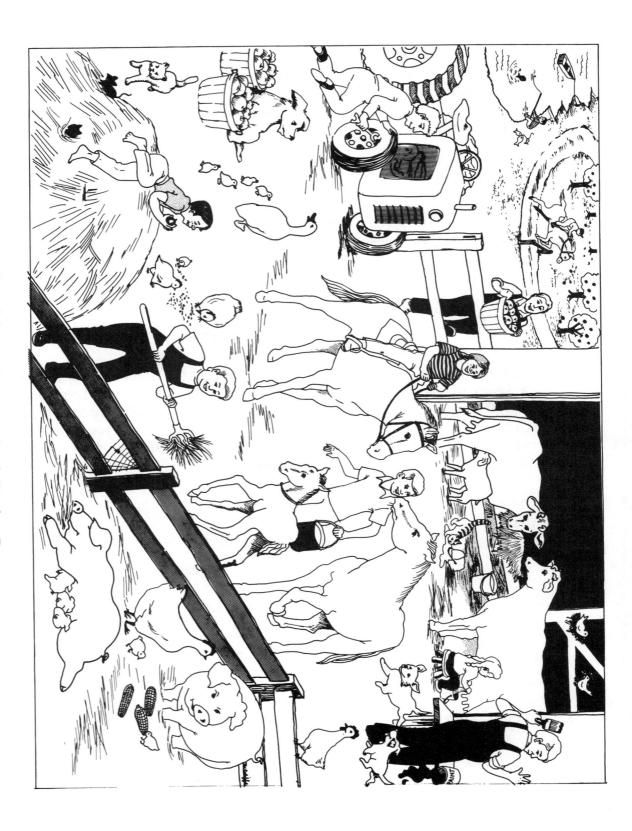

Figure 4–1. *Speech-Language Sample Stimulus—Farm*

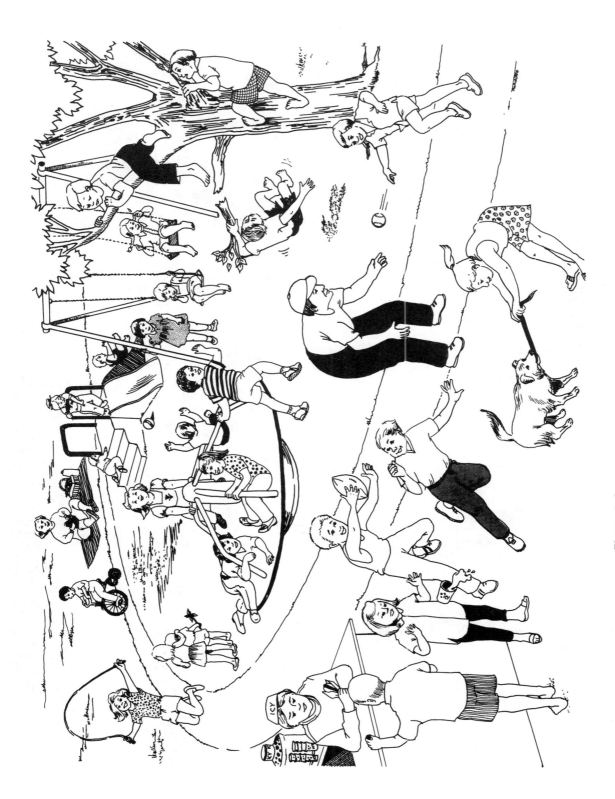

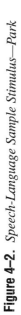

Figure 4–2. *Speech-Language Sample Stimulus—Park*

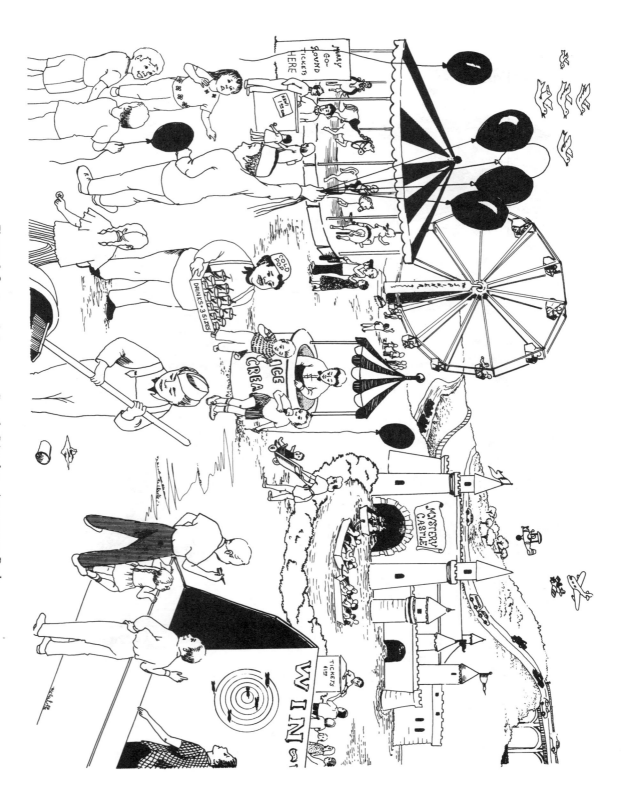

Figure 4–3. *Speech-Language Sample Stimulus—Amusement Park*

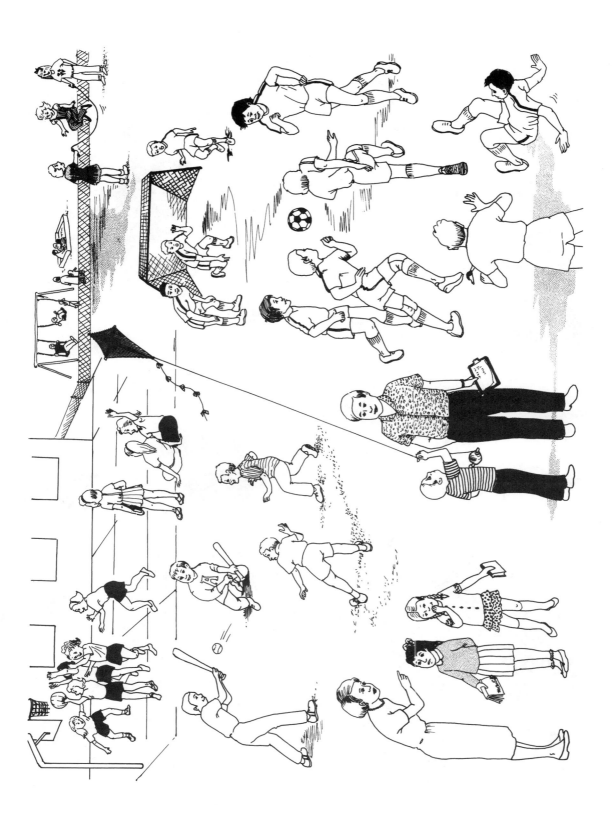

Figure 4-4. *Speech-Language Sample Stimulus—Playground*

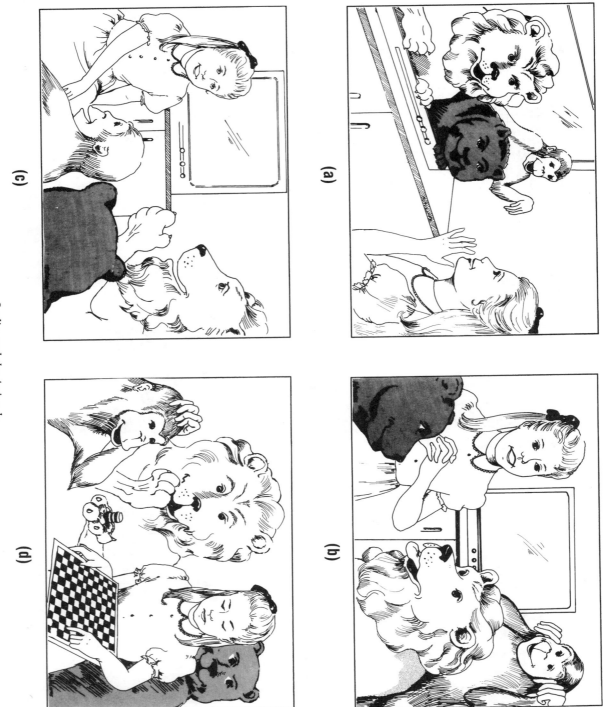

Lydia and the Animals

Figure 4–5

Lydia and the Animals

(a). One day when Lydia was watching television, an amazing thing happened. The animals on the screen came to life in her living room! A bear, a monkey, and a lion were looking right at her. Lydia was very scared. She tried to yell for her mom, but nothing came out of her mouth.

(b). Then the animals started talking to each other in a funny animal language Lydia did not understand. Finally, in a quiet voice she said, "Where did you come from?"

(c). Much to her amazement, the lion spoke English. The lion pointed to the TV and said, "We came from your television set. We want to play with you." She could tell from his voice that he was a friendly lion. She wasn't afraid anymore.

(d). "Let's play checkers!" Lydia said. All the animals looked at each other and nodded. Lydia got out the checker game and taught them how to play.

(continued)

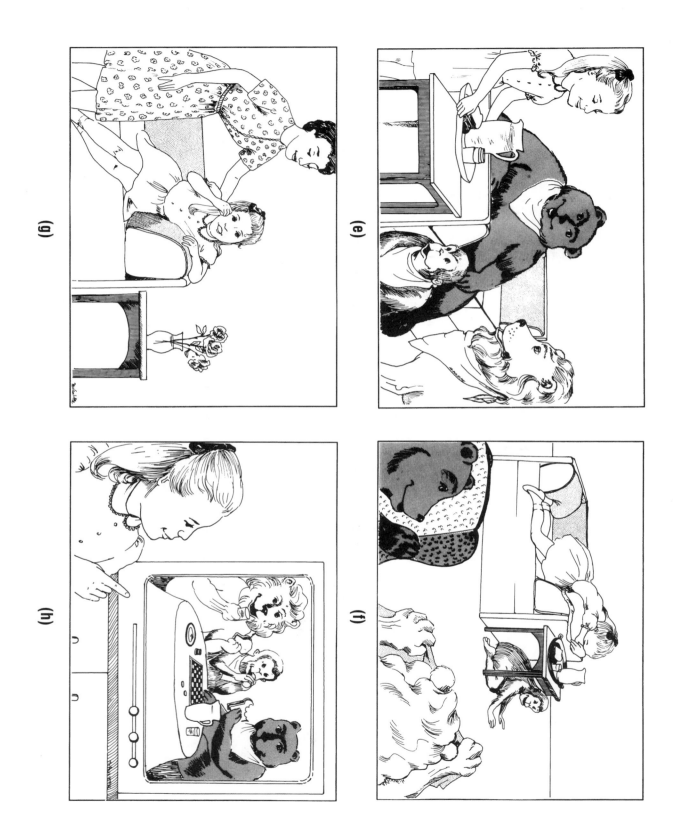

Figure 4–5

Lydia and the Animals (continued)

(e). After they played checkers, Lydia asked, "Are you hungry? I'll bring you some sandwiches." The animals nodded yes, so Lydia and the animals all sat down and ate peanut butter and jelly sandwiches and drank lemonade.

(f). Next, they decided to play hide-and-go-seek. Lydia was "it." "Stay in this room," she said, "I don't want my mom to see you!" While the animals were hiding, she fell asleep.

(g). A little while later, Lydia's mom came in and woke her up. Lydia looked around the room. The TV was on, the checkerboard was put away, and there were no cups and plates on the table. Was it all a dream?

(h). Then Lydia looked at the television. There she saw the animals giggling as they gazed up at her. The bear, monkey, and lion were drinking lemonade, eating sandwiches, and playing checkers on TV!

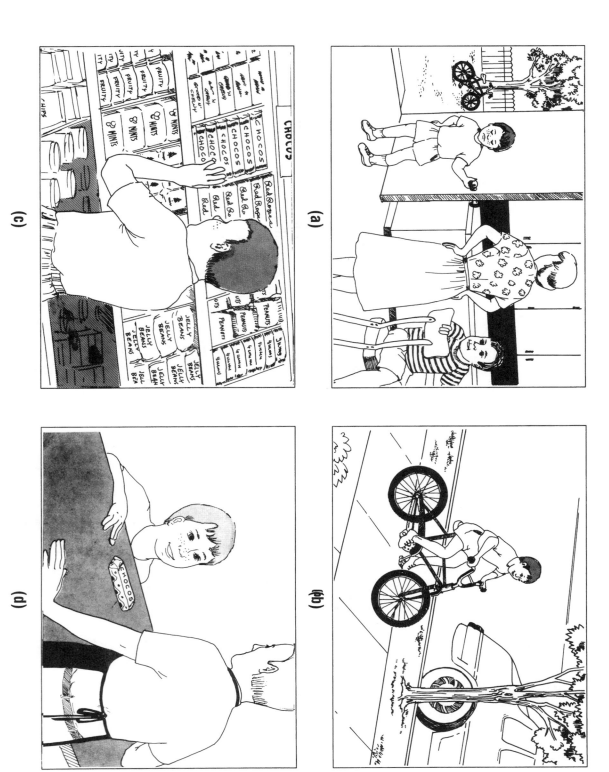

Jacob's Day

Figure 4–6

Jacob's Day

(a). Jacob was a young boy who had two big brothers and one big sister. He didn't like being the smallest boy in the family because he never got to do things by himself. One day Jacob asked his mom if he could go to the store to buy a candy bar. Of course she said, "Not by yourself, Jacob." That made Jacob very mad. Jacob sadly said, "Okay, I guess I'll go play outside."

(b). Once Jacob got outside, he got an idea. He thought, "I'll just go by myself anyway. I can get there and back without Mom ever knowing I was gone." So Jacob counted the money in his pocket to make sure he had enough and then got on his bicycle and pedaled to the store as fast as he could.

(c) He went inside the store and looked for the candy bar aisle. "Oh, look at all the choices!" he thought to himself. He was so excited! Jacob finally picked his favorite candy bar and stepped toward the counter.

(d). As he was paying for the candy the cashier asked, "Aren't you a little young to be here alone?" "Oh no, I'm older than I look," he said with a smile. He felt so grown up.

(continued)

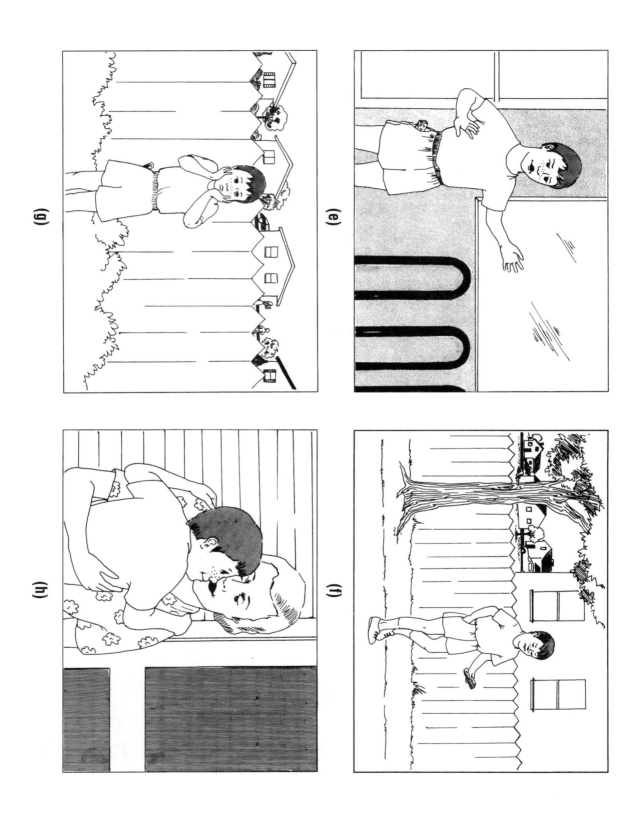

Figure 4–6

Jacob's Day (continued)

(e). Well, Jacob's excitement suddenly turned into fear when he went outside to go home. His bike was gone! How could he get home before his mom found out he had left? Jacob looked all around for his bike, but it was nowhere to be found. Somebody had stolen it.

(f). It was a long walk home for Jacob. He knew he was in big trouble. Somehow he didn't feel very grown up anymore. And he no longer wanted to eat his candy bar.

(g). When he turned onto the street where his house was, he could hear his mother calling out his name. Even though he was afraid to tell his mom what happened, he suddenly felt very scared.

(h). Jacob realized that he really was too young to be out alone and started running toward home. His mother gave him a big hug and said, "Where did you go? I was so worried!" Jacob cried as he told his story. After that, he didn't mind it so much that he never got to do things by himself.

EVALUATING RATE OF SPEECH

A client's speech rate can directly affect articulation, intelligibility, voice production, and/or fluency. With some clients, obtaining periodic rates will be necessary as a measure of improvement (e.g., such as with fluency) or deterioration (e.g., such as intelligibility associated with myasthenia gravis) over time. Since speech rates vary tremendously among normal speakers, it is difficult to assign a standard word-per-minute (WPM) index. As a general guideline, Calvert and Silverman (1983) reported that adults produce an average of 270 words per minute during conversational speech, and 160–180 words per minute during oral reading. Weiner (1984) reported that the speaking rate of a normal adult ranges from 220–410 words per minute during uninterrupted discourse.

Speech rates of children tend to be slower than those of adults. Purcell and Runyan (1980) measured the speaking rates of children in the first through fifth grades, and found a slight increase in their average rate at each grade level. The first graders averaged 125 words per minute, and the fifth graders averaged 142 words per minute.

Again, we need to emphasize that normal speaking rates vary tremendously among adults and children. Some people who use seemingly slow speech rates have excellent speech, while others with the same rate struggle with a communicative disorder. Some people who speak exceedingly fast may have excellent intelligibility and control of their speech, while others exhibit severe communicative impairments due to the rapid speech rate.

The importance of measuring the speech rate is not to compare it with preestablished norms, which only indicate whether the speech rate is normal, faster than normal, or slower than normal. The value of assessing rate of speech is that it allows you to evaluate its effect on the client's communicative abilities. Consider the rate of speech and its effects on the articulation of sounds, intelligibility, voice production, and fluency. Will the use of a faster or slower rate result in better communication? Can a better speech rate be elicited? Can it be maintained? These are important questions to consider when assessing the implications of speech rate on communication.

Determining Speech Rate

To determine a client's speech rate, tape record a sample of connected speech that is devoid of significant pausing in oral reading, in conversational speech, or both. In a 60-second interval, count the number of words produced and divide by 60 (or 120 for a 2-minute sample, 180 for a 3-minute sample, etc.). For example, 200 words produced in 60 seconds is 200 WPM. If there are no 60-second intervals of connected speech, follow the procedures below to calculate the speech rate. Use a stopwatch to time the speech intervals.

1. Time the sample (e.g., 20 seconds).
2. Count the number of words produced (e.g., 62 words).
3. Divide the number of seconds in a minute (60) by the number of seconds in the sample (20 seconds in the example): $60 \div 20 = 3$.
4. Multiply the number of words in the sample (62 in the example) by the number in Step 3 (3 in the example): $62 \times 3 = 186$. The WPM is 186.

Greater reliability in WPM calculations is possible by collecting several samples. The following is based on three samples.

1. The three samples are 20, 25, and 30 seconds, which equals a total of 75 seconds.

2. The number of words in the respective samples are 15, 20, and 25, which equals a total of 60 words.

3. The number of seconds in 3 minutes (60 seconds per minute times three samples) is 180 seconds. Divide the number of seconds (180) by the number of seconds in the three samples (75): $180 \div 75 = 2.4$.

4. Multiply the number of words in the sample (60) by the number in Step 3 (2.4): $60 \times 2.4 = 144$. The WPM is 144.

DETERMINING INTELLIGIBILITY

The speech-language sample not only allows you to assess rate of speech, it also allows you to determine your client's intelligibility. Calculating overall intelligibility is necessary when considering the need for treatment, identifying factors that contribute to poor intelligibility, selecting treatment goals, recording baseline information, and monitoring the effects of treatment over time. An "Intelligibility Assessment Worksheet," Form 4–3, is provided to help you calculate intelligibility.

Naturally, the speech-language sample you use must be an adequate, representative sample of the client's speech in order to calculate a valid intelligibility rating. If you have difficulty obtaining an adequate sample, refer to "Speech and Language Sampling" on page 97 and "Conversation Starters for Eliciting a Speech-Language Sample" on pages 98–99 for specific suggestions and stimuli. We recommend that you audiotape or videotape the sample for analysis and future comparison. The speech-language sample you use can be from a clinical session, from the client's home, or from another environment (e.g., classroom, workplace, etc.). For some clients, you may wish to obtain representative samples from several different environments.

As you assess your client's speech-language sample, realize that there are many factors that can negatively influence intelligibility. These include:

☐ The number of sound errors. Generally, the greater the number of sound errors, the poorer the intelligibility.

☐ The type of sound errors. For example, omissions and additions sometimes result in poorer intelligibility than substitutions or distortions.

☐ Inconsistency of errors.

☐ Vowel errors.

☐ The rate of speech, especially if it is excessively slow or fast.

☐ A typical prosodic characteristic of speech, such as abnormal intonation or stress.

☐ The length and linguistic complexity of the words and utterances used.

☐ Insufficient vocal intensity.

☐ Dysfluencies, particularly severe dysfluencies that disrupt the context.

☐ The lack of gestures or other paralinguistic cues that assist understanding.

☐ The testing environment (such as at home versus in the clinic).

☐ The client's anxiety about the testing situation.

☐ The client's lack of familiarity with the stimulus materials.

☐ The client's level of fatigue. Fatigue particularly affects very young children, elderly clients, or clients with certain neurological disorders.

☐ The clinician's ability to understand "less intelligible" speech.

☐ The clinician's familiarity with the client and the client's speaking context.

In most cases, there are multiple factors—some client-related, some clinician-related, and some environmentally related—that influence overall intelligibility. This means that clinicians need to:

☐ Identify factors that affect intelligibility.

☐ View the intelligibility rating as being approximate, rather than absolute or definitive.

☐ Take more than one speech-language sample, and seek varied environments when possible.

☐ Secure a representative sample of speech. The client or the client's caregiver can usually help you determine whether a particular sample was a typical representation of the client's speech.

We also recommend that clinicians:

☐ Use a high quality tape, and a tape recorder with an external microphone to prevent recording motor noise.

☐ Avoid stimulus items that tend to elicit play rather than talk (e.g., blocks, doll houses, puzzles, etc.).

☐ Use open-ended stimuli (e.g., "Tell me about the car.") rather than closed-ended stimuli (e.g., "What is that?" "What color is it?" "What is it used for?" etc.).

☐ Consider reporting intelligibility in ranges (e.g., 65–75%), particularly when intelligibility varies. For example, a child may be 90–100% intelligible when speaking in utterances of one to three syllables. However, the same child may be only 50% intelligible in utterances of four or more syllables.

☐ Compare intelligibility on word-by-word and utterance-by-utterance bases. For some clients, the results will be very similar. For others, they may be considerably different. For example, a client whose loudness and articulation deteriorate in longer utterances may have many intelligible words, particularly at the beginning of individual utterances. But the end of their utterances may be unintelligible. A child with a pragmatic or organizational language disorder may produce many intelligible words, but the connected discourse may be unintelligible. Jargon aphasic speech may also contain many intelligible words, but be contextually illogical.

Form 4–3. Assessing Intelligibility Worksheet

Name:_____ Age:_____ Date:_____

Examiner:_____

Testing Situation:

Stimuli (conversation, materials used, etc.): _____

Client's level of anxiety:_____

Talkative/Not talkative: _____

Prompts used: _____

Representativeness of sample: _____

Instructions:

1. Write out each word in each utterance (use phonetics if possible).

2. Use a dash (—) to indicate each unintelligible word.

3. An utterance is considered intelligible only if the entire utterance can be understood.

4. Calculate intelligibility for words and utterances.

Example:

Utterances	# Intelligible Words	Total Words	# Intelligible Utterances	Total Utterances
1. hi wɛnt hom	3	3	1	1
2. ɑr ju — tu go	4	5	0	1
3. — — θɪn	1	3	0	1
4. pwiz pwe wɪf mi	4	4	1	1
5. ɑɪ wɑnt tu go hom	5	5	1	1
Totals	**171**	**201**	**3**	**5**

$$\frac{\text{intelligible words:}\ 17}{\text{total words:}\ 20} = 85\%$$ $$\frac{\text{intelligible utterances:}\ 3}{\text{total utterances:}\ 5} = 60\%$$

(continued)

Form 4–3 *(continued)*

Utterances	# Intelligible Words	Total Words	# Intelligible Utterances	Total Utterances
11. _____	____	____	____	1
12. _____	____	____	____	1
13. _____	____	____	____	1
14. _____	____	____	____	1
15. _____	____	____	____	1
16. _____	____	____	____	1
17. _____	____	____	____	1
18. _____	____	____	____	1
19. _____	____	____	____	1
10. _____	____	____	____	1
11. _____	____	____	____	1
12. _____	____	____	____	1
13. _____	____	____	____	1
14. _____	____	____	____	1
15. _____	____	____	____	1
16. _____	____	____	____	1
17. _____	____	____	____	1
18. _____	____	____	____	1
19. _____	____	____	____	1
20. _____	____	____	____	1
21. _____	____	____	____	1
22. _____	____	____	____	1
23. _____	____	____	____	1
24. _____	____	____	____	1
25. _____	____	____	____	1
26. _____	____	____	____	1
27. _____	____	____	____	1
28. _____	____	____	____	1
29. _____	____	____	____	1

(continued)

Utterances	# Intelligible Words	Total Words	# Intelligible Utterances	Total Utterances
30. _____	_____	_____	_____	1
31. _____	_____	_____	_____	1
32. _____	_____	_____	_____	1
33 _____	_____	_____	_____	1
34. _____	_____	_____	_____	1
35. _____	_____	_____	_____	1
36. _____	_____	_____	_____	1
37. _____	_____	_____	_____	1
38. _____	_____	_____	_____	1
39. _____	_____	_____	_____	1
40. _____	_____	_____	_____	1
41. _____	_____	_____	_____	1
42. _____	_____	_____	_____	1
43. _____	_____	_____	_____	1
44. _____	_____	_____	_____	1
45. _____	_____	_____	_____	1
46. _____	_____	_____	_____	1
47. _____	_____	_____	_____	1
48. _____	_____	_____	_____	1
49. _____	_____	_____	_____	1
50. _____	_____	_____	_____	1

Totals
_____ _____ _____ _____

Findings

Average # Words per Utterance _____

% Intelligibility—Words _____

% Intelligibiligy—Utterances _____

Factors contributing to reduced intelligibility: _____

_____

_____

SYLLABLE-BY-SYLLABLE STIMULUS PHRASES

Clinicians use verbal phrases as stimuli for a variety of sampling tasks. They are especially valuable for evaluating stimulability, assessing the maintenance of newly learned target behaviors in the clinical setting, and determining the client's maximum phrase length for optimal speech production. Syllable-by-syllable phrases are useful with many disorders. The following are just a few examples of clinical questions that can be answered by using syllable-by-syllable phrases:

- ☐ Can the hyponasal (denasal) client maintain appropriate nasal resonance across increasingly longer phrases containing nasal sounds?

- ☐ Can the hypernasal client produce the nonnasal phrases without nasality?

- ☐ What speech rate is optimal for the client to be able to articulate all sounds correctly in phrases of increasing length?

- ☐ Are there specific syllable lengths at which the speech of the client with apraxia begins to deteriorate?

- ☐ Are there specific syllable lengths at which the articulation of the client with dysarthria becomes less intelligible?

- ☐ Can fluency be maintained in increasingly longer phrases?

- ☐ Can a desired voice quality (e.g., nonhoarse) be maintained in increasingly longer phrases?

You can see from the few examples above that syllable-by-syllable phrases are versatile and can be used with different disorders. Articulation, rate, prosody, inflection, and intonation can all be sampled across a variety of disorders using these phrase lists. The phrases in Table 4–1 can be imitated from the clinician's model, read by the client, or both. Note the syllable lengths at which the desired behavior (e.g., fluent speech, appropriate voice, articulatory accuracy, etc.) can be maintained, as well as the lengths at which the desired behavior cannot be maintained. Also identify contexts that may be either easier or more difficult for the client. The phrase levels where breakdowns occur are often good starting points for treatment when therapy is initiated.

Table 4–1. Syllable-by-Syllable Stimulus Phrases

Two-syllable Phrases

With Nasals	*Without Nasals*
at noon	back up
brown car	big boy
come in	blue sky
down please	dog house
front door	hot dog
I'm fine	keep out
in here	pull hard
my jam	push it
show me	red car
thank you	too slow

Three-syllable Phrases

With Nasals	*Without Nasals*
good morning	apple pie
hot and cold	catch the bus
jumping rope	far to go
make it up	How are you?
moon and stars	hurry up
more and more	laugh loudly
please call me	leave the house
run and jump	red roses
shoes and socks	see the cat
yes or no	slept all day

Four-syllable Phrases

With Nasals	*Without Nasals*
bacon and eggs	after he left
do it right now	do it this way
do it for him	he has a coat
It's a fine day	here is the key
leave him alone	I like to read
my hands were cold	I told you so
open it up	keep to the left
salt and pepper	show her the way
table and chairs	tell her okay
the meal was fine	the bus was full

(continued)

Table 4–1. *(continued)*

Five-syllable Phrases

With Nasals	*Without Nasals*
a piece of candy	a pair of scissors
a long vacation	beware of the dog
he wants the money	Did you hit the ball?
look out the window	he would if he could
my mother said no	How did you do it?
please open the door	let's go to the park
she is very nice	she is very shy
the dogs are barking	the car was dirty
the weather is fine	the weather is cold
we cut down the tree	we sat by the trees

Six-syllable Phrases

With Nasals	*Without Nasals*
a nickel and a dime	Are you ready to go?
give them each a muffin	Do you have the address?
How much more will it cost?	go to the library
I haven't heard from them	he rushed to catch the bus
just beyond the corner	he is very happy
leave the window open	I have lost the car keys
put everything away	the potatoes were cold
shut the door behind you	What size shoe do you wear?
the farmers needed rain	Where did you put her coat?
we can go after lunch	Will you keep it secret?

Seven-syllable Phrases

With Nasals	*Without Nasals*
come and see us when you can	Did you read today's paper?
come inside and close the door	he has a good idea
he wants more cake and ice cream	I thought it would start at four
I don't know what happened here	I would like a cup of tea
I wonder why she said that	put it back where you got it
Is it time for the movie?	she is a very good cook
please knock before you enter	they like to sit at the park
she is not very happy	Why did they go to the show?
What is it you want to know?	you did the best you could do
When does the next show begin?	you should tell her about it

(continued)

Table 4–1. *(continued)*

Eight-syllable Phrases

With Nasals	*Without Nasals*
Can you hear the television?	Did you see the keys to the car?
come over as soon as you can	give it to that boy over there
Do you want another one now?	he will pick you up after school
leave the window open tonight	I have a lot of work to do
the children are playing outside	I would like to do it for you
the melons are from our backyard	she has to buy food for supper
they are going to the movie	the letter arrived yesterday
we live just around the corner	they all ate breakfast together
we went to the animal farm	we already heard about it
When will you come to visit us?	we are so happy to see you

Source: The syllable lists are adapted from K. G. Shipley, *Systematic Assessment of Voice* (pp. 69–75). Oceanside, CA: Academic Communication Associates. Copyright © 1990 and used by permission.

READING PASSAGES

Information obtained during oral reading is valuable for making many assessment decisions as it allows you to observe your client's articulation, voice, fluency, and reading abilities. Compare your oral reading results with those from single-word or short-phrase evoked utterances and conversational speech samples. We have included seven reading passages that vary in difficulty and age appropriateness. The first four passages are intended for children. The reading grade levels presented below were determined by using the FullWrite Professional™ (Wiener & Young, 1988) software program. Use the grade-levels as guidelines only; they are not intended to assess reading skills of clients.

- *Kids Like Ice Cream*   First-grade level
- *Bears*   Third-grade level
- *The Spider's Home*   Fourth-grade level
- *The Toothbrush*   Fifth-grade level

There are three adult reading passages. The *Grandfather Passage* and *Rainbow Passage* have been used for clinical and research purposes in our field for many years. The third adult passage is a portion of the "Declaration of Independence." Two of the children's passages, *The Spider's Home* and *The Toothbrush*, are also appropriate for some adults. Other sources of reading materials for children and adults include children's books, grade-level readers, general textbooks, popular magazines, and newspapers.

Kids Like Ice Cream[1]

Ice cream is good! It comes in many colors. Some ice cream is pink. Some is brown. Some is white. The colors do not taste the same, but they are all very good. Ice cream tastes good by itself. It tastes even better with nuts and bananas on top. Some ice cream comes in a bowl. Some ice cream comes on a cone. It is always good! Ice cream is good on a hot summer day. It makes you cool and happy. You can eat it at the park. You can eat it at home. You can eat ice cream just about anywhere. It is also good to eat in the winter when you are in front of a warm fire. You can buy it at the grocery store or at an ice cream store. Kids like to eat ice cream!

Bears[2]

Have you ever seen a bear? Bears are big, furry animals that live in the mountains. Bears are awake and roam around the woods during the spring, summer, and fall. But in the winter they crawl into caves and sleep for several months before waking up. Bears usually eat the same foods that humans eat like berries, nuts, and fish. A bear's favorite food is honey. When a bear goes into a beehive to get honey, it is not even bothered by the angry bees that sting. A bear's skin is so shaggy that the bees' stings are not even noticed.

---

[1]From K. G. Shipley, *Systematic Assessment of Voice* (p. 95). Oceanside, CA Academic Communication Associates. Copyright © 1990 and used by permission.

[2] From K. G. Shipley, *Systematic Assessment of Voice* (p. 97). Oceanside, CA: Academic Communication Associates. Copyright © 1990 and used by permission.

A lot of people say that bears look soft and cuddly. But their looks can fool you! Bears are not usually harmful to people. But when they are mad, bears can be very harmful. They have long, sharp teeth and they will attack their enemies to protect their babies. If you are ever running from a bear, don't climb a tree because most bears climb trees faster than we can. They can also run much faster than we do. It is smart to make sure you never make a bear mad. If you ever see a bear in the woods, don't stick around to say hello. Just go the other way.

The Spider's Home

A spider is an amazing animal. It can build its own home and it doesn't even have to buy wood or a saw. Before the spider begins to build, it looks for the perfect spot. The spider likes to live in a grassy area where lots of insects can get caught in its web. Then the spider eats the insects for dinner. The spider also has to figure out which way the wind is blowing. The wind has to be on the spider's back before it is able to make its house.

After it finds a good place to live, it is ready to spin its webs. The spider has glands in its stomach that produce a silky liquid. It leaps from one side of the house and is carried by the wind to the other side. As it travels through the air, the liquid comes out. As soon as the liquid hits the air it becomes solid, making a fine, tough thread. The spider uses the first thread as a bridge to travel from one side to the other. Then it continues to build its web strand by strand until its home is complete.

The Toothbrush

Did you know that the toothbrush was invented in a prison? One morning in 1770, a man in an English jail woke up with a new idea. He thought it would be better if he could use a brush to clean his teeth, rather than wipe them with a rag. At dinner he took a bone from his meat and kept it. Then he told the prison guard about his idea. The guard gave him some bristles to use for the brush. The prisoner made holes in the bone and stuffed the bristles into the holes. It was a success! The prisoner was so excited about his new invention that he went into the toothbrush making business when he got out of jail.

For more than 200 years we have used toothbrushes similar to the one the prisoner invented. Toothbrushes are not made out of bones anymore. They come in all kinds of colors and sizes. The next time you brush your teeth, think about the prisoner in England who invented the toothbrush.

Grandfather

You wished to know all about my grandfather. Well, he is nearly ninety-three years old; he dresses himself in an ancient black frock coat, usually minus several buttons, yet he still thinks as swiftly as ever. A long, flowing beard clings to his chin, giving those who observe him a pronounced feeling of the utmost respect. When he speaks, his voice is just a bit cracked and quivers a trifle. Twice each day he plays skillfully and with zest upon our small organ. Except in winter when the ooze or snow or ice prevents, he slowly takes a short walk in the open air each day. We have often urged him to walk more and smoke less, but he always answers, "Banana oil!" Grandfather likes to be modern in his language.

Rainbow Passage

When the sunlight strikes raindrops in the air they act like a prism and form a rainbow. The rainbow is a division of white light into many beautiful colors. These take the shape of a long round arch, with its path high above, and its two ends apparently beyond the horizon. There is, according to legend, a boiling pot of gold at one end. People look, but no one ever finds it. When a man looks for something beyond his reach, his friends say he is looking for the pot of gold at the end of the rainbow.

Throughout the centuries men have explained the rainbow in various ways. Some have accepted it as a miracle without physical explanation. To the Hebrews it was a token that there would be no more universal floods. The Greeks used to imagine that it was a sign from the gods to foretell war or heavy rain. The Norsemen considered the rainbow as a bridge over which the gods passed from earth to their home in the sky. Other men have tried to explain the phenomenon physically. Aristotle thought that the rainbow was caused by reflection of the sun's rays by the rain. Since then physicists have found that it is not reflection, but refraction by the raindrops which causes the rainbow. Many complicated ideas about the rainbow have been formed. The difference in the rainbow depends considerably upon the size of the water drops, and the width of the colored band increases as the size of the drops increases. The actual primary rainbow observed is said to be the effect of superposition of a number of bows. If the red of the second bow falls upon the green of the first, the result is to give a bow with an abnormally wide yellow band, since red and green lights when mixed form yellow. This is a very common type of bow, one showing mainly red and yellow, with little or no green or blue.

Declaration of Independence

We hold these truths to be self-evident, that all men are created equal, that they are endowed by their Creator with certain unalienable rights, that among these are life, liberty and the pursuit of happiness. That to secure these rights, governments are instituted among men, deriving their just powers from the consent of the governed, that whenever any form of government becomes destructive of these ends, it is the right of the people to alter or abolish it, and to institute new government, laying its foundation on such principles and organizing its powers in such form, as to them shall seem most likely to effect their safety and happiness.

Prudence, indeed, will dictate that governments long established should not be changed for light and transient causes; and accordingly all experience has shown, that mankind are more disposed to suffer, while evils are sufferable, than to right themselves by abolishing the forms to which they are accustomed. But when a long train of abuses and usurpations, pursuing invariably the same object evinces a design to reduce them under absolute despotism, it is their right, it is their duty, to throw off such government, and to provide new guards for their future security.

CHARTING

Charting a client's behavior is useful both diagnostically and in treatment activities (Hegde, 1993; Mowrer, 1988). It allows you to score a client's responses and objectively identify the client's communicative abilities and deficits. You can chart desirable behaviors (e.g., correct sound productions, fluent speech, appropriate vocal productions) or undesirable behaviors (e.g., misarticulations, specific dysfluencies, instances of throat clearing). This information provides an assessment baseline for diagnostic decisions, and demonstrates progress in treatment. There are many behaviors you can chart during an assessment session, for example:

- Correct and incorrect productions of a particular sound at a specified syllable or word level;
- Frequency of specific dysfluency types;
- Instances of motor behaviors associated with stuttering (e.g., facial grimaces);
- Groping or pre-posturing behaviors in clients with apraxia;
- Specific language features (e.g., copula verbs, plural morphemes, verb phrases);
- Word-finding problems or circumlocutions in clients with aphasia;
- Correct phonatory behaviors, such as nonhoarse vocal productions;
- Inappropriate vocal behaviors, such as throat clearing or harsh phonatory onset.

Charting is also appropriate for behaviors that are important in treatment but not necessarily caused by the communicative disorder. For example, you can record each time a child responds to your stimulus, stays in the chair for 30 seconds, and so forth. There are several ways to chart behaviors, including:

1. *Note each time a preselected behavior is exhibited.* For example, record each instance of throat clearing, each associated motor behavior, every interjection (e.g., "OK" or "uh"), and so forth. In this method, opposite behaviors (e.g., the absence of throat clearing) are not recorded. The result is a count of the number of times a specified behavior occurred within the time interval sampled.

2. *Note each instance of both correct and incorrect behaviors.* Use a check (✔) or plus (+) for each desirable production, and a zero (0) or a minus (–) for every undesirable production. For example, after 10 productions of a given sound, perhaps 7 were correct and 3 were incorrect. This yields a percentage (70% in this case) that can be compared with previous or future results.

3. *Note behaviors according to one of several preselected criteria.* For example, when charting articulation a specified sound may be omitted (O), approximated (A), or produced correctly (C). Percentages can then be determined for each type of response.

There are a variety of forms available that are simple to use and appropriate for different clients. We have provided two such worksheets. Form 4–4 allows you to chart up to 200 responses. A different target response can be entered on each row, so you can monitor progress on different stimulus items. The worksheet is appropriate for charting children, adolescents, or adults.

Form 4–5 is designed especially for children. A total of 100 responses can be charted on the sheet. Children enjoy receiving a star, stamp, happy face, or sticker in each box when they correctly produce the target behavior. It is also an enjoyable way to teach children to chart their own responses.

Form 4–4. Charting Worksheet I

Name: _____ Age: _____ Date: _____

Examiner: _____

Charted Behavior: _____

Stimulus:	**Trials:**	**% Correct:**
_____	___, ___, ___, ___, ___, ___, ___, ___, ___, ___	_____
_____	___, ___, ___, ___, ___, ___, ___, ___, ___, ___	_____
_____	___, ___, ___, ___, ___, ___, ___, ___, ___, ___	_____
_____	___, ___, ___, ___, ___, ___, ___, ___, ___, ___	_____
_____	___, ___, ___, ___, ___, ___, ___, ___, ___, ___	_____
_____	___, ___, ___, ___, ___, ___, ___, ___, ___, ___	_____
_____	___, ___, ___, ___, ___, ___, ___, ___, ___, ___	_____
_____	___, ___, ___, ___, ___, ___, ___, ___, ___, ___	_____
_____	___, ___, ___, ___, ___, ___, ___, ___, ___, ___	_____
_____	___, ___, ___, ___, ___, ___, ___, ___, ___, ___	_____
_____	___, ___, ___, ___, ___, ___, ___, ___, ___, ___	_____
_____	___, ___, ___, ___, ___, ___, ___, ___, ___, ___	_____
_____	___, ___, ___, ___, ___, ___, ___, ___, ___, ___	_____
_____	___, ___, ___, ___, ___, ___, ___, ___, ___, ___	_____
_____	___, ___, ___, ___, ___, ___, ___, ___, ___, ___	_____
_____	___, ___, ___, ___, ___, ___, ___, ___, ___, ___	_____
_____	___, ___, ___, ___, ___, ___, ___, ___, ___, ___	_____
_____	___, ___, ___, ___, ___, ___, ___, ___, ___, ___	_____
_____	___, ___, ___, ___, ___, ___, ___, ___, ___, ___	_____
_____	___, ___, ___, ___, ___, ___, ___, ___, ___, ___	_____

Total Trials: _____ Total Correct: _____ % Correct: _____

Form 4–5. Charting Worksheet II

Name: _____

Date: _____
Clinician: _____

Target

CONCLUDING COMMENTS

The procedures described in this chapter are used across communicative disorders that affect articulation, language, fluency, voice, and resonance. Most of these procedures, or some variation of them, are included in many diagnostic sessions. This does not mean that each procedure has to be used during every assessment. For example, you may not formally evaluate a client's speech rate or include a reading task in every session, but you should be prepared to administer these tasks if necessary.

The procedures described here, while common to most communicative disorders, do not focus on specific problems associated with each disorder. The information and procedures applicable for specific disorders are found in Chapters 5 through 12. Thus, information from this chapter is to be used along with the material from the chapters that follow.

SOURCES OF ADDITIONAL INFORMATION

Oral-facial Evaluations and Diadochokinetic Rates

Dworkin, J., & Culatta, R. (1980). *Dworkin-Culatta oral mechanism examination.* Nicholasville, KY: Edgewood Press.

Fletcher, S. G. (1972). Time-by-count measurement of diadochokinetic syllable rate. *Journal of Speech and Hearing Research, 15*, 763–770.

Fletcher, S. G. (1978). *Time-by-count test measurement of diadochokinetic syllable rate*. Austin, TX: PRO-ED.

Hall, P. K. (1994). The oral mechanism. In J. B. Tomblin, H. L. Morris, & D. C. Spriestersbach (Eds.), *Diagnosis in speech-language pathology* (pp. 67–98). San Diego: Singular Publishing Group.

Hutchinson, B. B. (1979). Oral-peripheral and motor examination for speech. In B. B. Hutchinson, M. L. Hanson, & M. J. Mecham (Eds.), *Diagnostic handbook of speech pathology* (pp. 109–178). Baltimore: Williams & Wilkins.

Mason, R., & Simon, C. (1977). The orofacial examination checklist. *Language, Speech and Hearing Services in Schools, 8*, 155–163.

Meitus, I. J., & Weinberg, B. (1983a). Gathering clinical information. In I. J. Meitus & B. Weinberg (Eds.), *Diagnosis in speech-language pathology* (pp. 31–70). Austin, TX: PRO-ED.

Spriestersbach, D. C., Morris, H. L., & Darley, F. L. (1978). Examination of the speech mechanism. In F. L. Darley & D. C. Spriestersbach (Eds.), *Diagnostic methods in speech pathology* (2nd ed., pp. 322–345). New York: Harper & Row.

St. Louis, K., & Ruscello, D. (1987). *Oral speech mechanism screening examination* (rev. ed.). Austin, TX: PRO-ED.

Speech and Language Sampling

Bailey, D. B., & Wolery, M. (1989). *Assessing infants and preschoolers with handicaps*. Columbus, OH: Merrill.

Hubbell, R. D. (1988). *A handbook of English grammar and language sampling*. Englewood Cliffs, NJ: Prentice-Hall.

James, S. (1993). Assessing children with language disorders. In D. K Bernstein & E. Tiegerman (Eds.), *Language and communication disorders in children* (3rd ed., pp. 185–228). New York: Macmillan.

Lahey, M. (1988). *Language disorders and language development*. New York: Macmillan.

Lund, N. J., & Duchan, J. F. (1993). *Assessing children's language in naturalistic contexts* (3rd ed.). Englewood Cliffs, NJ: Prentice-Hall.

Miller, J. F. (1981). *Assessing language production in children*. Baltimore: University Park Press.

Owens, R. E. (1995). *Language disorders: A functional approach to assessment and intervention* (2nd ed.). Needham Heights, MA: Allyn & Bacon.

Reed, V. A. (1994). *An introduction to children with language disorders* (2nd ed.). New York: Macmillan.

Wiig, E. H., & Semel, E. (1984). *Language assessment and intervention for the learning disabled* (2nd ed.). Columbus, OH: Merrill.

Syllable-by-Syllable Stimuli

Blockcolsky, V. (1990). *Book of words: 1 7,000 words selected by vowels and diphthongs*. Tucson, AZ: Communication Skill Builders.

Blockcolsky, V. D., Frazer, J. M., & Frazer, D. H. (1987). *40,000 selected words organized by letter, sound, and syllable*. Tucson, AZ: Communication Skill Builders.

Shipley, K. G., Recor, D. B., & Nakamura, S.M. (1990). *Sourcebook of apraxia remediation activities* Oceanside, CA: Academic Communication Associates.

Charting

Hegde, M. N. (1993). *Treatment procedures in communicative disorders* (2nd ed.). Austin, TX: PRO-ED.

LaPointe, L. L. (1977). Base-10 programmed stimulation: Task specification, scoring and plotting performance in aphasia therapy. *Journal of Speech and Hearing Disorders, 42*, 90–105.

Mowrer, D. (1988). *Methods of modifying speech behaviors: Learning theory in speech pathology* (2nd ed.). Prospect Heights, IL: Waveland Press

Internet Sources

American Speech-Language-Hearing Association
http://www.asha.org
Listservers of Interest to Communication Disorders Folks
http://www.shc.uiowa.edu/wjshc/iiscdl.html

□ CHAPTER 5 □

Assessment of Articulation and Phonological Processes

OVERVIEW OF ASSESSMENT

Normal articulation is a series of complex actions. Accurate articulation requires exact placement, sequencing, timing, direction, and force of the articulators. These occur simultaneously with precise airstream alteration, initiation or halting of phonation, and velopharyngeal action. It is no wonder that the assessment of articulation is complex, requiring a good deal of skill and knowledge.

Articulatory problems result from organic (a known physical cause) or functional (no known physical cause) etiologies. Some organically based articulatory or phonological disorders are related to hearing loss, cleft lip or palate, cerebral palsy, ankylglossia (tongue-tie), acquired apraxia, dysarthria, and others. There are also many articulation disorders of a functional etiology. Clinicians attempt to identify physical causes, particularly during the oral-facial examination. However, in many cases, the precise cause of an articulatory difficulty is unknown.

The primary purposes of an assessment of articulation and phonological processes include:

☐ Describing the articulatory or phonological development and status of the client.

☐ Determining whether the individual's speech sufficiently deviates from normal expectations to warrant concern or intervention.

☐ Identifying factors that relate to the presence or maintenance of the speech disorder.

☐ Making prognostic judgments about change with and without intervention.

☐ Monitoring changes in articulatory or phonological abilities and performance across time. (Adapted from Bernthal & Bankson, 1988, pp. 200–201.)

The outline below identifies several important components of a complete evaluation of articulation and phonological processes.

History of the Client

    Procedures

        Written Case History
        Information-getting Interview
        Information from Other Professionals

    Contributing Factors

        Hearing Impairment
        Medical or Neurological Factors
        Dental Problems
        Maturation and Motor Development
        Intelligence, Sex, Birth Order, Motivation and Concern, Dialect

Assessment of Articulation and Phonological Processes[1]

Procedures

> Screening
> Articulation Tests
> Speech Sampling
> Stimulability of Errors

Analysis

> Number of Errors
> Error Types (substitutions, omissions, distortions, additions)
> Form of Errors (distinctive features, phonological processes)
> Consistency of Errors
> Intelligibility
> Rate of Speech
> Prosody

Oral-facial Examination

Hearing Assessment

Language Assessment

Determining the Diagnosis

Providing Information (written report, interview, etc.)

SCREENING

The purpose of a screen is to quickly identify those people who communicate within normal limits and those who *may* have a communicative disorder. People in the second group are seen or referred for a complete evaluation. A screen is not an in-depth assessment and should not take more than a few minutes. Screenings most commonly occur in the schools, where large numbers of children in the early grades are screened for problems.

An articulation screening test does not have to be formal. Many clinicians listen to the person's speech and have him or her perform simple tasks, such as counting, reciting the days of the week, reading, naming objects or colors, and so on. Other clinicians prefer to use published articulation screening tests. There are several available, including:

- *A Screening Deep Test of Articulation* (McDonald, 1976a)

- *Compton Speech and Language Screening Evaluation* (Compton, 1978)

- *Fluharty Preschool Speech and Language Screening Test* (Fluharty, 1978)

---

[1] Auditory discrimination is also listed by some authors (see Boone & Plante, 1993; Hegde, 1995b; McReynolds, 1990) for the sake of completeness. However, studies have shown that the relationship between speech-sound discrimination and articulation is equivocal. Professionals generally agree that there is no clear indication that auditory discrimination precedes articulatory production. Thus, we have not included it within the assessment process.

- *Predictive Screening Test for Articulation* (Van Riper & Erickson, 1973)

- *Templin–Darley Test of Articulation* (Templin & Darley, 1969)

You can easily develop your own screening instrument by using some of the resources in this manual, such as the "Reading Passages" (pp. 122–124) and the "Pictures" (pp. 99–103). If you choose to use picture stimuli, be sure to select pictures that will elicit the later-developing sounds. Refer to the developmental norms in Table 5–2 (p. 151) and "The Frequency of Occurrence of Consonants" in Table 5–3 (p. 155) in selecting appropriate target sounds when screening articulation.

ARTICULATION TESTS

There are many standard tests that clinicians use to identify articulation errors. Some of the more popular traditional tests include:

- *Arizona Articulation Proficiency Scale* (Fudala & Reynolds, 1986)

- *Fisher-Logemann Test of Articulation Competence* (Fisher & Logemann, 1971)

- *Goldman-Fristoe Test of Articulation* (Goldman & Fristoe, 1986)

- *Photo Articulation Test* (Pendergest, Dickey, Selmar, & Sudar, 1984)

- *Templin-Darley Tests of Articulation* (Templin & Darley, 1969)

These tests, and others like them, assess sounds in the initial, medial, and final positions (e.g., the /1/ in light, balloon, and ball), allowing the clinician to identify the number and types of errors.

Articulation tests are used to identify a client's articulation errors in a relatively quick and systematic fashion. They are popular and useful assessment tools. However, they do have limitations. For example, consider these drawbacks:

☐ These tests usually elicit phonemes in only one phonetic context within a preselected word. Even if the client produces the sound correctly, there may be other contexts and words in which the client cannot produce the target sound correctly. Or, an error may be elicited that is not reflective of a general pattern in other contexts.

☐ Most articulation tests elicit phonemes at the word level for the assessment of initial, medial, and final position productions. However, conversational speech is made up of complex, coarticulated movements in which discrete initial, medial, and final sounds may not occur. Thus, sound productions in single words may differ from those in spontaneous speech.

☐ Some articulation tests examine only consonants—yet accurately produced vowels are also important for well-developed speech.

☐ These tests provide only an inventory of the sounds sampled. They do not yield predictive information, such as whether a particular sound error might be outgrown.

☐ The reliability of findings may be questionable with disorders that result in variable sound productions. For example, a key feature of apraxia is inconsistently produced sounds. Many patients with apraxia produce a sound or word correctly one time, and incorrectly the next. With a variable disorder, the clinician who samples a given word once or only a few times may draw conclusions that are misleading.

A unique articulation test that differs from the tests described to this point is the *Deep Test of Articulation* (McDonald, 1976b), sometimes referred to as the "McDonald Deep." This test allows you to select a particular sound and examine it in up to 48 different phonetic contexts. Each sound is examined as it releases into, or terminates from, different sounds. This test is typically used after a more traditional articulation test has been administered. It is especially useful if there are only a few sound errors, or if you want to identify different contexts in which the sound is produced correctly or incorrectly.

The "Iowa Pressure Consonant Test" is a subtest of the *Templin-Darley Test of Articulation* (Templin & Darley, 1969). This test focuses on the 16 pressure consonants — /p/, /b/, /t/, /d/, /k/, /g/, /f/, /v/, /s/, /z/, /ʃ/, /tʃ/, /ʒ/, and /dʒ/. It is a useful assessment tool when velopharyngeal inadequacy is suspected as these pressure consonants require the build-up of intraoral pressure and, therefore, adequate velopharyngeal function.

When evaluating clients with moderate to severe articulation disorders, tests of phonological processes may prove more diagnostically valuable than traditional articulation tests. Phonological processes are described later in this chapter. Five tests commonly used to examine these processes are:

- *Assessment Link Between Phonology and Articulation* (Lowe, 1986)
- *Assessment of Phonological Processes* (Hodson, 1986)
- *Bankson-Bernthal Phonological Process Survey Test* (Bankson & Bernthal, 1990)
- *Compton-Hutton Phonological Assessment* (Compton & Hutton, 1978)
- *Phonological Process Analysis* (Weiner, 1979)

SPEECH SAMPLING

Collecting a speech-language sample was described in Chapter 4. The speech sample is especially important for accurately diagnosing disorders of speech sound production. After obtaining one or more representative samples of your client's speech, analyze the sample with a focus on the following behaviors:

☐ Number of errors;

☐ Error types;

☐ Consistency of errors between the speech sample and the articulation test, within the same speech sample, and between different speech samples;

☐ Correctly produced sounds;

☐ Intelligibility;

☐ Speech rate;

☐ Prosody.

Materials presented in other sections of this resource describe specific methods for analyzing speech samples. Refer to "Evaluating Rate of Speech" (pp. 112–113), "Determining Intelligibility" (pp. 113–117), "Comparison of Sound Errors from an Articulation Test and Connected Speech" (pp. 137–139), "Identifying Dysarthria" (pp. 291–292), or "Identifying Apraxia" (p. 300) for more information.

IDENTIFYING SOUND ERRORS

Most articulation tests allow for easy identification of sound errors. This is a more difficult task with speech samples because they may not elicit all of the phonetic sounds unless the sample is elicited in a systematic manner. To complete a thorough diagnostic evaluation, you will need to compare errors made during the articulation test to those errors made during connected speech. For some sounds, there may be multiple error types. Also inventory correctly produced sounds. Form 5–1 will allow you to identify the errors produced during the speech sample and then compare the results with errors identified on the articulation test. Typically, more sound errors will be found during the connected speech sample. Also note that initial, medial, and final sound positions are not as definitive in connected speech.

Form 5–1. Comparison of Sound Errors from an Articulation Test and Connected Speech

Name:_____ Age: _____ Date: _____

Examiner: _____

Instructions: Compare speech errors identified during an articulation test and connected speech. Here are recommended ways to mark errors:

Omission:	use a dash (—) or write *omit*
Distortion:	use diacritics; describe the error; or use a D or write *dist* and indicate severity with 1 (mild), 2 (moderate), or 3 (severe). For example, D^3 is a severe distortion.
Substitution:	transcribe the error
Addition:	transcribe the error
Stimulable:	use a (✔) or a (+); if the error is improved but not perfectly correct, mark an upward arrow (↑) or describe the nature of the improvement.
Not Stimulable:	use NS (not stimulable) or zero (0)

Then summarize your findings to identify error patterns.

	Articulation Test Errors			Connected Speech Errors		
Sound	**Initial**	**Medial**	**Final**	**Initial**	**Medial**	**Final**
p	_____	_____	_____	_____	_____	_____
b	_____	_____	_____	_____	_____	_____
t	_____	_____	_____	_____	_____	_____
k	_____	_____	_____	_____	_____	_____
g	_____	_____	_____	_____	_____	_____
f	_____	_____	_____	_____	_____	_____
v	_____	_____	_____	_____	_____	_____
θ	_____	_____	_____	_____	_____	_____
ð	_____	_____	_____	_____	_____	_____
s	_____	_____	_____	_____	_____	_____
z	_____	_____	_____	_____	_____	_____
ʃ	_____	_____	_____	_____	_____	_____

(continued)

Form 5–1. *(continued)*

Sound	Articulation Test Errors			Connected Speech Errors		
	Initial	Medial	Final	Initial	Medial	Final
ʒ	_____	_____	_____	_____	_____	_____
h	_____	_____	_____	_____	_____	_____
tʃ	_____	_____	_____	_____	_____	_____
dʒ	_____	_____	_____	_____	_____	_____
w	_____	_____	_____	_____	_____	_____
j	_____	_____	_____	_____	_____	_____
l	_____	_____	_____	_____	_____	_____
r	_____	_____	_____	_____	_____	_____
m	_____	_____	_____	_____	_____	_____
n	_____	_____	_____	_____	_____	_____
ŋ	_____	_____	_____	_____	_____	_____
i	_____	_____	_____	_____	_____	_____
ɪ	_____	_____	_____	_____	_____	_____
e	_____	_____	_____	_____	_____	_____
ɛ	_____	_____	_____	_____	_____	_____
æ	_____	_____	_____	_____	_____	_____
ɝ	_____	_____	_____	_____	_____	_____
ɚ	_____	_____	_____	_____	_____	_____
ə	_____	_____	_____	_____	_____	_____
ʌ	_____	_____	_____	_____	_____	_____
u	_____	_____	_____	_____	_____	_____
ʊ	_____	_____	_____	_____	_____	_____
o	_____	_____	_____	_____	_____	_____
ɔ	_____	_____	_____	_____	_____	_____
ɑ	_____	_____	_____	_____	_____	_____

Consistent Sound Errors:

Sounds Containing More Than One Error:

Patterns of Sound Errors:

Consistent Correct Sound Productions:

STIMULABILITY

Stimulability refers to a client's ability to produce a correct (or improved) production of an erred sound. The client attempts to imitate the clinician's correct production, often after receiving specific instructions regarding the articulatory placement or manner of sound production. For example, the clinician may hold the client's lips together to form a /p/, or touch the client's hard palate with a tongue depressor to show tongue placement for the production of /t/. In some cases, a mirror is helpful for eliciting the target sound.

The assessment of stimulability provides important prognostic information. If you are able to stimulate a target behavior at the sound level or word level during the diagnostic session, you can predict that the desired behavior may also be trainable at more complex levels. Those behaviors that are most easily stimulated provide excellent starting points in therapy as they often lead to treatment success quicker than other, less stimulable behaviors.

Your ability to stimulate erred sounds is based on a good working knowledge of phonetics. You must know what needs to be changed in order to improve the production. Also realize that, in some cases, there is more than one way to correctly articulate a sound. For example, a "textbook description" of /t/ will state that it is a lingua-alveolar sound produced by tapping the tongue on the hard palate. However, some people produce a good /t/ by tapping the tongue on the front teeth.

Another key to stimulability is visually observing the client's erred productions. Even though not *all* sounds are visible, many are. Beginning clinicians tend to *listen* to speech more than *watch* speech, but seeing an error can help you know what needs to change in order to produce a better sound.

There are resources that provide specific instructions for stimulating each phoneme. These are two that we recommend:

- *The Connection of Defective Consonant Sounds* (Nemoy & Davis, 1980)
- *Techniques for Articulatory Disorders* (Bosley, 1981)

Once a sound is stimulated at the sound or syllable level, sample it at the word and phrase levels. The next section, "Assessing Stimulability of Consonants," is provided for this purpose. The "Syllable-by-Syllable Stimulus Phrases" (pp. 119–121) can also be used to assess stimulability in phrases of increasing length.

Assessing Stimulability of Consonants

The words and sentences provided in Table 5–1 are designed for assessing stimulability of misarticulated phonemes. Three words and sentences are provided for each phoneme in the initial, medial, and final positions. For each sound, the single words contain a front vowel, a central vowel, and a back vowel for assessing consonant productions in different contexts. The normative age data in the left-hand column is from Prather, Hedrick, and Kern (1975), and it reflects the age at which 75% of the children they tested correctly produced the targeted sound in the initial and final positions. (Refer to the "Developmental Norms for Phonemes" on pp. 150–151 for more information on the use of norms.) Initial position blends are included following the singletons. Three words (each containing a front, central, and back vowel when possible) and a short phrase or sentence are provided for each blend.

Form 5–2 (pp. 148–149) can be used to summarize your stimulability assessment findings. In many cases, the form will help identify patterns of stimulable sounds at different levels, providing potential starting points for therapy. You may also get a clearer picture of specific error types that may be more amenable to earlier treatment (e.g., bilabials may be more stimulable than velars).

Table 5–1. Words and Phrases for Assessing Stimulability

Age	Sound	Initial	Medial	Final
2	/p/	pin	happy	sleep
		person	puppy	cup
		pool	soapy	soup
		Pie is good.	The hippo is big.	Let's move up.
		Pete didn't go.	What happened?	I found my cap.
		Peggy is nice.	It was a super effort.	Get the soap.
2–8	/b/	bake	rabbit	grab
		bird	cupboard	tub
		boot	robin	knob
		Bill is very tall.	It's above the sink.	She has a robe.
		Buy some milk.	The robber is quiet.	He needs a job.
		Bacon is good.	The label was torn.	He hurt his rib.
2–8	/t/	tan	guitar	sat
		tough	attend	mutt
		tooth	hotel	got
		Tim went home.	The motel was full.	They were late.
		Taste this.	No details are known.	Here's the boot.
		Tony is nice.	The cartoon is funny.	It's a goat.
2–4	/d/	dim	ladder	need
		dump	muddy	word
		duty	soda	food
		Do they know?	He's hiding in there.	It's too loud.
		Debbie went home.	The radio was loud.	Plant a seed.
		Dive right in.	The wedding is fun.	She has a braid.
2–4	/k/	cat	bacon	music
		cup	bucket	truck
		call	rocket	look
		Can I help you?	He's making a mess.	He saw a duck.
		Cake tastes good.	The pocket is full	It is black.
		Cut it out.	He's looking for her.	They like steak.
2–4	/g/	give	tiger	fig
		gum	again	rug
		ghost	soggy	dog
		Go away.	Read the magazine.	He found a frog.
		Get some more.	The sugar is sweet.	Sit on the rug.
		Good job.	It is foggy outside.	They like to dig.
2–4	/f/	fish	safety	stiff
		fun	muffin	rough
		fall	coffee	goof
		Find the other one.	Go before dinner.	Slice the loaf.
		Feel this paper.	It was safer inside.	Don't laugh.
		Food is good.	The cafe was full.	He likes beef.

(continued)

Table 5–1. *(continued)*

Age	Sound	Initial	Medial	Final
4	/v/	vase	beaver	have
		verdict	oven	curve
		vote	over	stove
		Visit him.	The movie was good.	They will arrive.
		Value your time.	It's a heavy box.	He wore a glove.
		Victory is sweet.	It's in the oval office.	He might move.
4	/θ/	thin	bathtub	math
		third	nothing	earth
		thought	author	tooth
		Think about it.	The athlete won.	I need a bath.
		Thank you.	Say something.	It's a myth.
		Thunder is loud.	The cathedral is big.	Tell the truth.
4	/ð/	that	feather	breathe
		there	mother	bathe
		those	bother	soothe
		These are old.	I would rather go.	He can breathe.
		They didn't like it.	The weather is hot.	It feels smooth.
		This is not right.	Her father is nice.	We sunbathe.
3	/s/	sand	hassle	chase
		sunny	mercy	fuss
		soap	bossy	moose
		Sip lemonade.	Leave a message.	It's a mess.
		Surprises are fun.	They saw a castle.	She has a horse.
		Soup is good.	They are chasing us.	His dog is loose.
4	/z/	zip	easy	peas
		zero	cousin	does
		zone	closet	chose
		Zip the coat.	They will visit us.	Touch the toes.
		Zoo trips are fun.	The closet was full.	He likes cheese.
		Zebras are big.	The dessert was good.	Hear the noise.
3–8	/ʃ/	ship	special	fish
		shirt	brushes	rush
		show	bushy	push
		Shall we go?	The dishes are dry.	He used cash.
		Shoes get lost.	The ocean is near.	It is fresh.
		Shells are pretty.	The machine broke.	Make a wish.
4	/ʒ/		measure	
			version	
			fusion	

(continued)

Table 5–1. *(continued)*

Age	Sound	Initial	Medial	Final
4	/ʒ/		Bury the treasure. Wear casual clothes. His vision is good.	
2	/h/	hiss hut hop Hurry for dinner. He is going. Have you done it?	behave rehearse forehead The playhouse is large. Go unhook it. Look behind you.	
3–8	/tʃ/	cheese chunk choose China is far away. Chuck is a friend. Chew your food.	matches merchant nachos The ketchup spilled. He is pitching. He's a natural.	beach much watch Sit on a couch. Strike a match. She ate a peach.
4	/dʒ/	jeep jug joke Jets are fast. Jump the fence. Jelly is good.	magic budget project The pigeon flew. The pajamas are red. It was a raging fire.	age budge dodge Turn the page. Cross a bridge. She likes fudge.
2–8	/w/	well won wood Winter is here. Wake up now. Why did he do it?	freeway away mower The sidewalk is hot. The reward was paid. He has a power saw.	
2–4	/j/	yell yummy yacht Yellow is bright. Yogurt is good. You can go now.	kayak royal coyote The tortilla was warm. He is a loyal friend. The lawyer called.	
3–4	/l/	leap learn look Linda went home. Lay it on the table. Let me see.	jelly color pillow She is silly. The palace was large. The jello was good.	fell pearl ball It is full. We will. Walk a mile.

(continued)

Table 5–1. *(continued)*

Age	Sound	Initial	Medial	Final
3–4	/r/	rip run row Rake the leaves. Rub it in. Ruth is nice.	erase carrot borrow The parade is today. He is sorry about it. Her earring was lost.	steer hair car It was not far. He ate the pear. Go to the store.
2	/m/	make money moon Meet me later. Mark is nice. My dog is brown.	hammer summer human It's lemon pie. He's coming back. Let Jimmy see it.	same hum boom You're welcome. Play the drum. They like ham.
2	/n/	net nothing new Never do that. Nancy said yes. Nobody was home.	many sunny phony He's a piano player. We cannot go. The bunny is white.	mean learn soon David is his son. Did you win? She has grown.
2	/ŋ/		finger hunger longer The singer is short. Put the hanger away. It's a jungle animal.	ring hung song He was young. He was wrong. Play on a swing.

Blend	Word	Phrase
/bl/	black blunt blue	a black shoe a blunt pencil the blue car
/br/	brave brush broke	the brave hero The brush fell. He broke it.
/dr/	drink drum draw	Don't drink it all. the drum beat Let's draw a picture.
/fr/	free front frog	set free in the front a big frog

(continued)

Table 5–1. (*continued*)

Blend	Word	Phrase
/fl/	fly	a fly swatter
	flurry	the snow flurry
	float	a root beer float
/gl/	glad	a glad boy
	glove	the glove box
	glue	sticky as glue
/gr/	green	the green tree
	grudge	hold a grudge
	grow	They grow corn.
/kl/	clam	a clam bake
	club	the clubhouse
	closet	the closet door
/kr/	cry	Do not cry.
	crumb	the crumb cake
	cruise	a cruise liner
/pl/	place	first-place ribbon
	plum	the plum pudding
	plot	The plot thickened.
/pr/	price	The price was high.
	protect	He will protect us.
	prove	Can you prove it?
/sk/	sky	The sky is blue.
	scare	Don't scare me.
	scoop	a scoop of ice cream
/skr/	screen	a screen door
	scrub	He will scrub the sink.
	scroll	the scroll cards
/sl/	slam	a slam dunk
	slush	The snow was slush.
	slow	She should slow down.
/sp/	spy	the secret spy
	spurt	a spurt of energy
	spoon	a soup spoon
/spl/	split	a banana split
	splurge	They splurged for it.
	splotch	the splotch of ink

(*continued*)

Table 5–1. *(continued)*

Blend	Word	Phrase
/spr/	spray	a spray bottle
	sprung	They sprung up.
	sprout	an alfalfa sprout
/sm/	smell	a nice smell
	smug	a smug look
	smooth	baby-smooth skin
/sn/	snack	The snack was good.
	snuggle	a snuggle bear
	snow	the snow shovel
/st/	stiff	a stiff shirt
	stunt	a tricky stunt
	stop	Don't stop yet.
/str/	stray	a stray dog
	struggle	a struggle to win
	strong	the strong man
/ʃr/	shrimp	The shrimp were large.
	shrunk	It shrunk in the wash.
	shrewd	He is shrewd.
/tr/	tray	the breakfast tray
	trumpet	a trumpet solo
	true	her true colors
/θr/	three	the three blind mice
	thrust	the initial thrust
	throw	Let's throw the ball.

Form 5–2. Sounds That Are Stimulable

Name: _____ Age: _____ Date: _____

Examiner: _____

Instructions: Record all stimulable sounds under the appropriate category using a check (✔) or plus (+). If a sound is stimulable at the phrase level, indicate the number of syllables in the phrase. For example:

p   ✔   ✔   ✔   _____   3   3   _____

Sound Level	**Word Level**			**Phrase Level**		
	Initial	**Medial**	**Final**	**Initial**	**Medial**	**Final**
p	_____	_____	_____	_____	_____	_____
b	_____	_____	_____	_____	_____	_____
t	_____	_____	_____	_____	_____	_____
d	_____	_____	_____	_____	_____	_____
k	_____	_____	_____	_____	_____	_____
g	_____	_____	_____	_____	_____	_____
f	_____	_____	_____	_____	_____	_____
v	_____	_____	_____	_____	_____	_____
θ	_____	_____	_____	_____	_____	_____
ð	_____	_____	_____	_____	_____	_____
s	_____	_____	_____	_____	_____	_____
z	_____	_____	_____	_____	_____	_____
ʃ	_____	_____	_____	_____	_____	_____
ʒ	_____	_____	_____	_____	_____	_____
h	_____	_____	_____	_____	_____	_____
tʃ	_____	_____	_____	_____	_____	_____
dʒ	_____	_____	_____	_____	_____	_____
w	_____	_____	_____	_____	_____	_____
j	_____	_____	_____	_____	_____	_____
l	_____	_____	_____	_____	_____	_____

SoundLevel	Word Level			Phrase Level		
	Initial	**Medial**	**Final**	**Initial**	**Medial**	**Final**
r	_____	_____	_____	_____	_____	_____	_____
m	_____	_____	_____	_____	_____	_____	_____
n	_____	_____	_____	_____	_____	_____	_____
ŋ	_____	_____	_____	_____	_____	_____	_____

	SoundLevel	**Word Level**	**Phrase Level**
i	_____	_____	_____
ɪ	_____	_____	_____
e	_____	_____	_____
ɛ	_____	_____	_____
æ	_____	_____	_____
ɝ	_____	_____	_____
ɚ	_____	_____	_____
ə	_____	_____	_____
ʌ	_____	_____	_____
u	_____	_____	_____
ʊ	_____	_____	_____
o	_____	_____	_____
ɔ	_____	_____	_____
ɑ	_____	_____	_____

DEVELOPMENTAL NORMS FOR PHONEMES

Clinicians often use normative data to determine whether or not a child is developing within normal expectations. Although norms are helpful, consider these limitations of over-relying on developmental norms.

☐ A norm is only an average age at which a behavior occurs. It refers, therefore, to a "hypothetical child" who does not and never did exist.

☐ True norms are collected from and apply to a normal, randomly selected sample. These exact representative samples rarely exist in the real world.

☐ Different norms are rarely in agreement with each other. The differences are caused by many factors, including: when the study was conducted, where the study was conducted, the size and characteristics of the sample, the research design followed, and the mastery criteria used.

Despite these limitations, norms are useful for estimating approximately how well a child's sounds are developing. In current practice, the more recent studies presented in Table 5–2 are referred to most frequently. Generally, the later studies indicate an earlier development of consonants than the earlier studies from the 1930s. The notes below are offered as a general introduction to the material in Table 5–2.

• Wellman, Case, Mengurt, and Bradbury's (1931) study represents the earliest age at which 75% of the 204 children tested (ages 2 to 6 years) correctly produced the consonant phoneme in the initial, medial, and final positions.

• Poole's (1934) study represents the earliest age at which 100% of the 140 children tested (ages 2:6 to 8:5) correctly produced the consonant phoneme in all three positions.

• Templin's (1957) study represents the earliest age at which 75% of the 480 children tested (ages 3 to 8) correctly produced the consonant phoneme in all three positions.

• Sander's (1972) data represent a reinterpretation of Templin's (1957) and Wellman et al.'s (1931) research based on a criterion of 51% accuracy in two out of three positions.

• Prather et al.'s (1975) study represents the earliest age at which 75% of the 147 children tested (ages 2 to 4) correctly produced the consonant in the initial and final positions.

Table 5–2. Five Commonly Cited Norms for Consonant Development

Consonant	Wellman et al. (1931)	Poole (1934)	Templin (1957)	Sander (1972)	Prather et al. (1975)
m	3	3^1/$_2$	3	before 2	2
n	3	4^1/$_2$	3	before 2	2
h	3	3^1/$_2$	3	before 2	2
p	4	3^1/$_2$	3	before 2	2
f	3	5^1/$_2$	3	3	2–4
w	3	3^1/$_2$	3	before 2	2–8
b	3	3^1/$_2$	4	before 2	2–8
ŋ		4^1/$_2$	3	2	2
j	4	4^1/$_2$	3^1/$_2$	3	2–4
k	4	4^1/$_2$	4	2	2–4
g	4	4^1/$_2$	4	2	2–4
l	4	6^1/$_2$	6	3	3–4
d	5	4^1/$_2$	4	2	2–4
t	5	4^1/$_2$	6	2	2–8
s	5	7^1/$_2$	4^1/$_2$	3	3
r	5	7^1/$_2$	4	3	3–4
tʃ	5		4^1/$_2$	4	3–8
v	5	6^1/$_2$	6	4	4
z	5	7^1/$_2$	7	4	4
ʒ	6	6^1/$_2$	7	6	4
θ		7^1/$_2$	6	5	4
dʒ			7	4	4
ʃ		6^1/$_2$	4^1/$_2$	4	3–8
ð		6^1/$_2$	7	5	4

Source: Reprinted with the permission of Merrill, an imprint of Macmillan Publishing Company from *Assessment and Remediation of Articulatory and Phonological Disorders*, Second Edition by Nancy A. Creaghead, Parley W. Newman, and Wayne A. Secord. Copyright © 1985 by Merrill Publishing Company (p. 47).

AGE RANGES OF NORMAL CONSONANT DEVELOPMENT

The data from the normative studies in Table 5–2 each resulted in a specific age of development, but these ages do not reflect normal and acceptable developmental variability. Sander (1972) reinterpreted the data collected by Templin (1957) and Wellman et al. (1931) and compiled the age ranges presented in Figure 5–1. It is important to view ranges, as they provide more useful information about developmental variations. For example, compare Table 5–2 with Figure 5–1. In Table 5–2, Sander suggests that /p/ develops before age 2. However, in Figure 5–1,you can see that he also found that /p/ in normal development may continue to develop until age 3.

Keep in mind that normative data only tell part of the story, as certain errors are developmentally appropriate while others are not. For example, consider two different errors involving /s/. A substitution of /t/ for /s/ is acceptable at age 2 but not at age 4, but a /θ/ for /s/ at age 4 may not be a concern. Remember to interpret normative data for individual sounds relative to their overall patterns.

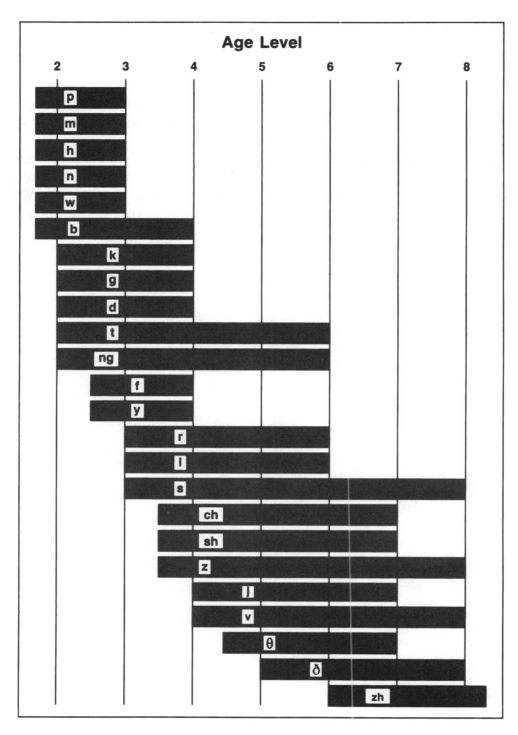

Figure 5–1. Age ranges of normal consonant development. Average age estimates and upper age limits of customary consonant production. The solid bar corresponding to each sound starts at the median age of customary articulation; it stops at an age level at which 90% of all children are customarily producing the sound (data from Templin, 1957; Wellman et al., 1931). (From E. Sander [1972], "When Are Speech Sounds Learned?" *Journal of Speech and Hearing Disorders, 37,* 55–63. Used by permission.)

FREQUENCIES OF OCCURRENCE OF CONSONANTS

Table 5–3 contains the percentages of occurrence of intended American English consonants in continuous speech. The information is from Shriberg and Kwiatkowski (1983), who summarized several studies of the frequency of consonant productions in natural speech. The studies they evaluated included data from children with normal and delayed speech development, as well as adults with normal speech.

A cumulative percentage of consonant occurrence is provided in the right-hand column of the table. Note that the sounds /n/, /t/, /s/, /r/, /d/, and /m/ cumulatively represent nearly one-half of the total consonants used. When misarticulated, these sounds will have a greater negative effect on speech than the less frequently occurring sounds such as /ʒ/, /tʃ/, /dʒ/, and /θ/.

Table 5–3. The Frequency of Occurrence of Individual English Consonants

Sound	Percentage of Occurrence	Cumulative Percentage
n	12.0	12.0
t	11.9	23.9
s	6.9	30.8
r	6.7	37.5
d	6.4	43.9
m	5.9	49.8
z	5.4	55.2
ð	5.3	60.5
l	5.3	65.8
k	5.1	70.9
w	4.9	75.8
h	4.4	80.2
b	3.3	83.5
p	3.1	86.6
g	3.1	89.7
f	2.1	91.8
ŋ	1.6	93.4
j	1.6	95.0
v	1.5	96.5
ʃ	0.9	97.4
θ	0.9	98.3
dʒ	0.6	98.9
tʃ	0.6	99.5
ʒ	<0.1	99.6

Source: From L. D. Shriberg and J. Kwiatkowski, "Computer-Assisted Natural Process Analysis (NPA): Recent Issues and Data," in *Seminars in Speech and Language.* 4(4), New York, 1983, Thieme Medical Publishers, Inc. Adapted by permission.

DESCRIPTIVE FEATURES OF PHONEMES

Phonemes of the English language can be grouped and separated according to similar and dissimilar features (Shriberg & Kent, 1995). Sounds are most commonly described according to place of articulation, manner of articulation, and voicing. An articulation test like the *Fisher-Logemann Test of Articulation* (Fisher & Logemann, 1971) is designed to identify errors of place, manner, and voicing, but these types of errors can be identified from any articulation test. Table 5-4 shows how sounds are described according to these categories. This information can serve as a reference for evaluating a client's articulatory behaviors. Take note of whether phoneme errors tend to occur within specific categories (e.g., errors of fricatives, errors of alveolars, errors of voicing, etc.).

Table 5–4. The Sounds of English Categorized by Place, Manner, and Voicing. Unvoiced Sounds Are Shown with an Asterisk.

Manner of Articulation	*Consonants* **Place of Articulation**						
	Bilabial	**Labiodental**	**Dental**	**Alveolar**	**Palatal**	**Velar**	**Glottal**
Stop	p*			t*		k*	
	b			d		g	
Fricative		f*	θ*	s*	ʃ*		h*
		v	ð	z	ʒ		
Affricate					tʃ*		
					dʒ		
Glide	w				j		
Liquid				l	r		
Nasal	m			n	ŋ		

	Vowels **Place of Articulation**		
	Front	**Center**	**Back**
High	i		u
(High)	ɪ		ʊ
	e	ɝ	
			o
Mid (Mid)	ɛ	ə ɚ	
		ʌ	ɔ
(Low)			
Low	æ		ɑ

DISTINCTIVE FEATURES OF CONSONANTS

Individual sounds consist of unique and distinct features that, when all features are present, make each sound different from all other sounds. For example, /f/ and /v/ are two sounds that share four distinctive features (consonantal, anterior, continuant, strident) but differ by one feature (voicing), which makes them separate sounds. Clinicians often use distinctive features to identify error patterns. Once the patterns are identified, therapy focuses on training the features that will improve speech productions. The advantage of the distinctive features approach is its ability to target one or more specific features that will help improve more than one sound at the same time.

The following examples show several distinctive feature patterns.

Example One:

/t/ for /k/   (*tup* for *cup*)
/d/ for /g/   (*dumb* for *gum*)
/n/ for /ŋ/   (*lawn* for *long*)

The erred feature in this example is an *anterior* placement. Sounds are produced in front of the mouth instead of the back

Example Two:

/d/ for /n/   (*dice* for *nice*)
/b/ for /m/   (*bake* for *make*)
/g/ for /ŋ/   (*lug* for *lung*)

The erred pattern involves *nasality*. Nonnasal sounds are substituted for nasal sounds.

Example Three:

/w/ for /f/   (*wine* for *fine*)
/l/ for /v/   (*lase* for *vase*)
/t/ for /s/   (*toap* for *soap*)
omissions of /s/, /ʃ/, /tʃ/, /ʒ/, and /dʒ/

While these errors do not initially appear related, the missing distinctive feature in all the sounds is *stridency.*

Table 5–5 is based on Chomsky and Halle's (1968) listing of the distinctive features of English consonants. For your reference, all terms are defined in the Glossary under "Distinctive Features."

Table 5–5. Distinctive Features of English Consonants

	b	m	w	f	v	θ	ð	t	d	s	z	n	l	ʃ	ʒ	j	r	tʃ	dʒ	k	g	ŋ	h	p
Voiced	+	+	+	−	+	−	+	−	+	−	+	+	+	−	+	+	+	−	+	−	+	+	−	−
Consonantal	+	+	−	+	+	+	+	+	+	+	+	+	+	+	+	+	−	+	+	+	+	+	−	+
Anterior	+	+	+	+	+	+	+	+	+	+	+	+	+	−	−	−	−	−	−	−	−	−	−	+
Coronal	−	−	−	−	−	+	+	+	+	+	+	+	+	+	+	−	+	+	+	−	−	−	−	−
Continuant	−	−	+	+	+	+	+	−	−	+	+	−	+	+	+	+	+	−	−	−	−	−	+	−
High	−	−	−	−	−	−	−	−	−	−	−	−	−	+	+	+	−	+	+	+	+	+	−	−
Low	−	−	−	−	−	−	−	−	−	−	−	−	−	−	−	−	−	−	−	−	−	−	+	−
Back	−	−	−	−	−	−	−	−	−	−	−	−	−	−	−	−	−	−	−	+	+	+	−	−
Nasal	−	+	−	−	−	−	−	−	−	−	−	+	−	−	−	−	−	−	−	−	−	+	−	−
Strident	−	−	−	+	+	−	−	−	−	+	+	−	−	+	+	−	−	+	+	−	−	−	−	−
Vocalic	−	−	−	−	−	−	−	−	−	−	−	−	+	−	−	−	+	−	−	−	−	−	−	−

Source: Based on N. Chomsky and M. Halle (1968), *The Sound Pattern of English* (pp. 176–177), New York: Harper & Row. From M. N. Hegde (1995), *Introduction to communicative disorders* (2nd ed., p. 120), Austin, TX: PRO-ED. Used by permission of both HarperCollins and PRO-ED.

PHONOLOGICAL PROCESSES

As stated previously, distinctive features refer to the characteristic features of individual sounds. Phonological processes, on the other hand, apply to larger segments which *include* individual sounds. A phonological process is more all encompassing and includes the changes that occur to individual sounds and their distinctive features. Phonological processes describe what children do in the normal developmental process of speech to simplify standard adult productions. When a child uses many different processes or uses processes that are not typically present during speech acquisition, intelligibility may be impaired.

Phonological process analysis compares a child's (or speech-impaired adult's) articulatory productions to normal adult productions. The advantage of using a phonological processes approach is that you can identify error patterns, and then target those patterns to remediate more than one sound at a time. For example, if a child exhibits a *final consonant deletion* pattern, you may choose to target final consonants in general rather than focus on only a few sounds in the final position. Some of the more commonly used assessment batteries for evaluating phonological processes include:

- *Assessment of Phonological Processes* (Hodson, 1986)
- *Assessment Link Between Phonology and Articulation* (Lowe, 1986)
- *Phonological Process Analysis* (Weiner, 1979)
- *Compton-Hutton Phonological Assessment* (Compton & Hutton, 1978)

Different authorities describe numerous phonological processes (see Hodson, 1986; Hodson & Paden, 1991; Ingram, 1981; Shriberg & Kwiatkowski, 1980; Stoel-Gammon & Dunn, 1985; Weiner, 1979; and others). We have provided descriptions and examples of 23 phonological processes (from Bernthal & Bankson, 1993; Creaghead, Newman, & Secord, 1989; Hodson, 1986; Lowe, 1986; Stoel-Gammon & Dunn, 1985). Refer to these descriptions or to the specific guidelines provided by the test you use when evaluating clients with multiple articulation errors. Realize that some of the examples below illustrate more than one process change.

Alveolarization

Substitution of an alveolar phoneme for a labial or linguadental phoneme:

/tæn/	for *pan*
/don/	for *bone*
/bæs/	for *bath*

Assimilation (Harmony)

Alteration of a consonant phoneme that is influenced by, and becomes more like, a surrounding phoneme:

/bɛb/	for *bed*
/dʌn/	for *gun*
/gɛnk/	for *thank*

Backing

Substitution of a more posteriorly produced phoneme for an anteriorly produced phoneme:

/kɑp/	for *top*
/bok/	for *boat*
/hup/	for *soup*

Cluster Reduction

Reduction of a cluster to a singleton:

/pen/	for *plane*
/tʌk/	for *truck*
/sip/	for *sleep*

Coalescence

Substitution of a single phoneme that is different from two adjacent target phonemes yet takes on features of the target:

/fok/	for *smoke*
/tufe/	for *Tuesday*
/læθ/	for *last*

Deaffrication

Substitution of a fricative for an affricate phoneme:

/ʃɪp/	for *chip*
/peʒ/	for *page*
/ʃiz/	for *cheese*

Denasalization

Substitution of a homorganic stop (similar place of articulation) for a nasal phoneme:

/do/	for *no*
/bæd/	for *man*
/sɪg/	for *sing*

Depalatalization

Substitution of an alveolar fricative or affricate for a palatal fricative or affricate:

/dʒu/	for *cue*
/wɑts/	for *wash*
/fɪs/	for *fish*

Diminutization

Addition of /i/ or consonant + /i/:

/lɛgi/	for *leg*
/hæti/	for *hat*
/mɑɪmi/	for *my*

Doubling

Repetition of a word:

/gogo/	for *go*
/dædæ/	for *dad*
/mimi/	for *me*

Epenthesis

Insertion of a new phoneme:

/bəlu/	for *blue*
/sθop/	for *soap*
/klələ˞/	for *color*

Final Consonant Deletion

Deletion of the final consonant:

/kʌ/	for *cup*
/dɑ/	for *doll*
/pu/	for *pool*

Fronting

Substitution of a more anteriorly produced phoneme:

/su/	for *shoe*
/frɔd/	for *frog*
/tændɪ/	for *candy*

Gliding

Substitution of a glide for a liquid:

/pwey/	for *play*
/wʌn/	for *run*
/jɛwo/	for *yellow*

Initial Consonant Deletion

Deletion of the initial singleton consonant:

/ʌp/	for *cup*
/æn/	for *man*
/ul/	for *pool*

Labialization

Substitution of a labial phoneme for a phoneme produced with the tip of the tongue:

/bɔg/	for *dog*
/hæf/	for *hat*
/fʌn/	for *sun*

Metathesis (Spoonerism)

Transposition of two phonemes:

/bəskɛtɪ/ for *spaghetti*
/faʊlɚ/ for *flower*
/lɪkstɪp/ for *lipstick*

Reduplication

Repetition of a complete or incomplete syllable:

/wɑwɑ/ for *water*
/dɑdɑ/ for *dog*
/wæwæ/ for *wagon*

Stopping

Substitution of a stop for a fricative or affricate:

/top/ for *soap*
/kæt/ for *catch*
/pʌdl/ for *puzzle*

Stridency Deletion

Omission of a strident or the substitution of a nonstrident consonant:

/op/ for *soap*
/wʌn/ for *fun*
/kɪθ/ for *kiss*

Unstressed Syllable Deletion

Deletion of an unstressed syllable:

/gɛdɪ/ for *spaghetti*
/maɪkwev/ for *microwave*
/nænə/ for *banana*

Voicing or Devoicing

Alteration in voicing influenced by a surrounding phoneme:

/dʒɑp/ for *job*
/beg/ for *bake*
/gʌp/ for *cup*

Vocalization (Vowelization)

Substitution of a vowel for a liquid phoneme in the final position:

/kʌvʊ/ for *cover*
/pipo/ for *people*
/hɛə/ for *hair*

Most phonological processes are seen in normal speech acquisition. Children typically outgrow them and learn to produce the correct adult targets by 8 years of age (Stoel-Gammon & Dunn, 1985). Research that identifies when specific patterns are outgrown is scarce. As a general indication of normal development, Stoel-Gammon and Dunn (1985) outline processes that disappear before age 3 and processes that persist after age 3:

Processes Disappearing by 3:0	**Processes Persisting after 3:0**
Unstressed Syllable Deletion	Cluster Reduction
Final Consonant Deletion	Epenthesis
Doubling	Gliding
Diminutization	Vocalization
Velar Fronting	Stopping
Consonant Assimilation	Depalatalization
Reduplication	Final Devoicing
Prevocalic Voicing	

They also note that some children never produce certain processes. The most common phonological processes that occur in normal speech acquisition are unstressed syllable deletion, final consonant deletion, gliding, and cluster reduction.

Form 5–3 is a worksheet for identifying phonological processes elicited during connected speech or on a formal test. An inventory of phonological processes is most valueable when working with children who have poor speech intelligibility due to multiple articulation errors. For children with only a few errors, use Form 5–1 (pp. 137–139), "Comparison of Sound Errors from an Articulation Test and Connected Speech."

Form 5—3. Phonological Processes Worksheet

Name:_____ Age: _____ Date: _____

Examiner: _____

Instructions: Record the child's exact articulatory productions and the indended target words. Then determine the phonological processes used for each error. If a process cannot be identified, leave the final column blank or write a question mark (?). Note which processes occur with the greatest frequency.

Child's Production	**Intended Production**	**Phonological Process**

Child's Production	Intended Production	Phonological Process

(continued)

Form 5–3. *(continued)*

Child's Production	Intended Production	Phonological Process
_____	_____	_____
_____	_____	_____
_____	_____	_____
_____	_____	_____
_____	_____	_____
_____	_____	_____
_____	_____	_____
_____	_____	_____
_____	_____	_____
_____	_____	_____
_____	_____	_____

Comments:

CONCLUDING COMMENTS

A variety of assessment materials and procedures were presented in this chapter. These ranged from articulation screening to administration of formal articulation tests, and from obtaining speech samples to assessing stimulability The resource materials included normative data, distinctive features, and phonological processes. Keep in mind that some of the resources in Chapter 4 are also useful for assessing disorders of articulation and phonological processes.

SOURCES OF ADDITIONAL INFORMATION

Screening

Compton, A. J., & Hutton, S. (1978). *Compton-Hutton phonological assessment.* San Francisco: Carousel House.

Drumwright, A. F. (1971). *Denver articulation screening examination.* Denver: University of Colorado Medical Center.

Fluharty, N. B. (1978). *Fluharty preschool speech and language screening test.* Boston: Teaching Resources Corporation.

McDonald, E. T. (1976a). *A screening deep test of articulation with longitudinal norms.* Tucson, AZ: Communication Skill Builders.

Neidecker, E. A. (1987). *School programs in speech-language: Organization and management* (2nd ed.). Englewood Cliffs, NJ: Prentice-Hall.

Taylor, J. S. (1992). *Speech-language pathology services in the schools* (2nd ed.). Needham Heights, MA: Allyn and Bacon.

Van Riper, C., & Erickson, R. L. (1973). *Predictive screening test of articulation* (3rd ed.). Kalamazoo: Western Michigan University.

Phonetic Inventories

Bernthal, J. E., & Bankson, N. W. (1993). *Articulation and phonological disorders* (3rd ed.). Englewood Cliffs, NJ: Prentice-Hall.

Creaghead, N. A., Newman, P. W., & Secord, W. (1989). *Assessment and remediation of articulatory and phonological disorders* (2nd ed.). Columbus, OH: Merrill.

Emerick, L. L., & Haynes, W. O. (1986). *Diagnosis and evaluation in speech pathology* (3rd ed.). Englewood Cliffs, NJ: Prentice-Hall.

Fisher, H. B., & Logemann, J. A. (1971). *The Fisher-Logemann test of articulation competence.* Boston: Houghton Mifflin.

Fudala, J. B., & Reynolds, W. M. (1986). *Arizona articulation proficiency scale* (2nd ed.). Los Angeles: Western Psychological Services.

Goldman, R., & Fristoe, M. (1986). *Goldman-Fristoe test of articulation.* Circle Pines, MN: American Guidance Service.

Haynes, W. O., Pindzola, R. H., & Emerick, L. L. (1992). *Diagnosis and evaluation in speech pathology* (4th ed.). Englewood Cliffs, NJ: Prentice-Hall.

McDonald, E. T. (1976b). *A deep test of articulation.* Tucson, AZ: Communication Skill Builders.

Pendergest, K., Dickey, S., Selmar, J., & Sudar, A. (1984). *Photo articulation test* (2nd ed.). Danville, IL: Interstate Printers & Publishers.

Peterson, H. A., & Marquardt, T. P. (1994). *Appraisal and diagnosis of speech and language disorders* (3rd ed.). Englewood Cliffs, NJ: Prentice-Hall.

Templin, M. C., & Darley, F. L. (1969). *Templin-Darley test of articulation* (2nd ed.). Iowa City: University of Iowa.

Stimulating Speech Sounds

Bernthal, J. E., & Bankson, N. W. (1988). *Articulation and phonological disorders* (2nd ed.). Englewood Cliffs, NJ: Prentice-Hall.

Bosley, E. C. (1981). *Techniques for articulatory disorders.* Springfield, IL: Charles C. Thomas.

Nemoy, E. M., & Davis, S. F. (1980). *The correction of defective consonant sounds* (16th printing). Londonberry, NH: Expression Co.

Distinctive Features and Phonological Processes

Bankson, N. W., & Bernthal, J. E. (1990). *Bankson-Bernthal phonological process survey test.* Tucson, AZ: Communication Skill Builders.

Bernthal, J. E., & Bankson, N. W. (1993). *Articulation and phonological disorders* (3rd ed.). Englewood Cliffs, NJ: Prentice-Hall.

Compton, A. J., & Hutton, S. (1978). *Compton-Hutton phonological assessment.* San Francisco: Carousel House.

Elbert, M., & Gierut, J. (1986). *Handbook of clinical phonology: Approaches to assessment and treatment.* San Diego: College-Hill Press.

Haynes, W. O., Pindzola, R. H., & Emerick, L. L. (1992). *Diagnosis and evaluation in speech pathology* (4th ed.). Englewood Cliffs, NJ: Prentice-Hall.

Hegde, M. N. (1995). *Introduction to communicative disorders* (2nd ed.). Austin, TX: PRO-ED.

Hodson, B. W. (1986). *Assessment of phonological processes* (rev. ed.). Danville, IL: Interstate Printers & Publishers.

Hodson, B. W., & Paden, E. P. (1991). *Targeting intelligible speech: A phonological approach to remediation* (2nd ed.). Austin, TX: PRO-ED.

Ingram, D. (1981). *Procedures for the phonological analysis of children's language.* Baltimore: University Park Press.

Lowe, R. J. (1986). *Assessment link between phonology and articulation (ALPHA).* East Moline, IL: LinguiSystems.

Lowe, R. J. (1989). *Workbook for the identification of phonological processes.* Danville, IL: Interstate Printers & Publishers.

Shriberg, L., & Kwiatkowski, J. (1980). *Natural process analysis.* New York: Wiley.

Stoel-Gammon, C., & Dunn, C. (1985). *Normal and disordered phonology in children.* Austin, TX: PRO-ED.

Weiner, F. F. (1979). *Phonological process analysis.* Austin, TX: PRO-ED.

Internet Sources

Listservers of Interest to Communication Disorders Folks
    http://www.shc.uiowa.edu/wjshc/iiscdl.html

□ CHAPTER 6 □

Assessment of Language

This chapter focuses on the evaluation of developmental language disorders. Those language disorders that result from neurological damage, specifically aphasia and cognitive impairments due to traumatic brain injury, are addressed in Chapter 9.

OVERVIEW OF ASSESSMENT

History of the Client

    Procedures

        Written Case History
        Information-getting Interview
        Specific Questions To Ask About Language Development/Disorder
        Information From Other Professionals

    Contributing Factors

        Hearing Impairment
        Medical or Neurological Factors
        Maturation and Motor Development
        Intelligence, Sex, Birth Order, Motivation, and Levels of Concern

Assessment of Language

    Procedures

        Screening
        Informal Tests
        Standardized Tests
        Speech Sampling

    Areas to Assess

        Pragmatics
        Semantics
        Syntax
        Morphology

    Analysis

        Error Types
        Form of Errors
        Consistency of Errors

Oral-facial Examination

Hearing Assessment

Determining the Diagnosis

Providing Information (written report, interview, etc.)

Assessment Approaches

The valid assessment of language is somewhat of an enigma for some clinicians. There is a vast array of procedures and tests available for the assessment of language. Even though there are a multitude of resources for assessment, language continues to be one of the most challenging disorders to evaluate. This is not surprising considering how varied and complex language really is. We have attempted to simplify this sometimes overwhelming task as much as possible in this manual.

Leonard (1990) writes that there are at least three ways to understand language disorders that children experience:

1. By comparing a child's language development and use to normal expectations; in effect, by making comparisons with normative information.
2. By identifying specific features or structures that are deficient and require attention.
3. By identifying conditions or etiologies (e.g., mental retardation) that are related to language impairment (adapted from pp. 162–166).

In practice, clinicians often use elements of each of these three approaches when assessing and treating language disorders.

Bernstein (1993) outlines two approaches for categorizing language problems: *etiological-categorical* and *descriptive-developmental*. Based on the work of McCormick and Schiefelbusch (1984, 1990), she describes five categories within the etiological-categorical classification. These are language and communicative disorders associated with:

1. Motor disorders such as motor deficits associated with language disorders due to brain pathology (e.g., cerebral palsy) or damage to the nervous system (e.g., spine bifida). Children in this category possess motor difficulties and may have mental retardation, visual or hearing impairment, and seizure disorders.
2. Sensory deficits such as those experienced by children with hearing and visual impairments.
3. Central nervous system damage. Children may be classified as learning disabled when the damage to the central nervous system is mild, or developmentally aphasic when damage is severe.
4. Severe emotional-social dysfunctions such as those experienced by children who are classified as psychotic, schizophrenic, and/or autistic. These children experience profound disruptions in the development of verbal and nonverbal interaction skills.
5. Cognitive disorders such as those experienced by children who are classified as mentally retarded (adapted from pp. 16–17).

The second approach described by Bernstein (1993), the developmental-descriptive approach, *describes* rather than classifies language problems. Based on the work of Bloom and Lahey (1978), five types of language disorders are identified:

1. Difficulties learning linguistic form, particularly phonologic, morphologic, and syntactic rules.

2. Difficulties conceptualizing and formulating ideas about events, objects, and relations, primarily in the area of semantics.

3. Difficulties using language, such as an inability to adapt language according to different speakers or events, or an inability to use language for a wide variety of functions. These are pragmatic disorders.

4. Difficulties integrating the form, content, and use of language.

5. Delayed language development. Language use is similar to that of younger children developing within normal expectations (adapted from pp. 18–19).

The *etiological-categorical* and the *descriptive-developmental* approaches both have advantages and limitations. From a practical standpoint, clinicians frequently identify etiological-categorical patterns that apply to a client through information from the case history, from other professionals, and by direct observation. The actual assessment of communicative functions and behaviors tends to focus on descriptive-developmental areas.

Understanding Language Deficiencies

Language problems can occur within many areas. For example, the following is a list of possible problems that are seen with some children with language disorders:

- ☐ Limited skills in understanding spoken language,
- ☐ Poor listening skills,
- ☐ Limited understanding of word meanings and meanings in general,
- ☐ Limited expressive language skills,
- ☐ Limited use or lack of use of morphologic elements of language,
- ☐ Limited use of sentence structures (limited syntacytic performance),
- ☐ Inappropriate use of language,
- ☐ Deficient use of language that has been learned,
- ☐ Limited conversational skills,
- ☐ Limited skills in narrating experiences.

In addition, some language-disordered children also experience:

- ☐ Limited cognitive skills,
- ☐ Later academic problems (reading and writing problems),
- ☐ Some abnormal patterns of language (Hegde, 1995, pp. 176–177).

SCREENING

Neidecker (1987) writes that the identification of language disorders in preschool and school-age children is sometimes a complicated, difficult, and frustrating task. This is true in some settings simply because of the number of children who need to be screened. Also, language is complex and multifaceted. Decisions must be made about which features of language to screen and at what developmental levels. The facets of receptive and expressive language to consider include phonologic, semantic, syntactic, and morphologic components. A variety of tests and scales are commercially available for screening purposes. Some of these include:

- *Boehm Test of Basic Concepts* (Boehm, 1986)
- *Receptive-Expressive Emergent Language Scale* (Bzoch & League, 1991)
- *Birth to Three Developmental Scales* (Bangs & Dodson, 1979)
- *Bankson Language Test* (Bankson, 1990)
- *Screening Test for Auditory Comprehension of Language* (Carrow, 1973)
- *Early Language Milestone Scale* (Coplan, 1987)
- *Kindergarten Language Screening Test* (Gauthier & Madison, 1983)
- *Fluharty Preschool Speech and Language Screening Test* (Fluharty, 1978)
- *Articulation and Language Screening Test* (Rodgers, 1976)
- *The Stephens Oral Language Screening Test* (Stephens, 1977)
- *CELF-R Screening Test (Clinical Evaluation of Language Fundamentals—Revised)* (Semel, Wiig, & Secord, 1989)
- *Preschool Language Scale* (Zimmerman, Steiner, & Pond, 1979)
- *Joliet 3-Minute Speech and Language Screening Test* (Kinzler & Johnson, 1983)
- *Merrill Language Screening Test* (Mumm, Secord, & Dykstra, 1980)
- *Screening Test for Adolescent Language* (Prather, Breecher, Stafford, & Wallace, 1980)

When selecting an appropriate screening tool, consider variables such as the amount of time necessary for administration and the areas of language that are sampled. Many clinicians develop their own screening instrument. Several items in this resource (such as Forms 6–1, 6–2, 6–5, and 6–7) can be adapted for screening purposes.

ASSESSING LANGUAGE

Because language is so broad, a thorough evaluation must explore a wide spectrum of features and aspects of language. James (1993) identifies these specific areas of language to assess:

VI. Semantics

    A. Word meaning

        1. Concrete words referring to observable objects, actions, attributes
        2. Relational words referring to dimensions, time, space

    B. Sentence meaning

        1. Semantic rules and relations within simple sentences
        2. Abstract relational meanings within complex sentences
        3. Meaning relations among sentences

    C. Nonliteral meaning

        1. Idioms
        2. Metaphors
        3. Proverbs

II. Grammar

    A. Grammatical morphemes

        1. Noun forms (plurals, possessive, prepositions, articles)
        2. Verb forms (progressive, past, third person singular, auxiliary, and copula)
        3. Adjective forms (comparative, superlative)
        4. Adverb forms (comparative, superlative)

    B. Syntax

        1. Clause structures (intransitive, transitive, equative)
        2. Noun phrase constituent
        3. Verb phrase constituent
        4. Negatives and questions
        5. Complex sentences (compound and embedded)

III. Pragmatics

    A. Communicative intentions

        1. Requesting information/action
        2. Conveying information
        3. Expressing attitude/emotion
        4. Regulating social interactions

    B. Conversational abilities

        1. Turn-taking
        2. Topic maintenance
        3. Presupposition (i.e., taking the other person into consideration when communicating)
        4. Narrative skills

IV. Metalinguistics (awareness of language)

    A. Phonological awareness

        1. Segmenting words into phonemes

    B. Word awareness

        1. Segmenting sentences into words
        2. Separating a word from its referent

    C. Grammatical awareness

        1. Judging the acceptability of sentences
        2. Detecting ambiguity in sentences

    D. Pragmatic awareness

        1. Judging message comprehensibility and adequacy
        2. Judging the appropriateness of communicative interactions (pp. 185–228)

Table 6–1 provides a list of basic evaluative procedures that are appropriate for assessing many of these elements of language.

Form 6–1, "Assessment of Language Development," is a worksheet that is useful for informally assessing all areas of language during observation or structured tasks.

Table 6–1. Basic Procedures for the Assessment of Language

	Receptive Abilities	**Expressive Abilities**
Semantics	Case History Information Observation Informal Tasks Formal Tests	Case History Information Observation Language Scales Language Samples Formal Tests
Syntax	Case History Information Observation Informal Tasks Formal Tests	Case History Information Observation Language Scales Language Samples Formal Tests
Morphology	Case History Information Observation Informal Tasks Formal Tests*	Case History Information Observation Language Scales Language Samples Formal Tests
Phonology	Case History Information Observation Informal Tasks Audiologic Testing Formal Tests	Case History Information Observation Language Scales Language Samples Formal Tests
Pragmatics	Case History Information Observation Informal Tasks	Case History Information Observation Language Scales Language Samples Formal Tests

*There is a methodologic problem clinicians often face when testing bound morphemes receptively. Children typically respond in the same manner whether the test presents a free morpheme (e.g., big) or a free and bound morpheme together (e.g., biggest). This precludes the ability to determine whether or not the client understood the free morpheme alone (Shipley, 1981).

Form 6–1. Assessment of Language Development

Name: _____ Age: _____ Date: _____

Examiner: _____

Instructions: Mark a plus (+) or a check (✔) if the child *does* exhibit the behavior, a minus (−) or a (0) if the child *does not* exhibit the behavior, and an *s* if the child exhibits the behavior *sometimes*. This form can be used during informal observation and/or completed by a parent or knowledgeable caregiver. Because children develop at different rates, avoid using strict application of the age approximations. The time intervals are provided only as a general guideline for age appropriateness.

0–6 Months

_____ startle response to sound

_____ repeats the same sounds

_____ frequently coos, gurgles, and makes pleasure sounds

_____ uses a different cry to express different needs

_____ smiles when spoken to

_____ recognizes voices

_____ localizes sound by turning the head

_____ quieted by the human voice

_____ listens to speech

_____ uses the phonemes /b/, /p/, and /m/ in babbling

_____ imitates sounds

_____ uses sounds or gestures to indicate wants

_____ varies pitch and loudness

7–12 Months

_____ understands *no* and *hot*

_____ understands and responds to own name

_____ listens to and imitates more sounds

_____ recognizes words for common items (e.g. cup, shoe, juice)

(continued)

Sources: The information contained here was compiled from a variety of sources, including American Speech-Language-Hearing Association (1983); Boone & Plante (1993); Gard, Gilman, and Gorman (1980); Hegde (1995); Kunz and Finkel (1987); Lane and Molyneaux (1992); and Lenneberg (1969).

7–12 Months

_____ babbles using long and short groups of sounds

_____ uses a song-like intonation pattern when babbling

_____ uses a large variety of sounds in babbling

_____ imitates some adult speech sounds and intonation patterns

_____ uses speech sounds rather than only crying to get attention

_____ listens when spoken to

_____ uses sound approximations

_____ begins to change babbling to jargon

_____ uses speech intentionally for the first time

_____ production of one or more words

_____ uses nouns almost exclusively

_____ has an expressive vocabulary of 1 to 3 words

_____ understands simple commands

13–18 Months

_____ uses adult-like intonation patterns

_____ uses echolalia and jargon

_____ uses jargon to fill gaps in fluency

_____ omits some initial consonants and almost all final consonants

_____ produces mostly unintelligible speech

_____ follows simple commands

_____ has an expressive vocabulary of 3 to 20 or more words (mostly nouns)

_____ produces 2-word phrases

_____ combines gestures and vocalizations

_____ requests more of desired items

19–24 Months

_____ uses words more frequently than jargon

_____ has an expressive vocabulary of 50–100 or more words

_____ has a receptive vocabulary of 300 or more words

_____ starts to combine nouns and verbs

19–24 Months

_____ begins to use pronouns (*I* and *mine*)

_____ maintains unstable voice control

_____ uses appropriate intonation for questions

_____ is approximately 25–50% intelligible to strangers

_____ answers "what's that?" questions

_____ enjoys listening to stories

_____ knows 5 body parts

_____ accurately names a few familiar objects

_____ follows 2-part commands

2–3 Years

_____ speech is 50–75% intelligible

_____ understands *one* and *all*

_____ verbalizes toilet needs (before, during, or after act)

_____ requests items by name

_____ responds to some yes/no questions

_____ names everyday objects

_____ points to pictures in a book when named

_____ identifies several body parts

_____ follows simple commands and answers simple questions

_____ enjoys listening to short stories, songs, and rhymes

_____ asks 1- to 2-word questions

_____ uses 3- to 4-word phrases

_____ uses some prepositions, articles, present progressive verbs, regular plurals, contractions, irregular past tense forms, and negation *no* or *not*

_____ uses some regular past tense verbs, possessive morphemes, pronouns, and imperatives

_____ uses words that are general in context

_____ produces several forms of questions

_____ understands *why*, *who*, *whose*, and *how many*

(continued)

2–3 Years

_____ continues use of echolalia when difficulties in speech are encountered

_____ has a receptive vocabulary of 500–900 or more words

_____ has an expressive vocabulary of 50–250 or more words (rapid growth during this period)

_____ exhibits multiple grammatical errors

_____ understands most things said to him or her

_____ frequently exhibits repetitions—especially starters, "I," and first syllables

_____ speaks with a loud voice

_____ increases range of pitch

_____ uses vowels correctly

_____ consistently uses initial consonants (although some are misarticulated)

_____ frequently omits medial consonants

_____ frequently omits or substitutes final consonants

_____ uses approximately 27 phonemes

_____ uses auxiliary _is_ including the contracted form

3–4 Years

_____ understands object functions

_____ understands differences in meanings (stop-go, in-on, big-little)

_____ follows 2- and 3-part commands

_____ asks and answers simple questions (who, what, where, why)

_____ frequently asks questions and often demands detail in responses

_____ produces simple verbal analogies

_____ uses language to express emotion

_____ uses 4 to 5 words in sentences

_____ repeats 6- to 13-syllable sentences accurately

_____ identifies objects by name

_____ manipulates adults and peers

_____ may continue to use echolalia

_____ uses up to 6 words in a sentence

_____ uses nouns and verbs most frequently

(continued)

3–4 Years

_____ is conscious of past and future

_____ has a 1,200–2,000 or more word receptive vocabulary

_____ has a 800–1,500 or more word expressive vocabulary

_____ may repeat self often, exhibiting blocks, disturbed breathing, and facial grimaces during speech

_____ increases speech rate

_____ whispers

_____ masters 50% of consonants and blends

_____ speech is 80% intelligible

_____ sentence grammar improves although some errors still persist

_____ appropriately uses *is*, *are*, and *am* in sentences

_____ tells two events in chronological order

_____ engages in long conversations

_____ uses some contractions, irregular plurals, future tense verbs, and conjunctions

_____ consistently uses regular plurals, possessives, and simple past tense verbs

4 Years

_____ imitatively counts to 5

_____ understands concept of numbers up to 3

_____ continues understanding of spatial concepts

_____ recognizes 1 to 3 colors

_____ has a receptive vocabulary of 2,800 or more words

_____ counts to 10 by rote

_____ listens to short simple stories

_____ answers questions about function

_____ uses grammatically correct sentences

_____ has an expressive vocabulary of 900–2,000 or more words

_____ uses sentences of 4 to 8 words

_____ answers complex 2-part questions

(continued)

4 Years

_____ asks for word definitions

_____ speaks at a rate of approximately 186 words per minute

_____ reduces total number of repetitions

_____ enjoys rhythms, rhymes, and nonsense syllables

_____ produces consonants with 90% accuracy

_____ significantly reduces number of persistent sound omissions and substitutions

_____ frequently omits medial consonants

_____ speech is usually intelligible to strangers

_____ talks about experiences at school, at friends' homes, etc.

_____ accurately relays a long story

_____ pays attention to a story and answers simple questions about it

_____ uses some irregular plurals, possessive pronouns, future tense, reflexive pronouns, and comparative morphemes in sentences

5–6 Years

_____ names 6 basic colors and 3 basic shapes

_____ follows instructions given to a group

_____ follows 3-part commands

_____ asks *how* questions

_____ answers verbally to *hi* and *how are you?*

_____ uses past tense and future tense appropriately

_____ uses conjunctions

_____ has a receptive vocabulary of approximately 13,000 words

_____ names opposites

_____ sequentially names days of the week

_____ counts to 30 by rote

_____ continues to drastically increase vocabulary

_____ reduces sentence length to 4 to 6 words

_____ reverses sounds occasionally

_____ exchanges information and asks questions

(continued)

5–6 Years

_____ uses sentences with detail

_____ uses grammatically complete sentences

_____ accurately relays a story

_____ sings entire songs and recites nursery rhymes

_____ communicates easily with adults and other children

_____ uses appropriate grammar in most cases

6–7 Years

_____ names some letters, numbers, and currencies

_____ sequences numbers

_____ understands *left* and *right*

_____ uses increasingly more complex descriptions

_____ engages in conversations

_____ has a receptive vocabulary of approximately 20,000 words

_____ uses a sentence length of approximately 6 words

_____ understands most temporal concepts

_____ recites the alphabet

_____ counts to 100 by rote

_____ uses most morphologic markers appropriately

_____ uses passive voice appropriately

OBSERVATION AND INFORMAL ASSESSMENT

Observation is an important clinical technique. It allows you, in a relatively informal and nonthreatening manner, to understand a client better and to identify specific language deficits. Wolery (1989) believes that observation is useful for assessment purposes because it allows the clinician to:

☐ Assess difficult-to-test behaviors;

☐ Validate information collected from other situations (e.g., formal testing);

☐ Extend assessment activities to other settings, circumstances, and tasks;

☐ Identify functional relationships between stimuli in the environment and the child's behavior;

☐ Monitor the effects of clinical interventions on an ongoing basis.

Observations can be made with or without direct interaction with the client. For example, you can observe from another room via a one-way mirror, in the same room but separated from the client, or in the same room seated closely to the client. There is no observation method that is inherently more effective or useful than the others. The method you use will depend on the purposes of your observation, the facilities available, and whether you are able to collect the information needed without having your presence adversely affect the child's behavior. Owens (1995) identified several features of language to be observed with children. They are:

☐ *Form of language.* Does the child use single words, phrases, or sentences primarily? Are the sentences of the subject-verb-object form exclusively? Are there mature negatives, interrogatives, and passive sentences? Does the child elaborate the noun or verb phrase? Is there evidence of embedding and conjoining?

☐ *Understanding of semantic intent.* Does the child respond appropriately to the various question forms (what, where, who, when, why, how)? Does the child confuse words from different semantic classes?

☐ *Language use.* Does the child display a range of illocutionary functions such as asking for information, help, and objects, replying, making statements, providing information? Does the child take conversational turns? Does the child introduce topics and maintain them through several turns? Does the child signal the status of the communication and make repairs?

☐ *Rate of speaking.* Is the rate inordinately slow or fast? Are there noticeable or lengthy pauses between the caregiver's and the child's turn? Are there noticeable or lengthy pauses between the child's adjacent utterances? Does the child use fillers frequently or pause before producing certain words? Are there frequent word substitutions?

☐ *Sequencing.* Does the child relate events in a sequential fashion based on the order of occurrence? Can the child discuss the recent past or recount stories? (p. 85)

Observations provide a general estimate of a child's language skills in comparison to normal expectations for language acquisition. Table 6–2 is one overview of the major milestones of language development. For a more detailed listing, see "Speech, Language, and Motor

Development" on pages 32–40. Also see Brown (1973) for a description of the stages of normal morphologic development.

Table 6–2. Major Milestones of Language Acquisition in Children

Age Range	Typical Language Behaviors
0–1 mos.	Startle response to sound; quieted by human voice.
2–3 mos.	Cooing; production of some vowel sounds; response to speech; babbling.
4–6 mos.	Babbling strings of syllables; imitation of sounds; variations in pitch and loudness.
7–9 mos.	Comprehension of some words and simple requests; increased imitation of speech sounds; may say or imitate "mama" or "dada."
10–12 mos.	Understanding of "No"; response to requests; response to own name; production of one or more words.
13–15 mos.	Production of 5–10 words, mostly nouns; appropriate pointing responses.
16–18 mos.	Following simple directions; production of two-word phrases; production of *I* and *mine*.
2.0–2.6 yrs.	Response to some yes/no questions; naming of everyday objects; production of phrases and incomplete sentences; production of the present progressive, prepositions, regular plural, and negation "no" or "not."
3.0–3.6 yrs.	Production of 3–4 word sentences; production of the possessive morpheme, several forms of questions, negatives "can't" and "don't"; comprehension of "why," "who," "whose," and "how many"; and initial productions of most grammatical morphemes.
3.6–5.0 yrs.	Greater mastery of articles, different tense forms, copula, auxiliary, third person singular, and other grammatical morphemes; production of grammatically complete sentences.

Source: From M. N. Hegde, *Introduction to Communicative Disorders* (2nd ed., p. 170). Austin, TX: PRO-ED. Copyright © 1995 and used by permission.

Informal tasks are sometimes used in conjunction with observation. These tasks allow you to assess specific features of language and identify specific abilities and deficits. Informal tasks can be receptively or expressively based. The following are examples of activities some clinicians use to sample language skills informally. Ask the child to:

☐ Stack blocks (to observe motor skills or the ability to follow directions).

☐ Follow oral commands. For example, ask the child to *point to the window* or *pick up the crayon.*

☐ Count, recite the alphabet, or perform another serial task.

☐ Point to pictures or items in the environment (to informally assess receptive vocabulary).

☐ Point to more than one of a named item (to sample basic morphologic comprehension). For example, *point to the pencils* (versus *pencil*).

☐ Tell you what one should say when someone does something nice for you (to sample pragmatic use).

☐ Put an object (e.g., a block) *over, under,* and *beside* the table (to sample basic prepositional understanding).

Form 6–2, the "Checklist for an Informal Assessment of Language," is provided to help you identify specific language behaviors a client exhibits during informal activities. You can use the worksheet during observation and/or during informal tasks. You can also ask a parent, caregiver, teacher, or other professional to complete the form in a nonclinical environment.

Form 6–2. Checklist for an Informal Assessment of Language

Name: _____ Age:_____ Date:_____

Examiner: _____

Instructions: Mark a plus (+) or a check (✔) if the child does exhibit the behavior, a minus (−) or a zero (0) if the child does not exhibit the behavior, and an *s* if the child exhibits the behavior *sometimes*. Make comments about what the child does on the right-hand side of the form. If a specific behavior is not assessed, leave the line blank. This form can be used during informal observation and/or completed by a parent or knowledgeable caregiver.

Comments

_____   the child takes turns during communication_____

   _____

_____   the child enjoys playing with other children   _____

   _____

_____   the child enjoys playing with his or her parents _____

   _____

_____   the child enjoys playing with his or her siblings _____

   _____

_____   the child usually plays alone   _____

   _____

_____   the child plays silently _____

   _____

_____   the child talks during play activities_____

   _____

_____   the child acts out common activities (e.g., plays house, plays store) _____

   _____

_____   the child uses play objects that are similar (in size, looks, etc.) to the true objects (e.g., a saucepan

   for a drum)   _____

   _____

(continued)

Form 6–2 *(continued)*

Comments

_____ the child uses play objects in a realistic manner (e.g., uses a toy dump truck in the way intended)

_____ the child looks at picture books page-by-page from front to back _____

_____ the child explores a variety of toys and does not repeatedly use the same item(s) _____

_____ the child uses coordinated motor movements _____

_____ the child uses complete sentences during play_____

_____ the child asks questions during play_____

_____ the child answers questions during play _____

_____ the child responds to requests _____

_____ the child primarily uses gestures to communicate _____

_____ the child uses gestures and speech to communicate_____

_____ the child looks at the listener when speaking _____

_____ the child uses appropriate vocabulary words _____

_____ the child relates real life experiences during conversation _____

_____ the child usually communicates in phrases of greater than 2 words _____

Comments

_____ the child usually communicates in phrases of greater than 3 words _____

_____

_____ the child usually communicates in phrases of greater than 4 words _____

_____

_____ the child initiates conversations or activities _____

_____

_____ the child dominates conversations _____

_____

_____ the child is able to follow conversational shifts _____

_____

_____ the child uses simple sentences _____

_____

_____ the child uses complex sentences _____

_____

_____ the child uses the correct word order when speaking _____

_____

_____ the child uses plurals (e.g, boys, animals) _____

_____

_____ the child uses more than one verb tense (e.g., present, past, future) _____

_____

_____ the child uses pronouns (e.g., he, she, I) _____

_____

_____ the child uses articles (e.g., the, an, a _____)

_____

_____ the child uses the verbs *is* and *are* _____

_____

_____ the child uses prepositions (e.g., on, in, under, beside) _____

_____

(continued)

Form 6–2 *(continued)*

Comments

_____ the child varies his or her communication depending on the listener _____

_____

_____ the child has good reading skills _____

_____

_____ the child has good writing skills _____

_____

_____ the child is able to follow the story line of a TV show _____

_____

How does the child's language differ from that of other children the same age?

How does the child's language differ from that of an adult?

FORMAL LANGUAGE TESTING

There are literally hundreds of formal language tests available for the assessment of language disorders. Some commonly used formal tests are listed in Table 6–3. The list in Table 6–3 is not all-inclusive. In fact, there are more than 200 different formal tests available for the assessment of language. For more information about formal language tests, consult:

- Bailey and Wolery (1989, pp. 359–365). They list 31 tests by the language area and age range assessed, format, and unique aspects of the test.
- Emerick and Haynes (1986, pp. 120–121). They outline 37 tests according to age range assessed.
- Haynes et al. (1992, pp. 388–391). These authors list 77 tests for assessing syntax by age ranges.
- Hutchinson, Hanson, and Mecham (1979, pp. 355–361). This resource includes an outline of 87 tests summarized by age level, administration time, standardization, area of emphasis, and the year the test was reviewed in the *Mental Measurements Yearbook*.
- James (1993, pp. 202–203). These authors summarize 22 tests by the type of scores available, age ranges, and whether the test samples language production, comprehension, or pragmatics.
- Lahey (1988, pp. 166–168). She summarizes 54 tests according to the language area assessed and whether the tests provide equivalent or standard scores.
- Lund and Duchan (1993, p. 339). These authors list 34 tests by general purpose, language areas emphasized, and whether the tests are receptively or expressively based.
- Nation and Aram (1991, pp. 317–347). They list 165 speech and language tests with information categorized into four categories: physical processing segments, behavioral correlates, speech product, and language product.
- Nicolosi, Harryman, and Krescheck (1996, pp. 338–350). This resource includes 114 tests, including the age range and a brief description of each test.
- Owens (1995, pp. 88–89). He summarizes 27 tests according to areas of language assessed, whether the tests are for screening or diagnosis, and whether they are receptively or expressively based. He also presents a brief description of 62 language tests for children with limited English proficiency (LEP) and different dialects and includes the address and cost of the instruments (pp. A–15—A–29).
- Owens, Haney, Giesow, Dooley, and Kelly (1983, pp. 101–111). They outline 17 tests by the grammatical or "other" features the tests sample.

One difficulty with selecting the best language test to use for diagnostic evaluation is that many of them are useful in different situations. There is no one test or even a set of tests that is right for all children or all clinicians (Lahey, 1988). You must be thoughtful when selecting appropriate testing instruments. Become familiar with various tests' uses, strengths, and weaknesses. See Appendix B at the end of the book for guidelines for evaluating assessment tests.

Table 6–3. Several Formal Tests for the Assessment of Language

Test	Author	Age/Grade	Receptive/ Expressive	Areas of Assessment
Assessment of Children's Language Comprehension (ACLC)	Foster, Giddan, & Stark (1983)	3:0–6:11	Receptive	Comprehension of words and phrases with 2–4 elements
Bankson Language Test	Bankson (1990)	4:1–8:0	Expressive	Includes semantic, syntactic, and morphologic areas
Boehm Test of Basic Concepts	Boehm (1970)	K–2nd	Receptive	Basic concepts, primarily semantic
Carrow Elicited Language Inventory (CELI)	Carrow (1974)	3:0–7:11	Expressive	Syntax through elicited imitation
Clinical Evaluation of Language Fundamentals— Revised (CELF-R)	Semel-Mintz & Wiig (1982)	K–12th	Both	Semantics, syntax, phonology, and memory
Compton Speech and Language Screening Evaluation	Compton (1978)	3:0–6:0	Both	Articulation, semantics, grammar, voice
Evaluating Communicative Competence	Simon (1986)	9:0–17:0	Both	Pragmatics
Expressive One-Word Picture Vocabulary Test	Gardner (1979)	2:0–11:11	Expressive	Vocabulary
Expressive One-Word Picture Vocabulary Test—Upper Extension	Gardner (1983)	12:0–15:0	Expressive	Vocabulary
Illinois Test of Psycholinguistic Abilities (ITPA)	Kirk, McCarthy, & Kirk (1968)	2:0–10:11	Both	Presumed psycholinguistic abilities associated with language development; some vocabulary and grammar
Peabody Picture Vocabulary Test— Revised (PPVT-R)	Dunn & Dunn (1981)	2:3–18:5	Receptive	Vocabulary

(continued)

Table 6–3. *(continued)*

Test	Author	Age/Grade	Receptive/ Expressive	Areas of Assessment
Receptive-Expressive Emergent Language Scale	Bzoch & League (1991)	0:1–3:0	Both	Interview scale for language development
Receptive One-Word Picture Vocabulary Test	Gardner (1985)	2:0–11:11	Receptive	Vocabulary
Test for Auditory Comprehension of Language-Revised (TACL-R)	Carrow-Woolfolk (1985)	3:0–9:11	Receptive	Word classes, grammatical morphemes, elaborated sentences (syntax)
Test of Adolescent Language (TOAL-2)	Hammill, Brown, Larsen, & Weiderholt (1987)	11:0–18:5	Both	Vocabulary grammar, reading, writing
Test for Examining Expressive Morphology (TEEM)	Shipley, Stone, & Sue (1983)	3:0–8:0	Expressive	Morphology
Test of Language Development-2 Intermediate (TOLD)	Newcomer & Hammill (1988a)	8:6–12:11	Both	Vocabulary and some aspects of grammar
Test of Language Development-2 Primary (TOLD-P)	Newcomer & Hammill (1988b)	4:0–8:11	Both	Vocabulary, articulation, and grammar

LANGUAGE SAMPLING

Language sampling is a vital part of a complete evaluation of language. Specific procedures for collecting a language sample are described in Chapter 4. There are several aspects of collecting a language sample that are especially important for assessing language disorders:

☐ Collect a representative sample, with a minimum of 50–100 utterances. Since language is so multifaceted, it may be necessary to sample your client's language for 30 minutes or even more (Bloom & Lahey, 1978; Miller, 1981).

☐ Vary the contexts and activities used to elicit the sample to assess different language features.

☐ If possible, ask others to interact with the client during the sample, such as another clinician, a peer, a parent or caregiver, or a teacher. Children commonly vary their language use depending on the audience.

☐ Collect multiple samples.

☐ Tape record or video tape (if possible) the sample for later analysis.

The following guidelines are adapted from Bloom and Lahey (1978), Hubbell (1988), Owens (1995), and Retherford (1993). These can be useful when transcribing the language sample:

☐ Transcribe the entire sample.

☐ Indicate the speaker for all utterances. For example, mark A for adult (or P for partner) and C for client or child. Create your own abbreviations as needed.

☐ Use phonetic symbols only to transcribe unintelligible or partially intelligible utterances. A dash (—) can also be used to indicate each unintelligible word. For example, "I want — —" indicates a four-word utterance with two unintelligible words.

☐ Capitalize only proper nouns and the pronoun *I*.

☐ Keep punctuation to a minimum.

☐ Indicate utterance endings with a slash (/).

☐ Number the client's utterances as you proceed.

☐ Transcribe utterances consecutively from the tape. The first few utterances may be omitted since this could be considered a "warming up" period.

Form 6–3 is a worksheet for recording the language sample.

Form 6–3. Worksheet for Recording a Language Sample

Name: _____ Age:_____ Date:_____

Examiner: _____

Instructions: List the utterance number in the first column and the speaker (C = child; A = adult) in the second column. The third column is for recording each utterance, and the fourth column is for recording the context of the utterance.

#	C/A	Utterance	Context
____	____	_____	_____
____	____	_____	_____
____	____	_____	_____
____	____	_____	_____
____	____	_____	_____
____	____	_____	_____
____	____	_____	_____
____	____	_____	_____
____	____	_____	_____
____	____	_____	_____
____	____	_____	_____
____	____	_____	_____
____	____	_____	_____
____	____	_____	_____
____	____	_____	_____
____	____	_____	_____
____	____	_____	_____
____	____	_____	_____
____	____	_____	_____
____	____	_____	_____
____	____	_____	_____
____	____	_____	_____
____	____	_____	_____

(continued)

Form 6–3 *(continued)*

#	C/A	Utterance	Context
___	___	_____	_____
___	___	_____	_____
___	___	_____	_____
___	___	_____	_____
___	___	_____	_____
___	___	_____	_____
___	___	_____	_____
___	___	_____	_____
___	___	_____	_____
___	___	_____	_____
___	___	_____	_____
___	___	_____	_____
___	___	_____	_____
___	___	_____	_____
___	___	_____	_____
___	___	_____	_____
___	___	_____	_____
___	___	_____	_____
___	___	_____	_____
___	___	_____	_____
___	___	_____	_____
___	___	_____	_____
___	___	_____	_____
___	___	_____	_____
___	___	_____	_____
___	___	_____	_____

DETERMINING THE MEAN LENGTH OF UTTERANCE

The mean length of utterance (MLU) is the average number of morphemes (or words, as will be described later) that a client produces in an utterance. MLU provides important information about language development, and it is one indicator of a language delay or disorder. Generally, a normal child's chronological age (up to age 5) will correspond closely to his or her MLU (Brown, 1973). For example, a normally developing 4-year, 3-month-old child will often exhibit an MLU of approximately 4.3 (plus or minus a few tenths). This method of interpretation is very general and must, of course, be used with caution when diagnosing or ruling out language disorders. Remember, children develop language at varying rates.

Roger Brown's (1973) classic study of three young children—Adam, Eve, and Sarah—provided the foundation for much of our current understanding of the relationship between mean length of utterance and language development. Brown's developmental stages are:

Stage	Age (years)	MLU
1.	1 to 2:2	1.0–2.0
II.	2:3 to 2:6	2.0–2.5
III.	2:7 to 2:10	2.5–3.0
IV.	2:11 to 3:4	3.0–3.75
V.	3:5 to 3:10	3.75–4.5
	3:11+	4.5+

Using a larger number of subjects, Miller and Chapman (1981) conducted a study in which MLUs from conversational speech samples were compared with children's chronological ages. Their findings are presented in Table 6-4. The table outlines predicted MLUs and standard deviations (SDs) for children 18 months through 5 years of age. The sample group in Miller and Chapman's study consisted of 123 middle to upperclass midwestern children in Madison, Wisconsin. As with any normative data, use caution when applying the information to children who are dissimilar to the population studied.

Table 6–4. Developmental Norms for Mean Length of Utterance (SD is standard deviation.)

Age (yr.–mo.)	Predicted MLU	Predicted MLU, 1 SD (middle 68%)	Predicted MLU, 2 SDs (middle 95%)
1–6	1.31	1.99 — 1.64	1.66 — 1.96
1–9	1.62	1.23 — 2.01	1.85 — 2.39
2–0	1.92	1.47 — 2.37	1.02 — 2 82
2–3	2.23	1.72 — 2.74	1.21 — 3.25
2–6	2.54	1.97 — 3.11	1.40 — 3.68
2–9	2.85	2.22 — 3.48	1.58 — 4.12
3–0	3.16	2.47 — 3.85	1.77 — 4.55
3–3	3.47	2.71 — 4.23	1.96 — 4.98
3–6	3.78	2.96 — 4.60	2.15 — 5.41
3–9	4.09	3.21 — 4.97	2.33 — 5.85
4–0	4.40	3.46 — 5.34	2.52 — 6.28
4–3	4.71	3.71 — 5.71	2.71 — 6.71
4–6	5.02	3.96 — 6.08	2.90 — 7.15
4–9	5.32	4.20 — 6.45	3.07 — 7.57
5–0	5.63	4.44 — 6.82	3.26 — 8.00

Source: From J. F. Miller and R. Chapman (1981). "The Relation Between Age and Mean Length of Utterance in Morphemes," *Journal of Speech and Hearing Research, 24,* 154–161. Adapted by permission of the American Speech-Language-Hearing Association.

Once the language sample is transcribed, you are ready to calculate your client's MLU. The first step is counting the morphemes in each utterance. Lund and Duchan (1993) outline specific do's and don'ts for computing mean length of utterance:[3]

Exclude from your count:

11. *Imitations* which immediately follow the model utterance and which give the impression that the child would not have said the utterance spontaneously.

12. *Elliptical answers* to questions which give the impression that the utterance would have been more complete if there had been no eliciting question (e.g., "Do you want this?" "Yes." "What do you have?" "*My dolls*").

13. *Partial utterances* which are interrupted by outside events or shifts in the child's focus (e.g., "That's my—oops").

14. *Unintelligible utterances* that contain unintelligible segments. If a major portion of a child's sample is unintelligible, a syllable count by utterance can be substituted for morpheme count.

15. *Rote passages* such as nursery rhymes, songs, or prose passages which have been memorized and which may not be fully processed linguistically by the child.

16. *False starts and reformulations* within utterances which may either be self-repetitions or changes in the original formulation (e.g., "I have one [just like] almost like that"; "[We] we can't").

17. *Noises* unless they are integrated into meaningful verbal material such as "He went xx."

18. *Discourse markers* such as *um, oh, you know* not integrated into the meaning of the utterance (e.g., "[Well] it was [you know] [like] a party or something").

19. *Identical utterances* that the child says anywhere in the sample. Only one occurrence of each utterance is counted. If there is even a minor change, however, the second utterance is also counted.

10. *Counting or other sequences of enumeration* (e.g., "blue, green, yellow, red, purple").

11. *Single words or phrases* such as "hi," "thank you," "here," "know what?"

Count as one morpheme:

11. Uninflected lexical morphemes (e.g., *run, fall*) and grammatical morphemes that are whole words (articles, auxiliary verbs, prepositions).

12. Contractions when individual segments do not occur elsewhere in the sample apart from the contraction. If either of the constituent parts of the contraction are found elsewhere, the contraction is counted as two rather than one morpheme (e.g., *I'll, it's, can't*).

13. Catentatives such as *wanna, gonna, hafta* and the infinitive models that have the same meanings (e.g., *going to* go). This eliminates the problem of judging a

---

[3]From N. Lund and J. Duchan, *Assessing Children's Language in Naturalistic Contexts*, 3rd ed., © 1993, pp. 205–206. Adapted by permission of Prentice-Hall, Englewood Cliffs, NJ.

morpheme count on the basis of the child's pronunciation. Thus *am gonna* is counted as two morphemes.

14. Phrases, compound words, diminutives, reduplicated words which occur as inseparable linguistic units for the child or represent single items (e.g., *oh boy*; *all right*; *once upon a time*; *a lot of*; *let's*; *big wheel*; *horsie*).

15. Irregular past tense. The convention is to count these as single morphemes because children's first meanings for them seem to be distinct from the present tense counterparts (e.g., *did, was*).

16. Plurals which do not occur in singular form (e.g., *pants*; *clothes*), including plural pronouns (*us*; *them*).

17. Gerunds and participles that are not part of the verb phrase (*Swimming* is fun; He was *tired*; That is the *cooking* place).

Count as more than one morpheme:

11. Inflected forms: regular and irregular plural nouns; possessive nouns; third person singular verb; present participle and past participle when part of the verb phrase; regular past tense verb; reflexive pronoun; comparative and superlative adverbs and adjectives.

12. Contractions when one or both of the individual segments occur separately anywhere in the child's sample (e.g., *It's* if *it* or *is* occurs elsewhere).

After you have counted all the morphemes, you are ready to calculate the MLU. The traditional method of calculating MLU is dividing the number of morphemes by the number of utterances. For example:

$$\frac{150 \text{ morphemes}}{50 \text{ utterances}} = 3.0 \text{ MLU}$$

Many clinicians also calculate the MLU for words by dividing the number of words by the number of utterances. This calculation does *not* reflect the use of bound morphemes (e.g., *-ing, -ed, -s*, etc.); therefore, the MLU for words will always be equal to or smaller than the MLU for morphemes. For example, the same 100-word sample might have:

$$\frac{100 \text{ words}}{50 \text{ utterances}} = 2.0 \text{ MLU-words}$$

$$\frac{120 \text{ morphemes}}{50 \text{ utterances}} = 2.4 \text{ MLU-morphemes}$$

MLU is a gross but reasonably accurate index of grammatical development up to four-to-five morphemes (Brown 1973; James, 1993). It is considered gross because the MLU is a general measure which tells us nothing about specific forms or structures used. However, the use of both free and bound morphemes is needed for utterance lengths to increase.

ASSESSMENT OF PRAGMATIC SKILLS

Pragmatics is the study of the use of language in communicative interactions. Pragmatic behaviors are situationally and environmentally specific; therefore, it is helpful to assess pragmatic skills in a variety of situations. Form 6–4, "Assessment of Pragmatic Skills," allows you to assess 15 pragmatic behaviors in a semi-structured manner. Several suggestions are provided for each behavior for eliciting pragmatic responses.

Form 6–4. Assessment of Pragmatic Skills

Name: _____ Age:_____ Date:_____

Examiner: _____

Instructions: Use activities such as those suggested in the right-hand column to elicit the desired pragmatic behaviors. Mark a plus (+) or a check (✔) if the response is correct or appropriate and a minus (−) or a zero (0) if the response is incorrect, not present, or inappropriate.

Pragmatic Behavior:	*Sample Activities:*
_____ respond to greetings	Observe the client's response when you say, "Hi! How are you?"
	Put your hand out to shake hands.
_____ make requests	Ask the client to draw a circle but don't immediately provide a pencil.
	Ask "What would you say to your mom if you were in the grocery store and wanted a candy bar?"
_____ describe events	Ask the client what he or she did this morning.
	Ask the client to tell you about a holiday or a special occasion.
_____ take turns	Ask the client to alternately count or recite the alphabet with you (e.g., you say *a*, client says *b*, you say *c*, client says *d*, etc.).
	Take turns telling 1–2 lines of *The Three Bears* or another children's story.
_____ follow commands	Ask the client to turn his or her paper over and draw a happy face or a square.
	Say to the client, "Touch your ears, then clap your hands twice."
_____ make eye contact	Consider whether the client has maintained normal eye contact during other parts of this assessment.
	Ask the client to tell you his or her address and/or phone number.
_____ repeat	Ask the client to repeat the following sentences:
	Michael is 7 years old.
	The oven door was open.
	She got a new book for her birthday.
_____ attend to tasks	Consider how the client has attended to this assessment.
	Ask the client to describe a picture you provide.

Pragmatic Behavior:

Sample Activities:

_____ maintain topic

Ask the client to tell you about a recent movie or TV show he or she has watched.

Ask the client to describe a hotdog.

_____ role-play

Ask the client to be the "teacher" for a while and give you things to complete.

Pretend you are in a fast-food restaurant. Tell the client to be the cashier while you pretend to be the customer.

_____ sequence actions

Ask the client to describe the steps involved in making the bed, buying groceries, or writing a letter.

Ask the client to describe how to make a hamburger or salad, or prepare breakfast.

_____ define words

Ask the client to define words such as:

    scissors
    kitchen
    computer

_____ categorize

Ask the client if the following words are days or months:

    Sunday
    June
    April
    Wednesday

Ask the client to name several farm animals, foods, or sports.

_____ understand object functions

Ask the client to show you how to use scissors.

Ask what a ruler is used for.

_____ initiate activity or dialogue

Place an odd-looking object on the table and see if the client asks what it is.

Observe the client with his or her parents, teacher, or with other children.

ASSESSMENT OF SEMANTIC SKILLS

Semantics is the study of language meaning, which can be expressed verbally, vocally, and/or gesturally. Meaning is complex and strongly influenced by context. Word definitions, syntactic structures, environmental situations, speaker relationships, pragmatic behaviors, and suprsegmental aspects of language intertwine to give language its meaning. Imagine greeting a friend by saying *starch* instead of *hi*. Even though your friend knows what the word starch means, it would have no meaning in such a social context.

One simple method for semantic analysis is described in the section entitled "Determining the Type-token Ratio." The TTR analysis provides information about vocabulary skills and allows you to identify the variety of word types your client uses. A more in-depth analysis involves assessing utterances by semantic categories. Based on the language sample, the clinician looks for examples of each semantic category from the child's utterances. Table 6–5 can be used as a basis for evaluating semantic relations.

Table 6–5. Common Semantic Relations (N indicates noun; V indicates verb)

Relation	Example	Structure
Nomination	That ball	Demonstrative + N
Nonexistence	No ball	No (all gone) + N
Agent-object	Roll ball	V + N
Action-agent	Baby cry	N + V
Recurrence	More cookie	More (another) + N
Action + locative	Jump [on] chair	V + N
	Roll here	V + Locative
Entity + locative	Ball [in] chair	N + N
	Mommy here	N + Locative
Possessor-possession	Baby ball	N + N
Agent-object	Baby [roll] ball	N + N
Entity-attributive	Pretty ball	Attribute + N
	Ball pretty	N + Attribute
Notice	Hi ball	Hi + N
Instrumental	Cut [with] knife	V + N
Action-indirect object	Give [to] doggie	V + N
Conjunction	Coat hat	N + N

Source: Reprinted with permission of Macmillan Publishing Company from *An Introduction to Children With Language Disorders* (2nd ed.), by Vicki Reed. Copyright © 1994 by Macmillan Publishing Company. (p. 65)

Determining The Type-token Ratio

The type-token ratio (TTR) is an easy-to-calculate measure of functional vocabulary skills. The ratio reflects the diversity of words used by the client during the language sample. Templin (1957) reported that normally developing children between the ages of 3 and 8 years have TTRs of .45–.50. A substandard TTR is one indicator of an expressive language delay or disorder. Remember, though, you must avoid using this kind of normative data as a single or primary method for establishing a diagnosis.

After you have transcribed the language sample, number every new word produced by the child. The last number you write is the number of different words produced. To calculate the TTR, divide the number of different words by the total number of words in the sample. For example:

$$\frac{100 \text{ different words}}{200 \text{ total words}} = .50 \text{ TTR}$$

Retherford (1993) presents a modification of the TTR. Rather than count all the different words, count the different *types* of words used in the sample. She uses eight different word types: nouns, verbs, adjectives, adverbs, prepositions, pronouns, conjunctions, afffirmatives (*yeah, okay,* etc.) and negatives (*no, not,* etc.), articles, and wh- words (*who, where,* etc.). Calculations are made by dividing the number of each different type of word by the total number of words in the sample. This method allows you to evaluate the diversity of word types used by your client. Form 6–5, "Type-token Ratio for Assessment of Semantic Skills," is a worksheet you can use to itemize word-type frequencies for the TTR calculation. Under the appropriate column, record first-time productions of each word noted during the language sample. Each time your client uses a word already recorded, tally the repeated production next to the original entry. For example:

go   (1 production of this word)
in   ✔   (2 productions)
me ✔✔✔   (4 productions)
no ✔✔✔✔✔✔   (7 productions)

Form 6–5. Type-token Ratio for the Analysis of Semantic Skills[1]

Name: _____ Age: _____ Date: _____

Examiner: _____

Instructions: Under the appropriate word-type column, record first-time utterances of every word. Repeated productions of the same word are marked with a tally next to the original entry. Count total productions of every different word and total productions of every different word type and enter in the summary section.

Nouns	Verbs	Adjectives	Adverbs	Prepositions

(continued)

---

[1]Excluding the identifying information and instructions sections, this form is from K. Retherford (1993), *Guide to Analysis of Language Transcripts* (2nd ed., pp. 80–81). Eau Claire, WI: Thinking Publications. Used by permission.

Form 6–5 *(continued)*

Pronouns	Conjunctions	Negative/ Affirmative	Articles	Wh- Words

Summary

Total Number of Different: _____   Total Number of:

Nouns _____   Nouns _____

Verbs _____   Verbs _____

Adjectives _____   Adjectives _____

Adverbs _____   Adverbs _____

Prepositions _____   Prepositions _____

Pronouns _____   Pronouns _____

Conjunctions _____   Conjunctions _____

Negative/Affirmative _____   Negative/Affirmative _____

Articles _____   Articles _____

Wh- Words _____   Wh- Words _____

Total Number of Different Words _____   **Total Number of Words** _____

$$\frac{\text{Total Number of Different Words}}{\text{Total Number of Words}} = \text{_____} = \text{Type token Ratio (TTR)}$$

ASSESSMENT OF SYNTACTIC SKILLS

Syntax refers to sentence structure. Our English language is based on many syntactic structures, making syntax a difficultt area to assess. Wiig and Semel (1984) described a general developmental sequence of syntactic forms. Their sequence is presented in Table 6–6.

Table 6–6. Developmental Stages in Early Syntactic Acquisition

Stage	Developmental Features	MLU
I	*Semantic roles and syntactic relations*: characterized by thematic relationships among multiple single words and by true word combinations (agent + action, action + object, agent + object, action +locative, entity + locative, possessor + possession, entity + attribute, demonstrative + entity)	1.0–2.0
II	*Modulated relations*: characterized by the emerging use of grammatical morphemes (present progressive, plural –s, in)	2.0–2.5
III	*Modalities of simple sentences*: characterized by the emergence of simple clauses and further acquisition of grammatical morphemes (possessive, on)	2.4–3.25
IV	*Advanced sentence modalities (embedding)*: characterized by multiple clause-utterances formed with connectives (e.g., *and*), or through complementation (e.g., "I wanna [want to] . . .") or relativization (e.g., *that*)	3.25–3.75
V	*Categorization (coordination)*: characterized by further differentiation of words within word classes (mass/count noun, transitive/intransitive, verbs, pronouns, prepositions) and acquisition of grammatical morphemes (articles, irregular past, regular past, contractile copula "be," regular third person singular)	3.75–4.0+
Vl (V+)	*Complex structures*: characterized by further acquisition of grammatical morphemes (contractible auxiliary "be," uncontractible copula "be," irregular third person singular, uncontractible auxiliary "be"), complex structures and sentence transformations, and ability to deal with structural ambiguities	4.0+

Source: Reprinted with permission from Merrill, an imprint of Macmillan Publishing Company from *Language Assessment and Intervention for the Learning Disabled*, Second Edition by Elisabeth Hemmersmith Wing and Eleanor Semel. Copyright © 1984, 1980 by Bell & Howell Company. (p. 297)

The most thorough and valid method of assessing syntactic development is through careful analysis of the language sample. Look specifically for syntactic structures at the phrase, clause, and sentence levels. The basic phrase structures described by Lund and Duchan (1988) include:

Noun phrases:

- Modifier + noun or pronoun

  Initiator + noun (only boys)
  Determiner + noun (the boy)
  Ordinal + noun (third boy)
  Quantifier + noun (two boys)
  Adjective + noun (big boy)
  Combina,tions of above (only the two big boys)

- Post-noun modifiers

  Prepositional phrases (the girl *in front* or a tree *in the park*)
  Relative clauses including a verb (*the girl who won the race* or the store *where we bought it*)
  Combination of above (*the girl in front who won the race*)

- Modifier + noun + post-noun modifiers

  Combinations (*only the girl who won the race*)

Examples of the elements of noun phrases are presented in more detail in Table 6–7.

To assess verb phrases adequately you must have an understanding of verbs and their functions. The following definitions may be helpful:

- **Lexical verbs.** These verbs add content to the utterance by indicating action or state (*she studies*; *he feels*).

  Transitive verbs. Verbs that need an object, person, or idea to be complete (*she broke it*; *he likes her*).

  Intransitive verbs. Verbs that do not need an object (*she fell*; *they are running*).

  Equative verbs. Copula verbs + noun, adjective, or adverb (*he is six*; *she was fast*).

- **Copula verbs.** "To be" verbs used to link the subject with a predicate, noun, adjective, or adverb (*he is a teacher*; *she was angry*).

- **Auxiliary verbs.** "To be," "have," or modal verbs that precede another verb (*he is talking*; *they have been shopping*).

- **Modal verbs.** Verbs that express attitudes or intentions that occur with lexical verbs (i.e., *can, may, shall, should, would, could, might,* and *must*).

- **Perfect (or perplexive) tense.** These are forms of "have" verbs used to convey action that has been or will be completed by a certain time.

Different elements of verb phrases are presented in Table 6–8.

Table 6–7. Elements of the Noun Phrase

Initiator	+	Determiner	+	Adjective	+	Noun	+	Post-noun Modifier
Only, a few of, just, at least, less than, nearly, especially, partially, even merely, almost		**Quantifier:** All both, half, no, one-tenth, some, any, either, each, every, twice, triple **Article:** The, a, an **Possessive:** My, your, his, her, its, our, your, their **Demonstrative:** This, that, these, those **Numerical Term:** One, two, thirty, one thousand		**Possessive: Nouns:** Mommy's children's **Ordinal:** First, next, next to last, last, final, second **Adjective:** Blue, big, little, fat, old, fast, circular, challenging **Descriptor:** *Shopping* (center), *baseball* (game), *hot dog* (stand)		**Pronoun:** I, you, he, she, it, we, you, they, mine, yours, his, hers, its, ours, theirs **Noun:** Boys, dog, feet, sheet, men and women, city of New York, Port of Chicago, leap of faith, matter of conscience		**Prepositional Phrase:** On the car, in the box, in the gray flannel suit **Adjectival:** Next door, pictured by Renoir, eaten by Martians, loved by her friends **Adverb:** Here, there **Embedded Clause:** Who went with you, that you saw

Examples:

Nearly	all of the one hundred	old college	alumni	attending the event

Almost all of	her thirty	former	clients	

Nearly	half of your	brother's old baseball	uniforms	in the closet

Source: Reprinted with permission of Allyn & Bacon from *Language Disorders: A Functional Approach to Assessment and Intervention* (2nd ed.), by Robert E. Owens, Jr. Copyright © 1995 by Allyn & Bacon. (p. 214)

Table 6–8. Elements of the Verb Phrase

Modal Auxillary	Perfect Auxillary	Verb to be	Negative[†]	Passive	Verb	Prepositional Phrase, Noun Phrase, Noun Complement, Adverbial Phrase
May, can, shall, will, must, might, should, would, could	Have, has, had	Am, is, are, was, were, be, been	Not	Been, being	Run, walk, eat, throw, see, write	On the floor, the ball, our old friend, a doctor, on time, late

Examples:

Transitive (may have direct object)

May . . . . have . . . . wanted . . . . . a cookie

Should . . . . not . . . . throw . . . . the ball in the house

Intransitive (does not take direct object)

Might . . . . have . . . . been . . . . walking . . . . to the inn

Could . . . . not . . . . talk . . . . with you

Equative (verb *to be* as main verb)

. . . . is . . . . not . . . . a doctor

. . . . was . . . . late

. . . . were . . . . on the sofa

May . . . . be ill

[†] When modal auxiliaries are used, the negative is placed between the modal and other auxiliary forms, for example, "Might not have been going."

Source: Reprinted with permission of Allyn & Bacon from *Language Disorders: A Functional Approach to Assessment and Intervention* (2nd ed.), by Robert E. Owens, Jr. Copyright © 1995 by Allyn & Bacon. (p. 216)

Clauses require a subject and a predicate (noun + verb phrase).

- **Independent clause.** A clause that can stand alone (*he ate*; *she ran home*).
- **Dependent clause.** A clause that cannot stand alone (*that he wanted*; *which was yellow*).

Each of these clauses contains a noun and a verb. The difference between these two clauses is that the independent clause has a noun-verb relationship; the dependent clause does not. Clauses also occur joined together.

- **Conjoining clauses.** These are two independent clauses joined together (*He arrived and she went home*).
- **Embedded clauses.** These contain a dependent clause joined to an independent clause (*He found what he wanted*).

Many clausal structures are possible (see Dever, 1978; Hannah, 1977; Hubbell, 1988; or others). Owen's (1991) overview of several clausal structures is presented below:

I. Complex verb phrases

   A. Object Clauses

     I hope *that you are ready to go*.
     She told me *Amy was coming*.

   B. Embedded questions

     I wonder *who she called*.
     That is *what I want*.

   C. Reduced embedded questions

     I wonder *who to call*.
     She asked me *what to wear*.

   D. Infinitive clauses

     I want *you to be there*.
     It is *for you to sit on*.

II. Adverbial clauses

   A. Introductory adverbial clauses

     Since I can't go, Jo will bring the equipment.
     In order for you to win, you have to work harder.

   B. Noninitial adverbial clauses

     Jo will bring the equipment *since I can't go*.
     You will have to *in order for you to win*.

III. Subject clauses

    A. *That* clauses

        That she is happy is obvious.
        That he is sick defies denial.

    B. Embedded questions

        Why she left is the real question.
        What the book said is beside the point.

    C. Infinitive clauses

        For me to be there would be a pleasure.
        To go slowly is safer.

IV. Relative clauses

    A. Subject modifiers

        The dog *that followed me home* is a setter.
        James *who has the new bike* gave me a ride.

    B. Object/complement modifiers

        I held the fish *that she caught.*
        That is the one *I like best.*

V. Compound clauses

    A. Complete clauses

        Harry called and then Jack showed up.
        I tried but I couldn't remember her name.

    B. Forward deletion and pronominalization clauses

        I tried but couldn't do it.
        Harry called and then he showed up. (p. 102)

A sentence by definition is an independent clause. It may also contain one or more dependent clauses and/or additional independent clauses. There are three primary types of sentences. They are:

1. Declaratives: statements (e.g., He is 3 years old.)

2. Imperatives: commands (e.g., Go away!)

3. Interrogatives: questions (e.g., Is that right?)

Some authors include a fourth type, which is *negatives* (e.g., She is not home.), although other authors point out that declaratives, imperatives, and interrogatives can all be positive or negative. For example:

	Positive	*Negative*
Declarative:	He is 3.	He isn't 3 yet.
Imperative:	Go away!	Don't go!
Interrogative:	Is she done?	She's not done?

Regardless of your view, it is important to incorporate negative sentences into the assessment of syntactic skills.

Form 6–6 is a worksheet for the assessment of syntactic skills. The form allows you to identify various phrase, clausal, and sentence structures used by your client.

Form 6–6. Assessment of Syntactic Skills

Name: _____ Age: _____

Examiner: _____ Date: _____

Instructions: Check each syntactic structure present for each utterance recorded in the language sample. (N = noun, V = verb, Prep = Prepositional, Phr = phrase, Adv = Adverb, and Comp = complement.)

Utterance	Noun Phrase					Verb Phrase									Clause							Sentence			
	Initiator	Determiner	Adjective	Noun/Pronoun	Post-N Modifier	Modal Auxiliary	Perfect Auxiliary	"To be" Verb	Negative	Passive	Verb	Prep Phr/N Phr	N Comp/Adv Phr	Independent	Dependent	Complex V Phr	Adverbial	Subject	Relative	Compound	Declarative	Imperative	Interrogative	Negative

(continued)

Form 6—6. *(continued)*

Utterance	Initiator	Determiner	Adjective	Noun/Pronoun	Post-N Modifier	Modal Auxiliary	Perfect Auxiliary	"To be" Verb	Negative	Passive	Verb	Prep Phr/N Phr	N Comp/Adv Phr	Independent	Dependent	Complex V Phr	Adverbial	Subject	Relative	Compound	Declarative	Interrogative	Interrogative	Negative

ASSESSMENT OF MORPHOLOGIC SKILLS

Morphology is the study of how morphemes (the smallest units of meaning) are combined to form meaning. Free morphemes are words that can stand alone to convey meaning (e.g, *case* or *boy*), while bound morphemes (e.g, *–s* or *–ing*) are word segments that must be attached to a free morpheme to convey meaning. Grammatic morphemes are free or bound morphemes with little or no meaning when produced by themselves, such as articles (*a, the*, etc.), prepositions (*in, at*, etc.), and grammatical word segments (*–ing, –ed*, etc.).

Bound morphemes can be either derivational or inflectional. Derivational morphemes are those that change the meaning and grammatical class of a word (e.g., the verb *vote* to the noun *voter*, or the adjective *quick* to the adverb *quickly*). Inflectional morphemes are those that affect nuances of meaning but not the basic meaning or grammatical class of a word (e.g., the noun *apple* still refers to the same fruit when an *–s* is added to form *apples*). An extensive list of bound morphemes is presented in Table 6–9. The morphemes that are most frequently sampled during diagnostic evaluations are indicated in bold print. You can use the information

Table 6–9. Derivational and Inflectional Morphemes (The most frequently assessed morphemes are in bold print.)

	Suffixes	
Prefixes	**Derivational**	**Inflectional**
a– (in, on, into, in a manner)	–able (ability, tendency, likelihood)	**–ed** (past)
bi– (twice, two)	–al (pertaining to, like, action, process)	**–ing** (at present)
de– (negative, descent, reversal)	–ance (action, state)	**–s** (plural)
ex– (out of, from, thoroughly)	–ation (denoting action in a noun)	**–s** (third person marker)
inner– (reciprocal, between, together)	**–en** (used to form verbs from adjectives)	**–'s** (possession)
mis– (ill, negative, wrong)	–ence (action, state)	
out– (extra, beyond, not)	**–er** (used as an agentive ending)	
over– (over)	**–est** (superlative)	
post– (behind, after)	–ful (full, tending)	
pre– (to, before)	–ible (ability, tendency, likelihood)	
pro– (in favor of)	–ish (belonging to)	
re– (again, backward motion)	–ism (doctrine, state, practice)	
semi– (half)	**–ist** (one who does something)	
super– (superior)	–ity (used for abstract nouns)	
trans– (across, beyond)	–ive (tendency or connection)	
tri– (three)	–ize (action, policy)	
un– (not, reversal)	–less (without)	
under– (under)	**–ly** (used to form adverbs)	
	–meet (action, product, means, state)	
	–ness (quality, state)	
	–or (used as an agentive ending)	
	–ous (full of, having, like)	
	–y (inclined to)	

Source: Reprinted with permission of Merrill, an imprint of Macmillan Publishing Company from *Language Disorders: A Functional Approach to Assessment and Intervention* (2nd ed.), by Robert E. Owens, Jr. Copyright © 1995 byAllyn &Bacon. (p. A–62)

in this table to identify which features your client is using appropriately, and which features are not used or have not yet been sampled.

The "Assessment of Morphologic Features," Form 6–7, is provided to help you identify the morphologic structures your client uses correctly and incorrectly. This is a challenging task since it is difficult, at times, to structure opportunities to produce the various target features. We recommend that you use the language sample to identify as many forms as possible, then use structured questions to elicit those forms that were not sampled through the language sample.

Form 6–7. Assessment of Morphologic Features

Name: _____ Age: _____ Date: _____

Examiner: _____

Instructions: Analyze your client's language sample and/or ask structured questions to assess morphologic features. Mark a plus (+) or a check (✔) if the client's attempt is correct and a minus (–) or a zero (0) if the attempt is incorrect. Make additional comments in the right-hand column.

Plurals   **Comments**

_____ /z/ as in *trees* _____

_____ /s/ as in *books* _____

_____ /vz/ as in *wolves* _____

_____ /əz/ as in *dishes* _____

_____ irregular such as *feet* _____

Possessive

_____ /z/ as in *boy's* _____

_____ /s/ as in *cat's* _____

_____ /əz/ as in *mouse's* _____

Articles

_____ a _____

_____ the _____

Present progressive tense

_____ /ɪŋ/ as in *eating* _____

Past tense

_____ /d/ as in *spilled* _____

_____ /t/ as in *dropped* _____

_____ /əd/ as in *melted* _____

_____ irregular such as *broke* _____

Third person singular

_____ /z/ as in *moves* _____

(continued)

Form 6–7. *(continued)*

Third person singular

_____ /s/ as in *walks* _____

_____ /əz/ as in *pushes* _____

Comparatives/superlatives

_____ /ə/ as in *softer* _____

_____ /əst/ as in *smallest* _____

_____ irregular such as *best* _____

Negation

_____ /ʌn/ as in ***un**happy* _____

_____ not as in *not now* _____

Reflexive pronouns

_____ /sɛlvz/ as in *them**selves*** _____

_____ /sɛlf/ as in *my**self*** _____

Prepositions

_____ in _____

_____ on _____

_____ under _____

_____ behind _____

_____ beside _____

_____ between _____

_____ in front _____

MAKING A DIAGNOSIS

As stated previously, children develop language skills at different rates. Such a wide range of normal makes it difficult to make an accurate diagnosis and appropriate recommendations in some cases. Lucas (1980) outlined some general guidelines to help you determine whether your client is exhibiting a delay that warrants clinical attention:

- ☐ If a 3-year-old child is not talking, or if the child is showing other problems in addition to language delay, then a complete diagnostic evaluation and probable therapeutic intervention is indicated.

- ☐ If a 3- to 4-year-old child shows a 12-month delay or signs of a disorder, then intervention (based on the child's other developmental behaviors and developmental history) may be indicated. Although the order of language acquisition for most children is relatively invariant for syntax and morphology, the rate varies greatly among preschool children.

- ☐ If a child between 5 and 8 years of age shows a 6- to 12-month delay and/or signs of disorders with or without other areas of developmental delay, remediation or intervention is probably warranted.

- ☐ If a child older than 8 has not developed basic syntactic and morphologic skills and/or shows signs of language disorders, intervention is most likely warranted. (p. 124)

Lucas' suggestions are general only and should not be applied to every child. For example, in some cases children as young as 18–24 months who are not talking may already be evidencing the need for clinical intervention. Or, a 3 year old who exhibits a 12-month language delay is already functioning about one-third behind normal expectations, which is a considerable discrepancy. An emphasis on early detection and on the prevention of the development of further discrepancies suggests the need for more aggressive detection of need and appropriate intervention.

CONCLUDING COMMENTS

Language is complex, varied, and often difficult to evaluate. Fortunately, many formal tests are available to examine a child's language abilities. Formal tests are nearly always administered as part of the assessment process. Language samples are also invaluable for evaluating language. A representative language sample allows the clinician to examine pragmatic, semantic, syntactic, and morphologic components. Even though language sampling is often a time-consuming process if done properly, the sample will yield a wealth of information for making clinical decisions. A thorough language evaluation is indeed extensive, but certainly necessary for adequately meeting the needs of the client.

SOURCES OF ADDITIONAL INFORMATION

Language Development and Disorders

Arwood, E. L. (1991). *Semantic and pragmatic language disorders* (2nd ed.). Gaithersburg, MD: Aspen.

Bailey, D. B., & Wolery, M. (Eds.). (1989). *Assessing infants and preschoolers with handicaps.* Columbus, OH: Merrill.

Bernstein, D. K, & Tiegerman, E. (Eds.). (1993). *Language and communication disorders in children* (3rd ed.). New York: Macmillan.

Bloom, L., & Lahey, M. (1978). *Language development and language disorders.* New York: John Wiley & Sons.

Brown, R. (1973). *A first language.* Cambridge, MA: Harvard University.

Gleason, J. Berko. (Ed.). (1993). *The development of language* (3rd ed.). New York: Macmillan.

Holland, A. L. (Ed.). (1984). *Language disorders in children.* San Diego: College-Hill Press.

James, S. (1990). *Normal language acquisition.* Boston: Little, Brown and Co.

Lahey, M. (1988). *Language disorders and language development.* New York: Macmillan.

Lane, V. W., & Molyneaux, D. (1992). *The dynamics of communicative development.* Englewood Cliffs, NJ: Prentice-Hall.

Lund, N. J., & Duchan, J. F. (1993). *Assessing children's language in naturalistic contexts* (3rd ed.). Englewood Cliffs, NJ: Prentice-Hall.

McCormick, L., & Schiefelbusch, R. L. (1990). *Early language intervention* (2nd ed.). Columbus, OH: Merrill.

Owens, R. E. (1995). *Language disorders: A functional approach to assessment and intervention* (2nd ed.). Needham Heights, MA: Allyn & Bacon.

Owens, R. E. (1996). *Language development: An introduction* (4th ed.). Needham Heights, MA: Allyn & Bacon.

Reed, V. A. (1994). *An introduction to children with language disorders* (2nd ed.). New York: Macmillan.

Reich, P. A. (1986). *Language development.* Englewood Cliffs, NJ: Prentice-Hall.

Wiig, E. H., & Semel, E. (1984). *Language assessment and intervention for the learning disabled* (2nd ed.). Columbus, OH: Merrill.

Language Sampling Procedures

Crystal, D. (Ed.). (1979). *Working with the LARSP.* New York: Elsevier.

Crystal, D., Fletcher, P., & Garman, M. (1989). *Grammatical analysis of language disability* (2nd ed.). San Diego: Singular Publishing Group.

Dever, R. B. (1978). *Teaching the American language to kids* (TALK). Columbus, OH: Merrill.

Hannah, E. P. (1977). *Applied linguistic analysis II: Synthesis and analysis of language.* Pacific Palisades, CA: SenCom.

Hubbell, R. (1988). *A handbook of English grammar and language sampling.* Englewood Cliffs, NJ: Prentice-Hall.

James, S. (1993). Assessing children with language disorders. In Bernstein, D. K., & Tiegerman, E. (Eds.), *Language and communication disorders in children* (3rd ed., pp. 185–228). New York: Macmillan.

Lahey, M. (1988). *Language disorders and language development.* New York: Macmillan.

Lee, L. (1974). *Developmental sentence analysis.* Evanston, IL: Northwestern University Press.

Lund, N. J., & Duchan, J. F. (1993). *Assessing language in naturalistic settings* (3rd ed.). Englewood Cliffs, NJ: Prentice-Hall.

Miller, J. (1981). *Assessing language behavior: Experimental procedures.* Austin, TX: PRO-ED.

Miller, J., & Chapman, R. (1985). *Systematic analysis of language (SALT,* a computer program). Madison, WI: Weisman Center on Mental Retardation and Human Development.

Owens, R. E. (1995). *Language disorders: A functional approach to assessment and intervention* (2nd ed.). Needham Heights, MA: Allyn & Bacon.

Internet Sources

Listservers of Interest to Communication Disorders Folks
    http://www.shc.uiowa.edu/wjshc/iiscdl.html

□ CHAPTER 7 □

Assessment of Fluency

- Overview of Assessment
- Screening
- Speech Sampling
    Evaluating the Speech Sample
- Descriptions of Dysfluencies
- Dysfluency Indexes
- Associated Motor Behaviors
- Physiological Factors
- Speech Rate
- Assessing Feelings and Attitudes
    Parental Concern
    Avoidance and Expectancy
- Adaptation and Consistency Effects
- Criteria for Diagnosing Stuttering
    Estimating Severity
- Stimulability
- Cluttering
    Assessment
    Stimulability
- Concluding Comments
- Sources of Additional Information

Fluency is a speech pattern which flows in a rhythmic, smooth manner. Dysfluencies are disruptions or breaks in the smooth flow of speech. Even speakers who are normally fluent experience dysfluencies. A speaker is dysfluent when unintentionally repeating a word or phrase, forgetting a word mid-utterance, or interjecting too many "uhs" or "OKs" during speech. It is the speech-language pathologist's responsibility to differentiate between normal dysfluencies and a fluency disorder.

There are several communicative disorders that adversely affect speech fluency, some of which are addressed in other chapters. For example, the word-finding problems in aphasia, the groping behaviors in apraxia, and the laryngeal hypervalving in spastic dysphonia are all associated with reduced fluency. This chapter focuses on two specific communicative disorders associated with fluency problems—stuttering and cluttering.

Stuttering is one of the most extensively studied yet poorly understood communicative disorders. Authorities do not agree on a universal definition of stuttering or on its etiology. Hegde (1995b) lists 11 different theories of stuttering etiology:[1]

Organic Theories

- Genetic theory: Stuttering or a predisposition to stutter is inherited.
- Cerebral dominance theory: Stutterers lack cerebral dominance for language; interhemispheric conflict.
- Hemispheric processing problems: Stutterers process language in the right, hence the "wrong," hemisphere.
- Defective neural control of speech: Unstable nervous system does not properly control the speech mechanism.
- Defective auditory mechanism: There is a built-in delay or other problems.

Environmental Theories

- Diagnosogenic theory (Johnson): Parental diagnosis causes stuttering which is avoidance behavior.
- Conditioned avoidance (Wischner): Stutterers are conditioned to avoid negative listener reactions.
- Anticipatory struggle (Bloodstein): Stuttering is a response of tension and fragmentation.
- Operant view: Stuttering is an operantly learned behavior, affected by its consequences.
- Two factor theory (Brutton & Shoemaker): Stuttering is due to classically conditioned anxiety.
- Psychoanalysis (Freud): Stuttering is due to regression to earlier stages of libido.

Other etiological theories have also been suggested. Fortunately, the disagreements about causation do not significantly influence the assessment process, because it is possible to validly detect and assess stuttering regardless of presumed etiology.

---

[1]From M. N. Hegde, *Introduction to Communicative Disorders* (2nd ed., p. 237). Austin, TX: PRO-ED. Copyright © 1995 and presented by permission.

OVERVIEW OF ASSESSMENT

History of the Client

    Procedures

        Written Case History
        Information-getting interview
        Information from Other Professionals

    Contributing Factors

        Medical or Neurological Factors
        Family History
        Sex, Motivation, and Levels of Concern

Assessment of Fluency

    Procedures

        Screening
        Speech Sampling
        Stimulability

    Analysis

        Dysfluency Indexes
        Associated Motor Behaviors
        Other Physiological Factors
        Rate of Speech
        Feelings, Attitudes, and Reactions to Speech

Oral-facial Examination

Hearing Assessment

Determining the Diagnosis

Providing Information (written report, interview, etc.)

Hutchinson (1983) outlines four objectives for the assessment of stuttering:

1. Obtain sufficient background and history about the disorder and its development.
2. Obtain complete descriptions of the overt (observable) behaviors present and the client's reactions to them.
3. Identify secondary problems that are related to the fluency disorder. For example, associated motor behaviors, negative emotional responses, and mental constructs about stuttering (i.e., what the client believes has caused or is maintaining the behavior).
4. Determine whether treatment is warranted.

SCREENING

A spontaneous sample of the client's connected speech is necessary to screen for stuttering or cluttering. Many times, a brief 2- or 3-minute speech sample is sufficient to detect a disorder. You may also wish to ask the client to describe pictures or tell narratives to screen for stuttering or cluttering.

Stuttering behaviors vary in some clients. Keep in mind that many individuals are fluent on some occasions and dysfluent on others. This is particularly true among young children. Therefore, repeated samples at different times and under different circumstances may be necessary. Also talk with others who interact with the child, especially parents or teachers. Ask the informant to describe the child's stuttering difficulty, especially the types of dysfluencies, their frequencies, the presence or absence of associated motor behaviors, and the degree of concern the child and the informant have toward the speech pattern. Older children are usually able to provide this information.

A screening of cluttering should also include a sample of conversational speech. Listen for an excessive speech rate and its effects on articulation. A language screen is also advisable. The descriptions of cluttering in Table 7–3 and on Form 7–8 may help you screen for a disorder of cluttering.

SPEECH SAMPLING

The most important procedure for any evaluation of stuttering is a speech sample. We strongly recommend obtaining speech samples from more than one session and, if possible, from more than one setting in order to obtain the most representative sample possible. Attempt to obtain samples that contain the fewest dysfluencies, the most dysfluencies, and the typical number of dysfluencies present in the client's speech. The collection of an adequate sample is critical, as it is the primary basis on which most analyses and judgments about fluency are made. If it is not possible to obtain samples in different settings, ask your client or a significant other to tape record a sample of the client's speech for you.

Collect speech samples from:

- ☐ The clinic or testing site,
- ☐ Outside the assessment area but still in proximity to it,
- ☐ Home,
- ☐ Classroom,
- ☐ Playground,
- ☐ Work environment, and/or
- ☐ Other places the client spends time and interacts with others.

Specific procedures and a variety of stimulus materials for collecting and analyzing a speech sample were presented in Chapter 4. For the assessment of fluency, you may use the "Pictures" (pp. 99–103), "Narratives With Pictures" (pp. 104–111), "Reading Passages" (pp. 122–124), and "Syllable-by-Syllable Stimulus Phrases" (pp. 118–121).

Evaluating the Speech Sample

After you have obtained a thorough, representative sample of your client's speech, you are ready to start the next phase of the assessment—analysis. Specifically, determine:

- ☐ Total number of dysfluencies,
- ☐ Frequencies of different types of dysfluencies,
- ☐ Duration of individual instances of dysfluency, and
- ☐ Types and frequencies of associated motor behaviors.

DESCRIPTIONS OF DYSFLUENCIES

The major dysfluency types are as follows.[2]

Example

☐ **Repetitions**
Part-word repetitions   "What t-t-t time is it'?"
Whole-word repetitions   *"What-what-what are you doing?"*
Phrase repetitions   *"I want to-I want to-I want to do it."*

☐ **Prolongations**
Sound/syllable prolongations   *"Lllllllet me do it."*
Silent prolongations   A struggling attempt to say a word when there is no sound.

☐ **Interjections**
Sound/syllable interjections   *"um . . . um I had a problem this morning."*
Whole-word interjections   "I had a *well* problem this morning."
Phrase interjections   "I had a *you know* problem this morning."

☐ **Silent Pauses**
A silent duration within speech considered abnormal   "I was going to the [pause] store."

☐ **Broken Words**
A silent pause within words   "It was won[pause]derful."

☐ **Incomplete Phrases**
Grammatically incomplete utterances   *"I don't know how to . . .* Let us go, guys."

☐ **Revisions**
Changed words, ideas   "I thought I will write a letter, card."

---

[2]From M. N. Hegde and D. Davis, *Clinical Methods and Practicum in Speech-Language Pathology* (2nd ed., p. 324). San Diego: Singular Publishing Group. Copyright © 1995 and used by permission.

DYSFLUENCY INDEXES

Dysfluency indexes refer to percentages of dysfluent speech present in the speech sample. Dysfluency indexes should be determined in several different environments (the therapy room, outside, at home, at work, etc.), within different modes of speech (reading, spontaneous speech, etc.), and across more than one assessment session. The "Fluency Charting Grid" (Form 7–1) and "Frequency Count for Dysfluencies" (Form 7–2) are methods for identifying and quantifying dysfluencies. Use Form 7–1 to count the total number of dysfluent and fluent productions and, for more sophisticated charting, to code each dysfluency type. Each grid allows you to tally up to 500 words. Form 7–2 can be used to tally occurrences of each type of dysfluency. Form 7–2 may be preferable for charting short samples, or for more informal charting such as screenings.

Form 7–3, "Calculating the Dysfluency Index," is provided to help you calculate the dysfluency indexes. When determining a dysfluency index, count each repetition of a sound, part of a word, whole word, or phrase only once. For example, *ba-ba-ba-ba-ball* is one dysfluency, *I-want-I want-I want to go* is one dysfluency, and *go-go-go-away* is also one dysfluency.[3]

The total dysfluency index reflects *all* dysfluencies produced by the client. For example, consider a 500-word sample with the following number of dysfluencies.

> 75 repetitions
> 50 pauses
> <u>25</u> sound prolongations
> 150 total dysfluencies

To calculate the Total Dysfluency Index:

1. Count the total number of words in the speech sample (500 in this example).
2. Count the total number of dysfluencies (150).
3. Divide the total dysfluencies by the total words. In this example: $150 \div 500 = .30$.
4. Change to a percentage: .30 = 30% Total Dysfluency Index.

Separate indexes can also be determined for individual dysfluency types. For example, to calculate a Total Repetitions Index (using the example above):

1. Count the total number of words in the speech sample (500 in this example).
2. Count the number of specified dysfluencies (75 repetitions in this example).
3. Divide the total specified dysfluency (repetitions) by the total words. In this example: $75 \div 500 = .15$.
4. Change to a percentage: .15 = 15% Total Repetitions index.

---

[3]There are times when counting the number of repetitions per dysfluency provides useful information. In the examples just provided, you can calculate the average number of repetitions per dysfluency. But again, for calculating a dysfluency index, do not count every repetition.

Of course, you can calculate indexes for any dysfluency type using the same method.

A third type of dysfluency index reflects the percentage of each dysfluency type based on the Total Dysfluency Index. For this calculation, base your computation on the total number of dysfluencies. Again, using the same example:

1. Count the total number of dysfluencies in the speech sample (150 in this example).
2. Count the number of specified dysfluencies (75 repetitions).
3. Divide the total specified dysfluency (repetitions) by the total dysfluencies. In this example: $75 \div 150 = .50$.
4. Change to a percentage: $.50 = 50\%$ of all dysfluencies present were repetitions.

Occasionally, a client will exhibit very few dysfluencies, resulting in a normal dysfluency index. However, some of the dysfluencies exhibited will be long in duration and therefore indicate a possible fluency disorder. In these cases, time the duration of the dysfluencies and determine a mean duration of dysfluency. Time each dysfluency with a stopwatch. Pauses or prolongations are most commonly measured, but the duration of repetitions can also be timed. For example, 10 dysfluencies resulting in a total of 42 seconds yields an average duration of 4.2 seconds.

Form 7–1. Fluency Charting Grid

Name: _____ Age: _____ Date: _____

Examiner: _____

Instructions: Make an appropriate mark in each square for every word uttered using the suggested symbols (or make up your own) to indicate the type of dysfluency present. The major categories of dysfluencies are in bold print.

(•)	**No Dysfluency**	**(1)**	**Interjection**
(R)	**Repetition**	(I-SS)	Sound/Syllable Interjection
(R-PW)	Part-word Repetition	(I-Wd)	Whole-word Interjection
(R-WW)	Whole-word Repetition	(I-Ph)	Phrase Interjection
(R-P)	Phrase Repetition	**(SP)**	**Silent Pause**
(P)	**Prolongation**	**(BW)**	**Broken Word**
(P-Sd)	Sound Prolongation	**(Inc)**	**Incomplete Phrase**
(P-Si)	Silent Prolongation	**(Rev)**	**Revision**

Form 7–2. Frequency Count for Dysfluencies

Name: _____ Age: _____ Date: _____

Examiner: _____

Instructions: Make a check (✔) on the appropriate line each time the corresponding dysfluency is produced.

Repetitions   **Totals**

    Part-word _____ _____

    Whole-word _____ _____

    Phrase _____ _____

Prolongations

    Sound _____ _____

    Silent _____ _____

Interjections

    Sound/Syllable _____ _____

    Whole-word _____ _____

    Phrase _____ _____

Silent Pauses _____ _____

Broken Words _____ _____

Incomplete Phrases _____ _____

Revisions _____ _____

Form 7–3. Calculating the Dysfluency Index

Name: _____ Age: _____ Date: _____

Examiner: _____

Instructions: Transfer your findings from the "Fluency Charting Grid" (Form 7–1) to the appropriate blanks below to determine the total dysfluency index and/or the index for specific dysfluency types. Calculate dysfluency indexes for general or specific dysfluency types. For example, *Repetitions* are general fluency types which consist of specific types: *Part-word, Whole-word,* and *Phrase Repetitions*. See pages 230–231 for calculation instructions.

Environment: _____

Sample Type: _____

Total Number of Words: _____

	Number of Dysfluencies	Dysfluency Index
Repetitions (R):	_____	_____
Part-word (R-PW):	_____	_____
Whole-word (R-WW):	_____	_____
Phrase (R-P):	_____	_____
Prolongations (P):	_____	_____
Sound (P-Sd):	_____	_____
Silent (P-Si):	_____	_____
Interjections (I):	_____	_____
Sound/Syllable (I-SS):	_____	_____
Whole-word (I-Wd):	_____	_____
Phrase (I-Ph):	_____	_____
Silent Pauses (SP):	_____	_____
Broken Words (BW):	_____	_____
Incomplete Phrases (Inc):	_____	_____
Revisions (Rev):	_____	_____
TOTAL NUMBER OF DYSFLUENCIES:	_____	_____

Comments:

ASSOCIATED MOTOR BEHAVIORS

Many stutterers exhibit extraneous body movements in association with their dysfluencies. These behaviors are present only during dysfluent speech; they do not occur when the stutterer is fluent or not speaking. Although such behaviors are common, not all stutterers exhibit associated motor behaviors.

These visible displays of tension usually involve parts of the oral-facial mechanism. They include such behaviors as eye blinking, wrinkling the forehead, sudden exhaustive exhaling, frowning, distorting the mouth, moving the head, and/or quivering the nostrils. Sometimes they include movements of body parts that are not normally associated with speech, such as moving the arms, hands, legs, feet, or torso (Bloodstein, 1987).

During the assessment session, it is important to note all unusual movements your client exhibits. Form 7–4, "Assessment of Associated Motor Behaviors," is designed to help you identify these extraneous movements. Please note that the form lists the most common behaviors; it is not an exhaustive list of all the possible behaviors clients may exhibit. Once the behaviors are identified, chart their frequency in the same manner you charted dysfluencies.

Form 7–4. Assessment of Associated Motor Behaviors

Name: _____ Age: _____ Date: _____

Examiner: _____

Instructions: Check all associated motor behaviors the client exhibits. Use the right-hand column to describe behaviors or record frequency counts.

Eyes

____ blinking _____

____ shutting _____

____ upward movement _____

____ downward movement _____

____ vertical movement _____

____ other (specify) _____

Nose

____ flaring _____

____ dilation _____

____ wrinkling _____

____ other (specify) _____

Forehead

____ wrinkling/creasing _____

____ other (specify) _____

Head

____ shaking _____

____ upward movement _____

____ downward movement _____

____ lateral movement to right _____

____ lateral movement to left _____

____ other (specify) _____

Lips

_____ quivering _____

_____ pursing _____

_____ invert lower lip _____

_____ other (specify) _____

Tongue

_____ clicking _____

_____ extraneous movement _____

_____ other (specify) _____

Teeth

_____ clenching _____

_____ grinding _____

_____ clicking _____

_____ other (specify) _____

Jaw

_____ clenching _____

_____ opening _____

_____ closing _____

_____ other (specify) _____

Neck

_____ tightening _____

_____ twitching _____

_____ upward movement _____

_____ downward movement _____

_____ lateral movement to the right _____

(continued)

Form 7–4 *(continued)*

Neck

_____   lateral movement to left   _____

_____   other (specify)   _____

Fingers

_____   tapping   _____

_____   rubbing   _____

_____   clenching   _____

_____   excessive movement   _____

_____   clicking   _____

_____   other (specify)   _____

Hands

_____   fist clenching   _____

_____   wringing   _____

_____   splaying   _____

_____   other (specify)   _____

Arms

_____   excessive movement   _____

_____   banging against side   _____

_____   banging against leg   _____

_____   jerky movement   _____

_____   tensing   _____

_____   other (specify)   _____

Leg

_____   tensing   _____

_____   kicking   _____

Leg

____ rapid movement _____

____ other (specify) _____

Breathing

____ speaking on little air _____

____ unnecessary inhalation _____

____ jerky breathing _____

____ audible inhalation _____

____ audible exhalation _____

____ dysrhythmic _____

____ other (specify) _____

Others (describe) _____

_____

_____

_____

_____

PHYSIOLOGICAL FACTORS

There are several factors, in addition to associated motor behaviors, that may be associated with stuttering. These include respiratory, phonatory, articulatory, and prosodic aspects of speech production. Form 7–5 is provided to help you identify pertinent factors associated with a stuttering pattern. Clinicians need to carefully examine whether these factors are present during fluent and dysfluent speech or only during dysfluencies.

Form 7–5. Assessment of Physiological Factors Associated with Stuttering[1]

Name: _____ Age: _____ Date: _____

Examiner: _____

Instructions: Check all behaviors the client exhibits. Use the right-hand column to clarify or make additional comments.

Respiratory Factors

_____ normal respiration at rest _____

_____ normal respiration during speech _____

_____ shallow breathing _____

_____ audible inhalation _____

_____ prolonged inhalation _____

_____ audible exhalation (nonspeech) _____

_____ gasping _____

_____ arhythmical breathing _____

_____ other (describe) _____

Phonatory Factors

_____ normal phonatory functions _____

_____ delays of phonatory onset _____

_____ hard glottal attacks _____

_____ pitch breaks _____

_____ excessive pitch variations _____

_____ too loud _____

_____ too soft _____

_____ alternating loudness _____

(continued)

[1]Based on G. Beverly Wells, *Stuttering Treatment: A Comprehensive Clinical Guide*, © 1987, p. 21. Adapted by permission of Prentice-Hall, Englewood Cliffs, NJ.

Form 7–5 *(continued)*

Phonatory Factors

_____ arhythmical breathing _____

_____ other (describe) _____

Articulatory Factors

_____ normal articulatory contacts _____

_____ easy articulatory contacts _____

_____ hard articulatory contacts _____

_____ normal articulation (place, manner) _____

_____ other (describe) _____

Prosodic Factors

_____ normal prosody _____

_____ prolonged sound productions _____

_____ excessive stressing _____

_____ atypical stressing _____

_____ other (describe) _____

Rate When Fluent

_____ appropriate _____

_____ excessively fast _____

_____ excessively slow _____

SPEECH RATE

Specific procedures for assessing rate of speech are provided in Chapter 4. Assessing speech rate is an especially important element of the evaluation of stuttering. It is important to determine whether you wish to evaluate:

- Overall rate (including dysfluencies), or
- Normal rate (excluding dysfluencies).

These two measures often produce very different results. For example, a stutterer may produce only a few words per minute when both fluent and dysfluent segments are measured. But, if you analyze only segments of fluent speech, the same stutterer may actually exhibit a very fast rate of speech. A rapid speech rate, which can go undetected if only the overall rate is assessed, may be a major contributor to the fluency disorder.

ASSESSING FEELINGS AND ATTITUDES

Stuttering is a debilitating handicap that can cause feelings of great pain, anguish, and frustration. The person who stutters may be corrected, teased, ridiculed, mocked, chastised, avoided, isolated, pitied, or scorned because of the speech disorder. Hegde (1995b) writes that "a person who stutters is bound to experience certain emotional and behavioral effects of this profound speech difficulty" (p. 224).

Erickson (1969) developed the *S-Scale*, a 39-item form used to assess stutterers attitudes about various speaking situations. This scale was later modified into a 24-item scale by Andrews and Cutler (1974) so that it could be readministered across time to assess progress. Researchers have reported conflicting results from studies of the *S-Scale* and its modified form (see Erickson, 1969; Guitar, 1979; Guitar & Bass, 1978; Ingham, 1979; Silverman, 1980; Ulliana & Ingham, 1984). One criticism is that the items are not exclusive to stutterers and, therefore, they are not fully discriminative between people with normal and disordered fluency. However, stutterers do answer "true" to items on the scale more often than nonstutterers.

We agree with Ham (1986) that understanding a stuttering client's feelings about his or her disorder is important. Using the modified *S-Scale* (Form 7–6) is a good way to begin addressing this information.

Form 7–6. The Modified S-Scale[1]

Instructions: Answer the following by circling "T" if the statement is generally true for you, or circle "F" if the statement is generally false for you. If the situation is unfamiliar or rare, judge it on a "If it was familiar . . ." basis.[2]

1.   T   F   I usually feel that I am making a favorable impression when I talk.

2.   T   F   I find it easy to talk with almost anyone.

3.   T   F   I find it very easy to look at my audience while talking in a group.

4.   T   F   A person who is my teacher or my boss is hard to talk to.

5.   T   F   Even the idea of giving a talk in public makes me afraid.

6.   T   F   Some words are harder than others for me to say.

7.   T   F   I forget all about myself shortly after I begin to give a speech.

8.   T   F   I am a good mixer.

9.   T   F   People sometimes seem uncomfortable when I am talking to them.

10.   T   F   I dislike introducing one person to another.

11.   T   F   I often ask questions in group discussions.

12.   T   F   I find it easy to keep control of my voice when speaking.

13.   T   F   I do not mind speaking before a group.

14.   T   F   I do not talk well enough to do the kind of work I'd really like to do.

15.   T   F   My speaking voice is rather pleasant and easy to listen to.

16.   T   F   I am sometimes embarrassed by the way I talk.

17.   T   F   I face most speaking situations with complete confidence.

18.   T   F   There are few people I can talk with easily.

19.   T   F   I talk better than I write.

20.   T   F   I often feel nervous while talking.

21.   T   F   I often find it hard to talk when I meet new people.

22.   T   F   I feel pretty confident about my speaking abilities.

23.   T   F   I wish I could say things as clearly as others do.

24.   T   F   Even though I knew the right answer, I have often failed to give it because I was afraid to speak out.

---

[1]From G. Andrews and J. Cutler (1974) "Stuttering therapy: The relation between changes in symptom level and attitudes." *Journal of Speech and Hearing Disorders*, 39, 312–319. Used by permission of the American Speech-Language-Hearing Association.

[2]Note that items 4, 5, 6, 9, 10, 14, 16, 18, 20, 21, 23, and 24 are presumed to be true for people who stutter; the other items are presumed to be false.

Parental Concern

One issue related to attitudes and feelings often addressed in our professional literature is parental concern, particularly for a child who stutters. Years ago, Wendell Johnson proposed that significant people in a child's environment (usually parents) reacted to their child's normally dysfluent speech, which caused the child to gain awareness and concern about dysfluency. This awareness, in combination with the inability to produce fluent speech, then led to the development and maintenance of a true stuttering pattern. (See Bloodstein, 1995; Johnson and Associates, 1959; Van Riper, 1971; and other sources for more information on Johnson's theory or other learning theories.)

This diagnosogenic theory (i.e., stuttering first diagnosed in the ear of the beholder) has not been established as the cause of stuttering, but neither has any other single theory of stuttering etiology. In a practical sense, it is extremely unlikely that a parent's concern "causes" stuttering, but it is important to keep in mind that parents do live with the problem. They live with the fears, anxieties, and concerns that surround their child as a result of a stuttering problem. Thus, in many cases, sampling parental attitudes is an important part of the evaluative process.

Questions from the "Modified S-Scale" (Form 7–6) are adaptable for use with parents. For example, change the remark "I find it easy to talk with almost anyone" to "*My child finds it easy to talk with almost anyone.*" You can also explore parental attitudes and feelings by asking similar questions during a parent interview. With parents of preschool-aged children, the "Parental Speech Chart" (Form 7–7) is useful for structured parental observations in the home.

Form 7–7. Parental Speech Chart

Child: _____   Age: _____

Informant: _____   Date: _____

Instructions: Indicate each dysfluency present and factors surrounding the dysfluency. This is a general worksheet; it does not need to be absolutely precise. Do the best you can, and write down any questions or thoughts you have, so you can mention them to the speech-language pathologist.

Date/Time	Type of difficulty (repeating sounds or words, prolongations, etc.)	Tension or struggle?	Reaction to dysfluency? Aware of difficulty?	Topic of conversation	Who was the child talking to? What did the other person do?	Did you notice anything that preceded the dysfluency?

Avoidance and Expectancy

Two specific responses to negative feelings about stuttering are *avoidance* and *expectancy*. Avoidance is a learned response to unpleasant stimuli. Just as people learn to avoid touching a hot stove because it is painful to get burned, many people who stutter learn to avoid certain sounds, words, or speaking situations that are especially difficult for them. Stuttering clients occasionally circumlocute—or talk around the subject—to avoid dysfluencies. Specifically, some stutterers tend to avoid difficult:

- Sounds,
- Words,
- Topics,
- People (e.g., employer, teacher, strangers, etc.),
- Situations (e.g., ordering in a restaurant, talking on the telephone, etc.),
- Communicative events (e.g., public speaking, speaking with members of the opposite sex, etc.).

During the assessment, pay particular attention to avoidance behaviors. Ask probing questions during the interview and observe the client's speech during the speech sample.

Avoidance behaviors can be described as primary or secondary. Primary avoidances refer to the client's attempts to alter the speaking act. Secondary avoidances are acts of reducing or ceasing attempts to talk. These types of avoidances include:

Primary Avoidances

- Starters: using words, sounds, gestures, or rituals to initiate speech.
- Postponements: silences (e.g, pretending to think), ritualistic acts (e.g, lip licking), or verbal stalling.
- Retrials: repeating a fluent utterance to "hurdle" a feared word or phrase.
- Circumlocutions: sound, word, or phrase substitutions.
- Antiexpectancies: altering the communicative text by speaking with an accent, imitating someone else's voice, overemphasizing articulation, speaking rhythmically, whispering, or singing.

Secondary Avoidances

- Reducing verbal output, or not talking at all.
- Relying on others to communicate for them.

Expectancy (or anticipation) is the expectation of a dysfluency before it occurs. Expectancies occur for sounds, words, people, or specific situations. Some clients respond to expectancy by "pushing forward" into the dysfluency. Others respond with avoidance behaviors. Obtain information about expectancy by observing and listening during speech tasks and interviews. Ask the client to tell you when he or she experiences expectancy. You can suspect its presence but confirmation comes only from the client or by repeated observation.

ADAPTATION AND CONSISTENCY EFFECTS

Some clinicians still evaluate the adaptation and consistency effects, which were first described in 1937 by Johnson and Knott. The adaptation effect refers to the reduction in dysfluencies on consecutive readings of the same passage. For example, during the first reading, a client may be 25% dysfluent; during the second reading, the client may be 13% dysfluent; and during the third reading, the client may be 10% dysfluent. The adaptation effect is 12% from the first to second reading (25% − 13% = 12%), and 15% from the first to third reading (25% − 10% = 15%).

The consistency effect is the occurrence of repeated dysfluencies on the same words during consecutive readings of the same passage. For example, during the first reading, a client may stutter 20 times; during the second reading, the client may stutter 10 times (adaptation effect) but all 10 dysfluencies occur on words that were also dysfluent during the first reading (10 dysfluencies ÷ 20 dysfluencies = 50%). The consistency effect is 50% from the first reading to the second. A study of consistency effect may help you identify words that are more difficult for your client to produce fluently.

The adaptation and consistency effects are sampled by some clinicians, presumably because they gain potentially useful information from either or both. We agree with Williams (1978) that there are not reasonable bases for routinely obtaining these measures as part of most assessments. Nevertheless, these effects were described here since they are still used by some clinicians.

CRITERIA FOR DIAGNOSING STUTTERING

As we stated earlier, not all authorities agree on a universal definition or the etiology of stuttering. Also, authorities do not agree on what constitutes a stuttering disorder as compared to normal nonfluent speech. Remember that even normal speakers have dysfluencies. This makes it difficult, in some cases, to diagnose a fluency disorder. Individual clinicians must use their professional judgment and experience to make an appropriate diagnosis. Several factors or criteria to consider both individually and collectively are:

- ☐ The total dysfluency index. Five percent (5%) or greater is usually considered a fluency disorder.
- ☐ The dysfluency indexes for repetitions, prolongations, and intralexical pauses. Three percent (3%) or greater is usually considered a fluency disorder.
- ☐ The duration of dysfluencies. Those that are 1 second or longer usually warrant a diagnosis of a fluency disorder.
- ☐ The presence of associated motor behaviors.
- ☐ The client's (or caregiver's) degree of concern about dysfluency.

Making a diagnosis is sometimes more complicated when the client is a young child. Most clinicians agree that many normally developing children experience a period of nonfluent speech. This typically occurs during the preschool years between 2 and 5 years of age. Experts have varying opinions about diagnosing a fluency disorder and recommending therapy for children who are stuttering. For example, Adams (1980) feels that a child's speech may be *normally nonfluent* if it:

☐ Is less than 9% dysfluent;

☐ Consists primarily of whole-word repetitions, phrase repetitions, and revisions;

☐ Is produced effortlessly and with no tension, particularly at the beginning of an utterance; and

☐ Does not substitute the schwa vowel /ə/ for the intended vowel in part-word repetitions.

Curlee (1984) believes that a diagnosis of stuttering (rather than normal nonfluency) can be made if any one of these behaviors is present:

☐ Part-word repetitions of two or more units per repetition on 2% or more of the words uttered. Increased tempo of repetitions, substitution of /ɔ/ or "uh" for appropriate vowels in syllable repetitions, and obvious vocal tension are additional danger signals.

☐ Prolongations longer than 1 second on 2% or more of the words uttered. Increases in loudness, pitch rises, and abrupt termination of prolongations are additional danger signs.

☐ Involuntary blockings or hesitations longer than 2 seconds in the flow of speech.

☐ Body movements, eye blinks, lip and jaw tremors, or other signs of struggle that are associated with instances of dysfluencies.

☐ Noticeable emotional reactions or avoidance behaviors associated with speaking.

☐ Complaints of not being able to perform satisfactorily because of speech.

☐ Marked variations in the frequency or severity of speech disruptions with changes in speaking situations or tasks (p. 16).

When assessing a nonfluent child, it is also important to consider his or her language, articulation, and oral-motor skills. In some cases, an apparent "fluency disorder" is actually a secondary behavior of another communicative disorder. If so, using only a traditional fluency treatment may not be of optimal benefit to the child, as it will not address the primary problem.

Estimating Severity

Speech-language pathologists often use the terms *mild, moderate,* and *severe* to estimate the severity of a client's disorder. Although these terms can be useful, realize they are subjective and based on personal judgment and opinion. One of the more popular severity scales for stuttering is Riley's (1986) *Stuttering Severity Instrument.* It is based on three-major measures: the frequency of repetitions and prolongations of sounds and syllables, the durations of the longest dysfluencies, and the severity of associated struggle behaviors. Riley's scale is useful for different ages and it yields a quick estimate of severity.

Wingate (1976) believed that subjective severity ratings were ineffective, so he developed objective standards for reporting the severity of stuttering. His Severity Rating Guide is presented in Table 7–1.

Table 7–1. Stuttering Severity Rating Guide

Rating	Total Dysfluency Index	Effort	Associated Motor Behaviors
Very Mild	1%	No perceptible tension	None
Mild	2%	Perceptible tension but "block" easily overcome	Minimal (staring; eyeblinks or eye movement or slight movement of the facial musculature)
Moderate	7%	Clear indication of tension or effort; lasts about 2 seconds	Noticeable movements of facial musculature
Severe	15%	Definite tension or effort; lasts about 2–4 seconds; frequent repeat attempts	Obvious muscular activity, facial or other
Very Severe	25%	Considerable effort; lasts 5 seconds or more; consistent repeat attempts	Vigorous muscular activity, facial or other

Source: From M. Wingate, *Stuttering Theory and Treatment* (p. 319). New York: Irvington Publishing Co. Copyright © 1976 and used by permission.

STIMULABILITY

Stimulability of fluency refers to a client's ability to produce fluent speech. Clinicians typically elicit fluent speech by using the same techniques that are used in treatment. Several of these techniques are described in Table 7–2. For more detail and additional procedures, see works such as Perkins (1984), Ham (1986), and Wells (1987).

Imitation and adequate instruction are key elements to successful stimulation. These techniques are used in combination with response-contingent management (specifically, positive or negative reinforcement of desired responses and punishment of undesired responses). Stimulation usually begins at the single-word level and increases in incremental steps. The "Syllable-by-Syllable Stimulus Phrases" on pp. 119–121 are especially useful for assessing stimulability of fluency in increasingly longer phrase lengths.

Table 7–2. Fluency Modification Techniques

Technique	Description
Prolonged Speech	The clinician seeks to prolong the client's duration of sounds, usually with a slow, well-controlled transition between sounds and syllables.
Gentle Onset/Airflow	The stutterer is directed to initiate vocalization with a stable egressive airflow and a gentle onset of phonation.
Reduced Speech Rate	The stutterer maintains a reduced rate of speech, usually beginning with single-word productions and advancing to longer, more complex utterances. Normal phrase boundaries and prosodic features are maintained.
Reduced Articulatory Effort	The client minimizes articulatory tension by bringing the specific articulatory patterns of ongoing speech into conscious attention.

Source: Adapted from J. M. Hutchinson (1983), "Diagnosis of fluency disorders." In I. J. Meitus and B. Weinberg (Eds.), *Diagnosis in Speech-Language Pathology* (p. 203). Baltimore: University Park Press. Used by permission of Allyn & Bacon, current copyright holder.

CLUTTERING

Cluttering is a communication disorder that can affect the four major areas of communication—articulation, language, voice, and fluency. It is presented in this chapter for several reasons:

- Cluttering affects fluency;
- Stuttering and cluttering are sometimes confused, particularly on initial observation and by less-experienced clinicians;
- Cluttering and stuttering can occur in the same client; and
- Most texts address cluttering in conjunction with fluency.

The information in this section is based on our own clinical experiences and the works of Boone and Plante (1993); Daly (1986); Ham (1986); Hegde (1995b); Shames (1990); St. Louis, Hinzman, and Hull (1985); and Weiss (1964).

The characteristics of cluttered speech vary from client to client, but a primary characteristic that is almost always found is an excessive speech rate. Ten of the most common characteristics of cluttering are:

☐ Excessive speech rate, which negatively affects other aspects of communication.

☐ Monotone voice.

☐ Indistinct, "mumbling" speech. Sound distortions and omissions are common.

☐ Errors present in connected speech that are less pronounced or not present during single-word articulation tests or during more slowly produced speech segments.

☐ Telescoped (compressed or omitted) errors. For example, "statistical" may become "stacal," or "refrigerator" may become "reor."

☐ Spoonerisms in which sounds are transposed in a word, phrase, or sentence. For example, "My Fair Lady" may become "My Lair Fady," "hit the books" may be produced as "bit the hooks," or "many people think so" may become "many thinkle peep so."

☐ Language deficiencies.

☐ Auditory processing difficulties.

☐ The client may be unaware of the speech disorder, at least initially. Clients who clutter are sometimes genuinely surprised when the disorder is diagnosed or when other people do not understand them.

☐ The disorder is difficult to treat. Establishing and maintaining a slower speech rate and generalizing treatment behaviors into everyday speech is often difficult.

As stated previously, clinicians sometimes confuse cluttering and stuttering disorders when making a diagnosis. Table 7–3 describes the differential characteristics of stuttering and cluttering. Some of the information is adapted from Ham (1986).

Table 7–3. Differential Characteristics of Stuttering and Cluttering

Stuttering	Cluttering
Client is aware of dysfluencies.	Client is unaware of dysfluencies.
Speech becomes less fluent when the client concentrates on being fluent.	Speech becomes more fluent when client concentrates on being fluent.
Spontaneous speech may be more fluent than oral reading or directed speech.	Spontaneous speech may be less fluent than oral reading or directed speech.
Speech is usually less fluent with strangers.	Speech is usually more fluent with strangers.
Brief verbalizations are often more difficult to control.	Brief verbalizations are often less difficult to control.
Structured retrials may not result in increased fluency.	Structured retrials may improve fluency.
More sound and syllable repetitions are present.	Fewer sound and syllable repetitions are present.
Fewer language problems (e.g., incomplete phrases, reduced linguistic complexity, etc.) are present.	More language problems are present.
Speech rate may be normal when dysfluencies are omitted from speech rate calculation.	Speech rate may be produced at a very rapid, "machine gun" rate.
Fewer articulation errors are present.	Multiple articulation errors may be present.

Assessment

Since cluttering affects all four primary aspects of communication—articulation, language, voice, and fluency—its assessment must also include each of these areas. The procedures that usually provide the best information for diagnosing cluttering are articulation testing and spontaneous speech sampling. A thorough examination of language is also recommended. You may wish to refer to the following procedures and stimulus materials for completing an assessment of cluttering:

- "Articulation Tests" (pp. 134–135)
- "Reading Passages" (pp. 122–124)
- "Speech and Language Sampling" (pp. 97–99)
- "Comparison of Sound Errors from an Articulation Test and Connected Speech" (pp. 137–139)
- "Evaluating Rate of Speech" (pp. 112–113)
- "Determining Intelligibility" (pp. 113–117)
- "Oral-facial Examination Form" (pp. 91–94)
- "Diadochokinetic Syllable Rates Worksheet" (p. 96)

The "Checklist of Cluttering Characteristics," Form 7–8, is designed to help you compile and evaluate your speech assessment findings. Realize, though, that a cluttering client will not necessarily exhibit every associated characteristic. You must consider the presenting behaviors in light of other assessment information to make an accurate diagnosis. Also be aware that some cases of apraxia or stuttering resemble cluttering, at least initially. It is important to be familiar with the differentiating characteristics of each disorder.

Form 7–8. Checklist of Cluttering Characteristics

Name: _____ Age: _____ Date: _____

Examiner: _____

Instructions: Check each characteristic your client exhibits. Include additional comments on the righthand side.

Comments

_____ Indistinct speech _____

_____ Minimal pitch variation _____

_____ Minimal stress variation _____

_____ Monotone voice _____

_____ More errors on longer units _____

_____ Rapid rate _____

_____ Sound distortions _____

_____ Spoonerisms _____

     _____ Within words _____

     _____ Within phrases/sentences _____

_____ Telescoping _____

     _____ Sounds _____

     _____ Words _____

     _____ Parts of phrases _____

_____ Speech improves when concentrating on fluency _____

_____ Speech improves when speech rate is reduced _____

_____ Speech improves during shorter intervals _____

_____ Structured retrials improve fluency _____

_____ Relatively few sound or syllable repetitions _____

_____ Presence of language problems _____

_____ Improved speech is somewhat difficult to stimulate _____

_____ Improved speech does not tend to generalize _____

_____ Client not very aware of speech problem _____

_____ Client not very concerned about speech problem _____

Stimulability

Once you have identified the characteristics of cluttering your client exhibits, it is important to see if the client can improve his or her speech. Two of the five techniques for eliciting improved fluency in Table 7–2 are also useful for cluttering, specifically *prolonged speech* and *reduced speech rate*. These are useful because excessive speech rate is a primary problem with a cluttering pattern. Another technique is borrowed from dysarthria therapy. Called *syllable-by-syllable attack*, it emphasizes that the client correctly produce every syllable in an utterance (see Darley, Aronson, & Brown, 1975; Rosenbek & LaPointe, 1985). To accomplish this, the client usually reduces his or her speech rate.

Even though the cluttering client usually exhibits errors of articulation, language, and voice, stimulation of all these deficits may not need to be the primary focus of your stimulability assessment. In many cases, reducing the speech rate to a slower, more manageable speed reduces or eliminates the effects of these secondary characteristics. As with other disorders, stimulability for flutterers should start at the most simple level and incrementally increase in complexity. The "Syllable-by-Syllable Stimulus Phrases" on pages 119–121 are especially useful for assessing stimulability across different syllable lengths.

CONCLUDING COMMENTS

The assessment of fluency disorders is an intriguing and challenging aspect of clinical work for speech-language pathologists. The behaviors exhibited vary considerably among individual clients, as do their reactions to these problems. The valid assessment of a fluency disorder is a prerequisite to effective clinical treatment. The clinician's understanding of the disorder, the patterns exhibited, and the client's (and/or caregiver's) reaction all enter into the diagnostic process. The absence of accurate knowledge and information precludes, or at least reduces, the chances of effectively diagnosing and treating the disorder.

SOURCES OF ADDITIONAL INFORMATION

Stuttering

Adams, M. (1980). The young stutterer: Diagnosis, treatment, and assessment of prognosis. *Seminars in Speech, Language, and Hearing, 1*, 289–299.
Bloodstein, O. (1995). *A Handbook on stuttering* (5th ed.). San Diego: Singular Publishing Group.
Curlee, R. F. (1984). A case selection strategy for young disfluent children. In W. H. Perkins (Ed.), *Stuttering disorders* (pp. 3–20). New York: Thieme-Stratton.
Curlee, R. F., & Perkins, W. H. (Eds.). (1984). *Nature and treatment of stuttering: New directions.* San Diego: College-Hill Press.
Erickson, R. L. (1969). Assessing communicative attitudes among stutterers. *Journal of Speech and Hearing Research, 12*, 711–724,
Ham, R. (1986). *Techniques of stuttering therapy.* Englewood Cliffs, NJ: Prentice-Hall.
Johnson, W., & Associates. (1959). *The onset of stuttering.* Minneapolis: University of Minnesota Press.

Lanyon, R. (1967). The measurement of stuttering therapy. *Journal of Speech and Hearing Research, 10*, 836–843.

Perkins, W. H. (Ed.). (1980). *Strategies in stuttering therapy.* New York: Thieme-Stratton.

Perkins, W. H. (Ed.). (1984). *Stuttering disorders.* New York: Thieme-Stratton.

Riley, G. D. (1981). *Stuttering prediction instrument.* Austin, TX: PRO-ED.

Riley, G. D. (1986). *Stuttering severity instrument.* Austin, TX: PRO-ED.

Shames, G. H., & Ramig, P. R. (1994). *Stuttering and other disorders of fluency.* In G. H. Shames, E. H. Wiig, & W. A. Secord (Eds.), *Human communication disorders: An Introduction* (4th ed., pp. 336–386). New York: Macmillan.

Shumak, I. C. (1955). A speech situation rating sheet for stutterers. In W. Johnson & R. R. Leutenegger (Eds.), *Stuttering in children and adults* (pp. 341–347). Minneapolis: University of Minnesota Press.

Silverman, F. H. (1980). Dimensions of improvement in stuttering. *Journal of Speech and Hearing Research, 23*, 137-151.

Starkweather, C. W. (1987). *Fluency and stuttering.* Englewood Cliffs, NJ: Prentice-Hall.

Starkweather, C. W., Gottwald, S. R., & Halfond, M. H. (1990). *Stuttering prevention: A clinical method.* Englewood Cliffs, NJ: Prentice-Hall.

Van Riper, C. (1971). *The nature of stuttering.* Englewood Cliffs, NJ: Prentice-Hall.

Van Riper, C. (1973). *The treatment of stuttering.* Englewood Cliffs, NJ: Prentice-Hall.

Wells, G. B. (1987). *Stuttering treatment: A comprehensive clinical guide.* Englewood Cliffs, NJ: Prentice-Hall.

Cluttering

Daly, D. A. (1986). The clutterer. In K. O. St. Louis (Ed.), *The atypical stutterer: Principles and practices of rehabilitation* (pp. 152–192). New York: Academic Press.

Diedrich, W. M. (1984). Cluttering: Its diagnosis. In H. Winitz (Ed.), *Treating articulation disorders* (pp. 307–323). Baltimore: University Park Press.

Ham, R. (1986). *Techniques of stuttering therapy.* Englewood Cliffs, NJ: Prentice-Hall.

Hegde, M. N. (1995). *Introduction to communicative disorders.* (2nd ed.) Austin, TX: PRO-ED.

Shames, G. H. & Ramig, P. R. (1994). *Stuttering and other disorders of fluency.* In G. H. Shames, E. H. Wiig, & Secord, W. A. (Eds.), *Human communication disorders: An introduction* (4th ed., pp. 336–386). New York: Macmillan.

St. Louis, K. O., Hinzman, A. R., & Hull, F. M. (1985). Studies of cluttering: Disfluency and language measures in young possible clutterers and stutterers. *Journal of Fluency Disorders, 10*, 151-172.

Weiss, D. A. (1964). *Cluttering.* Englewood Cliffs, NJ: Prentice-Hall.

Internet Sources

Australian Stuttering Research Centre
   http://www.cchs.usyd.edu.au/Academic/ASRC
Canadian Association for People Who Stutter
   http://www.webcon.net/~caps
Listservers of Interest to Communication Disorders Folks
   http://www.shc.uiowa.edu/wjshc/iiscdl.html
National Center for Stuttering
   http://www.stuttering.com

□ CHAPTER 8 □

Assessment of Voice and Resonance

Voice disorders are classified according to etiology or symptoms. The etiology is its cause, which is either organic or functional. Organic disorders are those that have a known physical cause (e.g., vocal fold paralysis). Functional disorders, which may result in physical changes, do not have a known physical etiology. Table 8–1 lists 27 voice problems categorized by organic or functional cause.

For assessment and treatment purposes, classifying voice disorders by vocal behaviors or symptoms provides the most clinically useful information for the speech-language pathologist. In this text, the features of voice are identified as *pitch, quality, loudness, nasal resonance,* and *oral resonance.*

Table 8–1. Twenty-Seven Voice Problems Related to Either Faulty Usage of the Vocal Mechanism or to Organic Changes of Vocal Mechanism

Functional Disorder	Organic Disorder
Contact Ulcers	Cancer
Diplophonia	Dysarthria
Falsetto	Endocrine changes
Functional aphonia	Granuloma
Functional dysphonia	Hemangioma
Phonation breaks (abductor spasms)	Hyperkeratosis
Pitch breaks	Infectious laryngitis
Spastic dysphonia[†]	Laryngectomy
Thickening (vocal fold)	Laryngofissure
Traumatic laryngitis	Leukoplakia
Ventricular dysphonia	Papilloma
Vocal nodules	Pubertal changes
Vocal polyps	Vocal fold paralysis
	Webbing

[†]The etiology of spastic dysphonia is unknown. It may be classified as a functional disorder by some authors. For a discussion of this disorder and its subtypes, see Watterson & McFarlane (1992) and Karnell (1992).

Source: From Daniel R. Boone and Stephen C. McFarlane, *The Voice and Voice Therapy*, 5th ed., © 1994 by Prentice-Hall, Englewood Cliffs, NJ, p. 62. Presented by permission of Allyn & Bacon, Needham Heights, MA, current copyright holder.

OVERVIEW OF ASSESSMENT

History of the Client

    Procedures

        Written Case History
        Information-getting Interview
        Information from Other Professionals

    Contributing Factors

        Environmental and Behavioral Factors
        Medical or Neurological Factors
        Motivation and Concern

Assessment of Voice (Pitch, Quality, Resonance, Loudness)

    Procedures

        Screening
        Serial Tasks
        Oral Reading
        Speech Sampling
        S/Z Ratio
        Velopharyngeal Function
        Stimulability of Improved Voice
        Use of Instrumentation

Oral-facial Examination

Hearing Assessment

Determining the Diagnosis

Providing Information (written report, interview, etc.)

SCREENING

A screen for voice disorders can be accomplished with a few quick and easy tasks. For example, have the client imitate words or phrases, count, recite the alphabet, read a short passage, or talk conversationally. Wilson (1987) recommends these four steps to screen children for voice disorders:

1. Count from 1 to 10.
2. Read orally for one minute.
3. Produce continuous speech for one minute.
4. Prolong the following vowels for five seconds each: /ɑ/, /ʌ/, /i/, /u/, /æ/.

This sample is then evaluated according to the screening guidelines in Table 8–2. Any rating of 2 or greater is an indication that further evaluative measures or a rescreen at a later time should be pursued.

Table 8–2. Buffalo III Voice Screening Profile

	Normal	Mild	Moderate	Severe	Very Severe
Laryngeal Tone Breathy Harsh Hoarse	1	2	3	4	5
Pitch Too High Too Low	1	2	3	4	5
Loudness Too Loud Too Soft	1	2	3	4	5
Nasal Resonance Hypernasal Hyponasal	1	2	3	4	5
Overall Voice Rating	1	2	3	4	5

Comments _____

_____

Follow-Up   No   Yes   If yes, dates _____

Source: From D. K Wilson, *Voice Problems of Children* (3rd ed.), p. 97. Baltimore: Williams & Wilkins. Copyright © 1987 and used by permission.

The screening procedure from the *Boone Voice Program for Children* (Boone, 1986) is also useful. Boone utilizes a 3-point scale to evaluate the basic parameters of voice, as shown in Table 8–3. If any response is not scored as normal, the client fails the screen and is referred for a complete voice evaluation. Boone also recommends completing an s/z ratio analysis for a thorough screen. The s/z ratio is described later in this chapter.

Other materials provided in this book are also helpful screening tools. We recommend one or more of the following:

- "Pictures" (pp. 100–103)
- "Narratives With Pictures" (pp. 104–111)
- "Reading Passages" (pp. 122–124)

Table 8–3. A Three-Point Scoring System for Screening Voice Disorders

	–	N	+
Pitch	Too low	Normal	Too high
Loudness	Inadequate	Normal	Too loud
Quality	Hoarse/Breathy	Normal	Tight/Harsh
Nasal Resonance	Denasal	Normal	Hypernasal
Oral Resonance	Excessive posterior tongue carriage resulting in inadequate oral resonance	Normal	Excessive front-of the-mouth tongue resulting in "thin" or "babyish" quality

Source: From D. R Boone, *The Boone Voice Program for Children: Screening, Evaluation, and Referral* (p. 6). Austin, TX: PRO-ED. Copyright © 1986 and used by permission.

NEED FOR MEDICAL EVALUATION

Boone and McFarlane (1988) suggest that:

> Occasional voice patients, such as those who do not talk loud enough or those who use aberrant pitch levels for what appear to be functional reasons, may not require medical evaluation. Patients with voice quality and resonance problems generally require some medical evaluation of the ears, nose, and throat as part of the total voice evaluation. . . . A laryngeal examination must be made before a patient can begin voice therapy for problems related to quality or resonance. . . . Voice therapy efforts should be deferred until a medical examination (which would include laryngoscopy) is concluded, because there are occasional laryngeal pathologies, such as papilloma or carcinoma, for which voice therapy would be strongly contraindicated. In such cases, the delay of accurate diagnosis of these pathologies could be life-threatening. (pp. 104–105).

Clearly, a medical evaluation is indicated for most clients with voice problems.

EXAMINING THE VOICE

To complete a thorough assessment of voice, it is important that you collect a representative sample of your client's speech. Specific procedures for collecting a speech sample were described in Chapter 4. The "Conversation Starters for Eliciting a Speech-Language Sample" (pp. 98-99), "Pictures" (pp. 100–103), "Narratives With Pictures" (pp. 104–111), and "Reading Passages" (pp. 122–124) are a few recommended speech sampling resource materials. You can also ask the client to perform serial tasks, such as count to 20, name the days of the week, name the months of the year, or recite the alphabet. Regardless of the procedure used to collect the sample, it is important that you focus on the following areas:

- Pitch, Intensity, and Quality;
- Resonance;
- Prosody;
- Vocal habits (including abusive behaviors); and
- Respiratory support for speech.

The "Vocally Abusive Behaviors Checklist" (Form 8–1) provides a list of many behaviors that lead to voice disorders. Evaluate these behaviors during speech sampling or during an information-getting interview. You can fill the form out yourself or ask your client to complete the form. Form 8–2, the "Vocal Characteristics Checklist," is designed to help you identify specific deficits of voice your client exhibits during speech.

Form 8–1. Vocally Abusive Behaviors Checklist

Name: _____ Age:_____ Date:_____

Examiner: _____

Instructions: Have the client evaluate each behavior according to the rating scale. Use the comments column on the right-hand side to add any additional, relevant information.

1 = never
2 = infrequently
3 = occasionally
4 = frequently
5 = always

Comments

_____ alcohol consumption _____

_____ arcade talking _____

_____ arguing with peers, siblings, others _____

_____ athletic activities involving yelling _____

_____ breathing through the mouth _____

_____ caffeine products used (coffee, chocolate, etc.) _____

_____ calling others from a distance _____

_____ cheerleading or pep squad participation _____

_____ coughing or sneezing loudly _____

_____ crying _____

_____ dairy products used _____

_____ debate team participation _____

_____ environmental irritants exposure _____

_____ grunting during exercise or lifting _____

_____ inhalants used _____

_____ laughing hard and abusively _____

_____ nightclub social talking _____

_____ participation in plays _____

(continued)

Form 8–1 *(continued)*

Comments

_____ singing in an abusive manner _____

_____ smoking _____

_____ speeches presented _____

_____ talking loudly during menstrual periods _____

_____ talking loudly during respiratory infections _____

_____ talking for extended periods of time _____

_____ talking in noisy environments _____

_____ talking in smoky environments _____

_____ talking while in the car _____

_____ teaching or instructing _____

_____ telephone used _____

_____ vocalizing toy or animal noises _____

_____ vocalizing under muscular tension _____

_____ yelling or screaming_____

_____ other _____

Form 8–2. Vocal Characteristics Checklist

Name: _____ Age:_____ Date:_____

Examiner: _____

Instructions: Check each characteristic your client exhibits and indicate severity. Make additional comments on the right-hand side of the page.

1 = mild
2 = moderate
3 = severe

Pitch   **Comments**

_____ too high_____

_____ too low _____

_____ monotone _____

_____ limited variation _____

_____ excessive variation _____

_____ pitch breaks _____

_____ diplophonia _____

Loudness

_____ too loud_____

_____ too soft or quiet _____

_____ monoloudness _____

_____ limited variation _____

_____ excessive variation _____

Phonatory-based Quality

_____ breathy voice _____

_____ shrill voice _____

_____ strident voice _____

_____ harsh voice _____

_____ hoarse voice _____

(continued)

Form 8–2 *(continued)*

Phonatory-based Quality   **Comments**

_____ quivering voice _____

_____ tremor in the voice _____

_____ weak voice _____

_____ loss of voice _____

_____ glottal fry _____

Nasal Resonance

_____ hypernasal _____

_____ nasal emission _____

_____ assimilation nasality _____

_____ hyponasal (denasal) _____

Oral Resonance

_____ cul-de-sac _____

_____ chesty _____

_____ thin, babyish voice _____

Other

_____ reverse phonation _____

_____ progressively weakening voice _____

_____ aggressive personality factors _____

_____ breathing through the mouth _____

_____ hard glottal attacks _____

_____ inadequate breath support _____

_____ throat clearing _____

_____ disordered intonational patterns _____

_____ disordered stress patterns _____

ASSESSMENT INSTRUMENTATION

Some professional settings are equipped with a variety of instruments and equipment for assessing and treating voice disorders. Other settings have little more than a knowledgeable clinician, a tape recorder and tape, some resource books, and a pencil and paper. Good instrumentation is truly an asset for working with voice, but the absence of it does not preclude offering effective, valuable service.

Some of the more common instruments and procedures used with voice are described briefly in this section. For further information about these and other voice assessment instruments, consult the "Sources of Additional Information" listing at the end of this chapter.

- ☐ *Endoscope*: An endoscope is a small, narrow instrument that is directed into the nares or oral cavity. The assessment procedure is called endoscopy. Oral endoscopy allows a direct view of the larynx or velopharynx. Nasal endoscopy allows a direct view of the larynx only. Videoendoscopy administered orally or nasally can yield a videotape of the observation for review by the clinician and/or client at a later time.

- ☐ *Phonatory Function Analyzer (Nagashima Medical Instruments)*: This instrument measures five parameters of voice: frequency, phonation, intensity, rate of air flow, and volume of air expired.

- ☐ *Visi-Pitch (Kay Elemetrics Corporation)*: A Visi-Pitch is used to evaluate aspects of pitch, including fundamental frequency, frequency range, optimal pitch, and habitual pitch. It can also measure intensity.

- ☐ *PM 100 Pitch Analyzer (Voice Identification, Inc.)*: Like the Visi-Pitch, this instrument measures aspects of pitch.

- ☐ *Fundamental Frequency Indicator (Special Instruments, America)*: This instrument indicates a client's fundamental frequency on a VU meter. It is used for diagnosis and treatment.

- ☐ *Nasometer (Kay Elemetrics Corporation)*: A nasometer provides a visual analysis of the oral-nasal resonance ratio.

- ☐ *Micro Speech Lab, CSpeech, and MacSpeech Lab*: Three computer software programs that are useful for the assessment and treatment of voice disorders.

NORMAL FUNDAMENTAL FREQUENCIES

The fundamental frequency, sometimes called habitual pitch, is the average pitch that a client uses during speaking and reading. A voice disorder is generally present if the client's habitual pitch is two or more tones away from the optimal pitch for his or her age and sex (Prater & Swift, 1984). Tables 8–4 and 8–5 present normal fundamental frequencies for males and females of various ages.

Several methods exist for determining a client's fundamental frequency. Instruments that objectively analyze habitual pitch, such as a Fundamental Frequency Indicator, are available commercially. If you do not have access to such a device, tape record a sample of

Table 8–4. Normal Fundamental Frequencies for Males

	Fundamental Frequency		Acceptable Range for Fundamental Frequency	
Age	Hz	Note	Hz	Notes
1–2	400	G_4	340–470	E_4–$A\#_4$
3	300	D_4	255–360	C_4–$F\#_4$
4	285	$C\#_4$	240–340	B_3–F_4
5	270	$C\#_4$	225–320	A_3–$D\#_4$
6	265	C_4	220–315	A_3–$D\#_4$
7	260	C_4	220–310	A_3–$D\#_4$
8	250	B_3	210–295	$G\#_3$–D_4
9	240	B_3	200–285	G_3–$C\#_4$
10	235	$A\#_3$	195–280	G_3–$C\#_4$
11	230	$A\#_3$	195–275	G_3–$C\#_4$
12	230	$A\#_3$	195–275	G_3–$C\#_4$
13 a[†]	230	$A\#_3$	195–275	G_3–$C\#_4$
13 b[‡]	175	F_3	140–215	$C\#_3$–A_3
14	175	F_3	140–215	$C\#_3$–A_3
15	165	E_3	135–205	D_3–$G\#_3$
16	150	D_3	125–180	B_2–$F\#_3$
17	135	$C\#_3$	115–165	$A\#_2$–E_3
18	125	B_2	105–160	$G\#_2$–D_3

[†]13a = less mature
[‡]13b = more mature

Source: From D. K. Wilson, *Voice Problems of Children* (3rd ed.), p. 119. Baltimore: Williams & Wilkins. Copyright © 1987 and used by permission.

the client's speech. Then use a musical instrument like a piano or pitch pipe to match the instrument's pitch with the client's pitch at several different places in the sample. An average can be determined from those pitches. If tape recordings are made, it is especially important to have a high-quality tape recorder with good batteries; otherwise the tape speed may be too slow, thus altering the client's actual pitches.

One of the quickest ways to *estimate* a client's habitual pitch for screening purposes is to ask a yes-no question and have the client respond with "mmm-hhmm" (yes) or "hhmmm-mmm" (no). The pitch that the client uses for the "mmm" syllable is often the client's habitual pitch.

Table 8–5. Normal Fundamental Frequencies for Females

Age	Fundamental Frequency		Acceptable Range for Fundamental Frequency	
	Hz	**Note**	**Hz**	**Notes**
1–2	400	G_4	340–470	E_4–$A\#_4$
3	300	D_4	255–360	C_4–$F\#_4$
4	285	$C\#_4$	240–340	B_3–F_4
5	270	$C\#_4$	230–325	$A\#_4$–$D\#_4$
6	265	C_4	225–315	A_3–$D\#_4$
7	260	C_4	220–310	A_3–$D\#_4$
8	255	C_4	215–300	A_3–D_4
9	245	B_3	205–290	$G\#_3$–D_4
10	245	B_3	205–290	$G\#_3$–D_4
11	240	B_3	200–285	G_3–$C\#_4$
12	240	B_3	200–280	G_3–$C\#_4$
13 a[†]	240	B_3	200–280	G_3–$C\#_4$
13 b[‡]	225	A_3	195–275	$F\#_3$–$C\#_4$
14	225	A_3	190–270	$F\#_3$–$C\#_4$
15	220	A_3	185–260	$F\#_3$–C_4
16	215	A_3	180–255	$F\#_3$–C_4
17	210	$G\#_3$	175–250	F_3–B_3
18	205	$G\#_3$	175–245	F_3–B_3

[†]13a = less mature
[‡]13b = more mature

Source: From D. K. Wilson, *Voice Problems of Children* (3rd ed.), p. 120. Baltimore: Williams & Wilkins. Copyright © 1987 and used by permission.

ASSESSING BREATHING AND BREATH SUPPORT

Good breath support is a critical element of a good voice. Some clients with voice disorders will have developed poor breathing habits. It is important to identify undesirable habits during the assessment process in order to complete a thorough diagnostic evaluation. People tend to use one of three breathing patterns when they speak:

1. *Clavicular.* This pattern primarily relies on the neck accessory muscles, providing very poor respiratory support for speech. The shoulders elevate during inhalation and breathing may be effortful. Clavicular breathing is the least efficient breathing pattern, particularly for speech.

2. *Thoracic.* This pattern relies on the thoracic muscles, which provide adequate respiratory support for speech. The chest usually expands and contracts on inhalation and exhalation. Thoracic breathing is the most common of the three breathing patterns.

3. *Diaphragmatic-thoracic.* This pattern utilizes the lower thoracic and abdominal muscles, providing optimal respiratory support for speech. Very little, if any, chest movement occurs. Most people do not use diaphragmatic-thoracic breathing naturally; those who do have often been trained in its use (e.g., during musical training).

Detecting a clearly identifiable pattern may be difficult with some clients. St. Louis and Ruscello (1987) question the reliability and accuracy of making judgments about the type of breathing used. In our view, these patterns are identifiable with many (but not all) clients, and the information is valuable in some instances. The "Identification of Breathing Patterns" worksheet (Form 8–3) is based in part on information from Boone and McFarlane (1994), Prater and Swift (1984), and Shipley (1990). Observe the client during any speech task (conversation, reading, reciting, etc.) and note the breathing pattern used most frequently. A section for assessing breath support in varying tasks is also included on the worksheet. A client with a breathing deficiency for speech will have increased difficulty with longer speech tasks.

Form 8–3. Identification of Breathing Patterns

Name: _____ Age:_____ Date:_____

Examiner: _____

Instructions: Identify the type of breathing your client exhibits in Part I. Then rate the behaviors listed in Part II according to severity, using the right-hand side for comments or observations.

PART I: TYPE OF BREATHING

Normal (Nonspeech)	**During Speech**	
_____	_____	*Clavicular*: The shoulders elevate during inhalation. The neck-accessory muscles are the primary muscles of inhalation. Effortful breathing (particularly on inhalation) may be noted.
_____	_____	*Diaphragmatic-thoracic*: The lower thoracic and abdominal muscles are used. There may be little, if any, chest movement.
_____	_____	*Thoracic*: Appears somewhere between clavicular and diaphragmatic-thoracic breathing. Chest movement may be noted.

PART II: BREATH SUPPORT FOR SPEECH

1 = mild difficulties
2 = moderate difficulties
3 = severe difficulties

Comments

_____ Count from 1 to 100_____

_____ Recite the alphabet _____

_____ Name the days of the week _____

_____ Name the months of the year _____

_____ Maintain gradual, slow inspiration _____

_____ Maintain gradual, slow expiration _____

_____ Sustain "ah" as long as possible _____

_____ Imitate phrases or sentences of increasing length _____

_____ Read phrases or sentences of increasing length _____

THE S/Z RATIO

An assessment task that helps assess a client's respiratory and phonatory efficiency is the s/z ratio (Boone & McFarlane, 1994; Eckel & Boone, 1981). Ask the client to sustain each phoneme as you use a stopwatch to calculate the maximum number of seconds your client is able to produce each sound. The normal, average sustained /s/ production is approximately 10 seconds in children and 20–25 seconds in adults (Prater & Swift, 1984). Instructions to the client are as follows:

"Take a breath and make the longest /s/ you can, like this, /s------------s/" (model the target response). After the patient produces the sustained /s/, say "Good! Now do it one more time, and see if you can make the /s/ even longer."

After the sustained /s/ production is measured a minimum of two times, repeat the instructions using /z/. Model the target response as before and obtain at least two productions.

Compare the longest /s/ production with the longest /z/ production. Determine an s/z ratio by dividing the /s/ by the /z/. For example:

$$\frac{\text{longest /s/} = 20 \text{ seconds}}{\text{longest /z/} = 20 \text{ seconds}} = 1.0 \text{ s/z ratio}$$

or

$$\frac{\text{longest /s/} = 15 \text{ seconds}}{\text{longest /z/} = 15 \text{ seconds}} = 1.25 \text{ s/z ratio}$$

Once you have obtained the s/z ratio, use the interpretation guidelines below to determine the ratio's clinical significance. This information is adapted from Prater and Swift (1984).

- A 1.0 ratio with normal duration of productions of /s/ and /z/ (approximately 10 seconds for children and 20–25 seconds for adults) suggests normal respiratory ability and the absence of a vocal fold pathology.

- A 1.0 ratio with reduced duration of /s/ and /z/ indicates possible respiratory inefficiency. The patient may have a reduced vital capacity or poor control of expiration.

- An s/z ratio of 1.2 or greater with normal duration of the /s/ production indicates possible vocal fold pathology. Unlike /s/, the voiced /z/ requires phonation. Therefore, unequal phonatory control of the /s/ and /z/ is indicative of a laryngeal pathology rather than a respiratory problem. The higher the s/z ratio is above 1.0, the greater the likelihood of laryngeal pathology. For example, Eckel and Boone (1981) reported that 95% of their subjects with vocal fold pathology scored 1.4 or greater while normal controls approximated a 1.0 ratio.

ASSESSING RESONANCE

The following speech tasks are provided to help you identify the presence of hypernasality, hyponasality, and/or assimilation nasality. These three resonance problems are often detected through careful listening. However, if you need more objective and reliable information, use instruments such as a nasometer, spirometer, or accelerometer.

We also recommend using a nasal listening tube when evaluating nasal resonance problems.[1] This inexpensive, easy-to-use device channels energy from the client's nasal cavity directly into the clinician's ear. The intensified sound makes it much easier to identify a resonance problem. A nasal listening tube also allows you to test each naris separately, so you can obtain more discriminative information.

Hypernasality

Occlude the client's nares and instruct him or her to recite *nonnasal* words and phrases such as the sample phrases below. If excessive nasal pressure is felt, or if nasopharyngeal "snorting" is heard, suspect hypernasality.

This horse eats grass.

I saw the teacher at church.

Sister Suzie sat by a thistle.

The nonnasal words and phrases provided in the "Pressure Consonants" section on pages 277–278 or in the "Syllable-by-Syllable Stimulus Phrases" on pages 119–121 can be used for a more complete assessment.

Methods for identifying hypernasality without occluding the nares also exist. For example, carefully listen for nasality or hold a mirror under the nostrils and look for clouding as air moves through the nose. These less invasive techniques are usually not as effective as occluding the nares.

Hyponasality

Instruct the client to recite each of the phrases with *nasal* sounds on the next page; then occlude the patient's nares and repeat the task. If the client's unoccluded and occluded productions sound the same, hyponasality (denasality) is present.

---

[1]A nasal listening tube can be made by attaching a nasal olive to each end of surgical tubing. The tubing (preferably 3/4" in diameter) is usually about 30" long. These supplies can be purchased for a few dollars through a medical/surgical supplier.

Manny made me mad.

My name means money.

Momma made some lemon jam.

Mommy made money on Monday.

To differentiate between hypernasality and hyponasality, instruct the patient to rapidly repeat the phrase below. If both words sound like maybe, hypernasality is present. If both words sound like baby, hyponasality is present (Boone & McFarlane, 1988). With the following phrase, the /m/ and /b/ is very discernible in normal speech. When the words all sound like "maybe," this usually indicates hypernasality. When all words sound like "baby," this is typically hyponasality.

maybe, baby, maybe, baby, maybe, baby

Assimilation Nasality

Assimilation nasality occurs when sounds that precede or follow a nasal consonant are also nasalized. To evaluate, instruct the client to recite the following words and phrases while listening carefully for the presence of assimilation nasality. Pay particular attention to the client's speech rate in relation to the severity of his or her resonance problem. Is the assimilation nasality more noticeable at a faster speech rate? Is it eliminated at a reduced speech rate?

Phrases with Nasal Sounds

mail
pan
him
alone
funny
honeycomb

alone again
another night
Mickey Mouse
midnight madness

next time he can
My neighbor is nice.
His son made a home run.
They cannot come tonight.
Can you make my lunch tomorrow?
The singer sang with the entire gang.

Phrases with Multiple Nasal Sounds

man
many
woman

many men
my mommy
many women
my imagination

man on the moon
home on the range
My mom made me mad.
Mickey and Minnie Mouse
Manny wouldn't mind singing.
My mommy made some lemon jam.
Manny's mommy made me mad on Monday.

ASSESSING VELOPHARYNGEAL FUNCTION

In most cases, valid estimates of velopharyngeal function can be made without the benefit of sophisticated instrumentation. Use the "Pressure Consonants" and the "Modified Tongue Anchor Procedure" to assess the function of the velopharyngeal mechanism. The 16 pressure consonants require a great amount of intraoral air pressure. Insufficient velopharyngeal abilities may result in nasal emissions and hypernasality, particularly on the pressure consonants (Boone & McFarlane, 1994; Morris, Spriestersbach, & Darley, 1961; Shipley, 1990).

The Pressure Consonants

Use the following nonnasal words, phrases, and sentences to detect nasal emissions and hypernasality.

/p/	paper	pepper	top
	Pass the pepper.	papa's puppy	up top
	Please put the supper up.		
/b/	Bob	baby	bib
	baby's tub	baby's bib	the bear cub
	Baby's bib is by the tub.		
/k/	cake	hockey	kick
	Kathy's cake	kid's breakfast	broke his truck
	Katie's breakfast was cake.		
/g/	gave	forgot	hug
	Give it here.	Go get the sugar.	big hog
	Gary gave sugar to the dog.		

/t/	two	guitar	hat
	tabletop	top hotel	hit the light
	Terry took the top hat.		

/d/	day	today	good
	Dave did it.	Ted cried	good bread
	Dick was louder with David.		

/f/	fall	laughter	off
	feed father	before relief	half a loaf
	Fred carefully fed his calf.		

/v/	view	review	five
	very evil	every cover	have to drive
	Vicki loves to drive.		

/s/	sit	icy	house
	Suzie said so.	It's icy.	It's rice.
	Sarah spilled the sausage by the box.		

/z/	zero	busy	his
	Zack is lazy.	Easy does it.	those eyes
	Zack was too busy to choose.		

/ʃ/	ship	ashes	wish
	ship-shape	wishy-washy	fresh radish
	She washed a bushel of fish.		

/ʒ/	visual	usual	prestige
	beige corsage	visual pleasure	usual prestige
	a casual corsage		

/tʃ/	chalk	teacher	batch
	child's chair	richest butcher	each pitch
	Chip reached for the teacher's watch.		

/θ/	thought	birthday	bath
	thirsty father	third birthday	through both
	Thought I'd get a toothbrush for both.		

/ð/	they	father	bathe
	their father	the leather	They bathe.
	Their other brother likes to bathe.		

The Modified Tongue Anchor Procedure

Fox and Johns (1970) described a simple procedure for assessing velopharyngeal function. Their approach is called the modified tongue anchor technique.

1. Tell the client to "puff up your cheeks like this." Then puff up your cheeks and hold the air in the oral cavity to model the behavior.
2. Tell the client to stick out his or her tongue as you hold the anterior portion with a sterile gauze pad.
3. While you are holding the tongue, tell the client to puff up the cheeks again. Say "Puff up your cheeks again, like you did the first time. I will help you by holding your nose so the air doesn't get out." Then gently pinch your client's nose closed.
4. Tell the client to continue holding the air in the cheeks as you release the nostrils.
5. As the nostrils are released, listen for nasal emission. Velopharyngeal seal is considered *adequate* if the air does not escape through the open nostrils. It is considered *inadequate* if air leaks out.
6. Complete a minimum of three trials to be sure the client understands the task and to verify your observations.

STIMULABILITY

Stimulability for the voice client focuses on the deficiencies identified on the "Vocal Characteristics Checklist" (Form 8–2). Stimulating normal voice may be difficult depending on the severity of the disorder. With more severe cases, you may only be able to stimulate improvements or approximations of the desired target behavior, which will then need to be refined and shaped in therapy. Boone and McFarlane (1994) and Prater and Swift (1984) are excellent resources for stimulation techniques. Other recommended resources are Case (1991), Colton and Casper (1996), Shipley (1990), and Wilson (1987).

CONCLUDING COMMENTS

There are multiple aspects to consider when evaluating voice and resonance. An adequate case history, which can be taken from a questionnaire or interview, is essential. Many disorders of voice or resonance are caused by an organic etiology that has a medically related history. Other disorders are functionally based, caused by "faulty usage"or behavioral histories. For most voice disorders, a medical evaluation that includes observation of the vocal folds is needed before commencing therapy.

The evaluation of voice and resonance is multifaceted. The clinician detects and identifies the vocal behaviors that are abnormal. These behaviors become the basis for determining whether a problem exists and, if so, what vocal behaviors require attention.

SOURCES OF ADDITIONAL INFORMATION

Evaluation and Therapy

Andrews, M. L. (1995). *Manual of voice treatment: Pediatrics through geriatrics*. San Diego: Singular Publishing Group.

Aronson, A. E. (1990). *Clinical voice disorders: An interdisciplinary approach* (3rd ed.). New York: Thieme.

Boone, D. R. (1986). *The Boone voice program for children: Screening, evaluation, and referral*. Austin, TX: PRO-ED.

Boone, D. R., & McFarlane, S. C. (1994). *The voice and voice therapy* (5th ed.). Englewood Cliffs, NJ: Prentice-Hall.

Brown, W. S., Vinson, B. P., & Crary, M. A. (Eds.). (1996). *Organic voice disorders: Assessment and treatment*. San Diego, Singular Publishing Group.

Case, J. L. (1991). *Clinical management of voice disorders* (2nd ed.). Austin, TX: PRO-ED.

Colton, R. H., & Casper, J. K. (1996). *Understanding voice problems: A physiological perspective for diagnosis and treatment* (2nd ed.). Baltimore: Williams & Wilkins.

Emerick, L. L., & Haynes, W. O. (1986). *Diagnosis and evaluation in speech pathology* (3rd ed.). Englewood Cliffs, NJ: Prentice-Hall.

Johnson, T. S. (1985). *Vocal abuse reduction program*. Austin, TX: PRO-ED.

Peterson, H. A., & Marquardt, T. P. (1994). *Appraisal and diagnosis of speech and language disorders* (3rd ed.). Englewood Cliffs, NJ: Prentice-Hall.

Shipley, K. G. (1990). *Systematic assessment of voice*. Oceanside, CA: Academic Communication Associates.

Stemple, J. C. (1992). *Clinical voice management: Techniques for children*. St. Louis: MosbyYear Book.

Stemple, J. C., Glaze, L. E., & Gerdeman, B. K. (1995). *Clinical voice pathology: Theory and management* (2nd ed.). San Diego: Singular Publishing Group.

Wilson, F. B., & Rice, M. (1977). *A programmed approach to voice therapy*. Allen, TX: DLM/Teaching Resources.

Wilson, D. K. (1987). *Voice problems of children* (3rd ed.). Baltimore: Williams & Wilkins.

Instrumentation & Equipment

Boone, D. R., & McFarlane, S. C. (1988). *The voice and voice therapy* (4th ed.). Englewood Cliffs, NJ: Prentice-Hall.

Colton, R. H., & Casper, J. K (1996). *Understanding voice problems: A physiological perspective for diagnosis and treatment* (2nd ed.). Baltimore: Williams & Wilkins.

Decker, T. N. (1990). *Instrumentation: An introduction for students in the speech and hearing sciences*. New York: Longman.

Stemple, J. C., Glaze, L. E., & Gerdeman, B. K. (1995). *Clinical voice pathology: Theory and management* (2nd ed.). San Diego: Singular Publishing Group.

Stimulability

Boone, D. R., & McFarlane, S. C. (1988). *The voice and voice therapy* (4th ed.). Englewood Cliffs, NJ: Prentice-Hall.

Brown, W. S., Vinson, B. P., & Crary, M. A. (Eds.). (1996). *Organic voice disorders: Assessment and treatment*. San Diego, Singular Publishing Group.

Case, J. L. (1991). *Clinical management of voice disorders* (2nd ed.). Austin, TX: PRO-ED.

Colton, R. H., & Casper, J. K. (1996). *Understanding voice problems: A physiological perspective for diagnosis and treatment* (2nd ed.). Baltimore: Williams & Wilkins.

Prater, R. J., & Swift, R. W. (1984). *Manual of voice therapy*. Boston: Little, Brown and Co.

Shipley, K. G. (1990). *Systematic assessment of voice*. Oceanside CA: Academic Communication Associates.

Wilson, D. K. (1987). *Voice problems of children* (3rd ed.). Baltimore: Williams & Wilkins.

Internet Sources

National Institute on Deafness and Other Communication Disorders
http://www.nih.gov/nidcd

□ CHAPTER 9 □

Assessment of Neurologically Based Communicative Disorders

- Overview of Assessment
- The Cranial Nerves
- Differential Characteristics of Dysarthria and Apraxia
- Assessment of Dysarthria
- Assessment of Apraxia
    Development Apraxia of Speech
- Assessment of Aphasia
- Appendix 9–A Evaluation of Aphasia
- Assessment of Right Hemisphere Dysfunction
- Assessment of Traumatic Brain Injury
- Assessment of Dementia
- Concluding Comments
- Sources of Additional Information

This chapter focuses on six types of neurologically based communicative disorders: dysarthria, apraxia, aphasia, traumatic brain injury, dementia, and right hemisphere dysfunction. Apraxia and dysarthria are motor speech disorders that affect expressive speech abilities. Aphasia is characterized by expressive and/or receptive language impairment. Disorders such as dysarthria and apraxia often occur simultaneously with aphasia.

As the name implies, traumatic brain injury (TBI) is a traumatic insult that occurs to the brain. The result of this injury is impairment of cortical function. Since the brain is the headquarters for all communicative abilities, various disruptions of communication occur.

OVERVIEW OF ASSESSMENT

History of the Client

    Procedures

        Written Case History
        Information-getting Interview
        Information from Other Professionals

    Contributing Factors

        Medical Diagnosis
        Pharmacological Factors
        Age
        Intelligence, Motivation, and Levels of Concern

Assessment of Dysarthria and Apraxia

    Procedures

        Screening
        Speech Sampling
        Motor-speech Assessment
        Stimulability of Errors
        Formal Testing

    Analysis

        Type of Errors
        Consistency of Errors
        Intelligibility
        Rate of Speech
        Prosody

Assessment of Aphasia

    Procedures

        Screening
        Speech and Language Sampling
        Formal Testing
        Cognitive Skills Evaluation

Analysis

    Expressive/Receptive Abilities
    Types of Errors
    Intelligibility

Assessment of Right Hemisphere Dysfunction

    Procedures

        Screening
        Speech and Language Sampling
        Formal Testing
        Cognitive Skills Evaluation

    Analysis

        Cognitive-Linguistic Abilities
        Types of Errors
        Visual-Perceptual Abilities

Assessment of Traumatic Brain Injury

    Procedures

        Screening
        Speech and Language Sampling
        Formal Testing
        Cognitive Skills Evaluation

    Analysis

        Expressive/Receptive Abilities
        Types of Errors
        Intelligibility

Assessment of Dementia

    Procedures
        Screening
        Behavioral Observations
        Formal Testing

    Analysis

        Expressive-Receptive Abilities
        Severity of Impairment
        Functional Potential

Oral-facial Examination

Hearing Assessment

Determining the Diagnosis

Providing Information (written report, interview, etc.)

THE CRANIAL NERVES

The 12 cranial nerves perform the critical task of sending sensory and motor information to all the muscles of the body. It is helpful to have an understanding of these nerves and their functions when assessing neurological impairments. Table 9–1 is based on information from Love and Webb (1992); Nicolosi, Harryman, and Kresheck (1989); and Palmer and Yantis (1990). The cranial nerves that are directly related to speech, language, swallowing, or hearing are indicated with an asterisk in the table.

Table 9–1. The Cranial Nerves—Types and Functions

Nerve	Type	Function	
I	Olfactory	Sensory	Smell
II	Optic	Sensory	Vision
III	Oculomotor	Motor	Movement of eyeball, pupil, upper eyelid
IV	Trochlear	Motor	Movement of superior oblique eye muscle
V*	Trigeminal	Mixed	Tactile facial sensation, movement of muscles for chewing
VI	Abducens	Motor	Open the eyes
VII*	Facial	Mixed	Taste, movement of facial muscles
VIII*	Acoustic	Sensory	Hearing and equilibrium
IX*	Glossopharyngeal	Mixed	Taste, gag, elevation of palate and larynx for swallow
X*	Vagus	Mixed	Taste, elevation of palate, movement of pharynx and larynx
XI*	Accessory	Motor	Turn head, shrug shoulders, movement of palate, pharynx, and larynx
XII*	Hypoglossal	Motor	Movement of tongue

*Indicates nerves that are most directly related to speech, language, swallowing, or hearing.

DIFFERENTIAL CHARACTERISTICS OF DYSARTHRIA AND APRAXIA

Dysarthria and apraxia are both motor speech disorders that affect verbal expression. These disorders are sometimes confused with one another, especially by beginning clinicians. However, their symptoms are actually quite different. It is important to understand the differences between the two disorders to make an appropriate diagnosis. The general differences between dysarthria and apraxia are outlined below. This information is based on information from Darley et al. (1975); Duffy (1995); LaPointe and Wertz (1974); Weiss, Gordon, and Lillywhite (1987); and Wertz, LaPointe, and Rosenbek (1991).

Dysarthria:

- All processes of speech are affected (including respiration, phonation, resonance, articulation, and prosody).

- There is a change in muscle tone secondary to neurologic involvement that results in difficulty with voluntary and involuntary motor tasks (such as swallowing, chewing, and licking).

- Speech errors result from a disruption in muscular control of the central and/or peripheral nervous systems.

- Errors of speech are consistent and predictable. There are no islands of clear speech.

- Articulatory errors are primarily distortions and omissions.

- Consonant productions are consistently imprecise; vowels may be neutralized.

Apraxia:

- The speech process for articulation is primarily affected. Prosody may also be abnormal.

- There is a change in motor programming for speech secondary to neurologic involvement, but muscle tone is not affected. Involuntary motor tasks typically are not affected.

- Speech errors result from a disruption of the message from the motor cortex to the oral musculature.

- Errors of speech are inconsistent and unpredictable. Islands of clear, well-articulated speech exist.

- Articulatory errors are primarily substitutions, repetitions, additions, transpositions, prolongations, omissions, and distortions (which are least common). Most errors are close approximations of the targeted phoneme. Errors are often perseveratory or anticipatory.

- Consonants are more difficult than vowels; blends are more difficult than singletons; initial consonants are more difficult than final consonants; fricatives and affricates are the most difficult consonants. Errors increase as the complexity of the motor pattern increases.

Dysarthria *(continued)*

- The speech rate is slow and labored; strain, tension, and poor breath support may be apparent.

- Speech intelligibility is reduced as the speaking rate increases.

- Increases in word/phrase complexity result in poorer articulatory performance.

Apraxia *(continued)*

- A prosodic disorder may occur as a result of compensatory behaviors (stopping, restarting, and difficulty initiating phonation and/or correct articulatory postures).

- Speech intelligibility sometimes increases as the speaking rate increases.

- Increases in word/phrase complexity result in poorer articulatory performance.

ASSESSMENT OF DYSARTHRIA

Dysarthria is a motor speech disorder that results from muscular impairment. Muscular weakness, slowness, or incoordination can affect all the basic processes of speech—respiration, phonation, resonance, articulation, and prosody. Articulation errors are the most common feature of dysarthria, followed by impairments of voice, resonance, and fluency. Dysarthria is sometimes confused with apraxia of speech, also a motor speech disorder associated with expressive speech impairment, but the two disorders are quite different. A primary differentiating characteristic is that dysarthria is associated with muscular impairment; apraxia of speech is not.

There are six types of dysarthria, each characterized by a different etiology and different speech behaviors. During a diagnostic evaluation, it is easy to confuse the dysarthrias, as many of their characteristics overlap and more than one type may be present. Drs. Arnold Aronson and Frederick Darley of the Mayo Clinic pioneered research into the differential characteristics of the dysarthrias. Their work has led to a standard classification system for identifying the different dysarthrias in clinical practice. A summary of their work and a listing of potential etiologies for each dysarthria are presented in Table 9–2.

Table 9–2. Differentiating the Six Dysarthrias

Type	Site of Lesion	Possible Causes	Primary Speech Characteristics
Flaccid	Lower motor neuron	Viral infection Tumor CVA Congenital conditions Disease Palsies Trauma	Hypernasality Imprecise consonants Breathiness Monopitch Nasal emission
Spastic	Upper motor neuron	CVA Tumor Infection Trauma Congenital condition	Imprecise consonants Monopitch Reduced stress Harsh voice quality Monoloudness Low pitch Slow rate Hypernasality Strained-strangled voice Short phrases
Mixed (flaccid and spastic)	Upper and lower motor neuron	Amyotrophic lateral sclerosis Trauma CVA	Imprecise consonants Hypernasality Harsh voice quality Slow rate Monopitch Short phrases Distorted vowels Low pitch Monoloudness Excess and equal stress Prolonged intervals
Ataxic	Cerebellar system	CVA Tumor Trauma Congenital condition Infection Toxic effects	Imprecise consonants Excess and equal stress Irregular articulatory breakdowns Distorted vowels Harsh voice Loudness control problems Variable nasality
Hypokinetic	Extrapyramidal system	Parkinsonism Drug-induced	Monopitch Reduced stress Monoloudness Imprecise consonants Inappropriate silences Short rushes of speech Harsh voice Breathy voice

(continued)

Table 9–2 *(continued)*

Type	Site of Lesion	Possible Causes	Primary Speech Characteristics
Hyperkinetic	Extrapyramidal system	Chorea Infection Gilles de la Tourette syndrome Ballism Athetosis CVA Tumor Dystonia Drug-induced Dyskinesia	Imprecise consonants Distorted vowels Harsh voice quality Irregular articulatory breakdowns Strained-strangled voice Monopitch Monoloudness

Source: Information based on material presented in Darley, Aronson, and Brown (1975). This table is from R. T. Wertz, "Neuropathologies of Speech and Language: An Introduction to Patient Management." In D. F. Johns (Ed.), *Clinical Management of Neurogenic Communication Disorders* (2nd ed., pp. 76–77). Boston: Little, Brown and Co. Copyright © 1985 and used by permission.

To complete an assessment of dysarthria, it is important to obtain a complete oral-facial examination and a good speech sample at structured levels (according to syllabic length) and in continuous speech. These samples will be the basis for identifying the primary speech characteristics your client exhibits. Suggestions for obtaining a speech sample are found in other sections of this book. We also recommend using the "Reading Passages" (pp. 122–124) and "Syllable-by-Syllable Stimulus Phrases" (pp. 119–121). Use Form 9–1, "Identifying Dysarthria," to analyze your client's speech and identify the type of dysarthria present. Formal tests such as Enderby's (1983) *Frenchay Dysarthria Assessment* or Yorkston, Beukelman, and Traynor's (1984) *Assessment of Intelligibility of Dysarthric Speech* are also useful.

Form 9–1. Identifying Dysarthria[1]

Name: _____ Age: _____ Date: _____

Examiner:_____

Instructions: Identify the speech characteristics noted during the speech sample.

Flaccid Dysarthria (lower motor neuron involvement)

_____ Hypernasality

_____ Imprecise consonants

_____ Breathiness

_____ Monopitch

_____ Nasal emission

Spastic Dysarthria (upper motor neuron involvement)

_____ Imprecise consonants

_____ Monopitch

_____ Reduced stress

_____ Harsh voice quality

_____ Monoloudness

_____ Low pitch

_____ Slow rate

_____ Hypernasality

_____ Strained-strangled voice quality

_____ Short phrases

Mixed Dysarthria (upper and lower motor neuron involvement)

_____ Imprecise consonants

_____ Hypernasality

_____ Harsh voice quality

_____ Slow rate

_____ Monopitch

_____ Short phrases

(continued)

---

[1]From J. C. Rosenbek and L. L. LaPointe, "The Dysarthrias: Diagnosis, Description, and Treatment." In D. F. Johns (Ed.), *Clinical Management of Neurogenic Communication Disorders* (2nd ed., p. 100). Boston: Little, Brown and Co. Copyright © 1985 and used by permission.

Form 9–1.   (*continued*)

_____ Distorted vowels

_____ Low pitch

_____ Monoloudness

_____ Excess and equal stress

_____ Prolonged intervals

Ataxic Dysarthria (cerebellar involvement)

_____ Imprecise consonants

_____ Excess and equal stress

_____ Irregular articulatory breakdowns

_____ Distorted vowels

_____ Harsh voice

_____ Loudness control problems

_____ Variable nasality

Hypokinetic Dysarthria (Parkinsonism)

_____ Monopitch

_____ Reduced stress

_____ Monoloudness

_____ Imprecise consonants

_____ Inappropriate silences

_____ Short rushes of speech

_____ Harsh voice

_____ Breathy voice

Hyperkinetic Dysarthria (Dystonia and Choreathetosis)

_____ Imprecise consonants

_____ Distorted vowels

_____ Harsh voice quality

_____ Irregular articulatory breakdowns

_____ Strained-strangled voice quality

_____ Monopitch

_____ Monoloudness

ASSESSMENT OF APRAXIA

Apraxia, sometimes referred to as *dyspraxia*, is a motor disorder resulting from neurological damage. It is characterized by an inability to execute volitional (purposeful) movements despite having normal muscle tone and coordination. In other words, the muscles are capable of normal functioning but faulty programming from the brain prevents the completion of precise, purposeful movements.

There are three types of apraxia: limb, oral, and verbal. Limb apraxia is associated with volitional movements of the arms and legs. The client may be unable to wave goodbye or make a fist on command (volitionally), even though the muscular strength and range of motion necessary to complete the tasks are present and the client is able to automatically (nonvolitionally) perform the tasks. The client with oral apraxia may be unable to protrude the tongue or smack the lips volitionally. Oral apraxia is sometimes confused with the third type, verbal apraxia, since they both involve oral-facial muscles, but they are not the same. Verbal apraxia is a disorder of motor programming for the production of speech. The client with verbal apraxia has difficulty positioning and sequencing muscles involved in the volitional production of phonemes. Clients may exhibit one, two, or all three types of apraxia. Verbal apraxia is the most common type and limb apraxia is the least common type. Form 9–2, "Checklists for Limb, Oral, and Verbal Apraxia," is provided to help you identify the type(s) of apraxia your client exhibits.

Most of this section on the assessment of apraxia focuses on the assessment of verbal apraxia, also called *apraxia of speech*. Many of the major features of apraxia of speech have been described by Darley (1982); Darley et al. (1975); Duffy (1995); Haynes (1985); Rosenbek (1985); Rosenbek, Kent, and LaPointe (1984); and others. Based in part on these works, Shipley, Recor, and Nakamura (1990) listed 25 characteristics of apraxia of speech with specific diagnostic features and treatment suggestions. Summarized excerpts from their work are presented below:[1]

☐ The number of misarticulations increases as the complexity of the speech task increases.

☐ Misarticulations occur on both consonants and vowels. Articulation errors occur more frequently on consonant clusters than on singletons. Vowels are misarticulated less frequently than consonants.

☐ Sounds in the initial position are affected more often than sounds in the medial or final positions.

☐ The frequency of specific sound errors is related, at least in part, to the frequency of occurrence in speech. More errors are noted with less frequently occurring sounds.

☐ Sound substitutions, omissions, distortions, and additions are all observed. The most frequent misarticulations are substitutions and omissions.

☐ Articulation errors and struggle behaviors increase as the length and complexity of the target word, phrase, or sentence increases.

---

[1]Adapted from K. G. Shipley, D. B. Recor, and S. M. Nakamura, *Sourcebook of Apraxia Remediation Activities* (pp. 2–5). Oceanside, CA: Academic Communication Associates. Copyright © 1990 and used by permission.

☐ Speech production is variable. It is common for a person with apraxia of speech to produce a sound, syllable, word, or phrase correctly on one occasion and then incorrectly on another. It is also common to observe several different misarticulations for the same target sound.

☐ Struggling behaviors (such as groping to position the articulators correctly) are observed in many patients with apraxia of speech.

☐ Automatic speech activities (such as counting to 10 or naming the days of the week) tend to be easier and more error-free than volitional speech. Reactive speech (such as "thank you" or "I'm fine") is also easier for clients with apraxia to produce.

☐ Metathetic errors (errors of sound or syllable transposition) are common. For example, the client may say *snapknack* for *knapsack* or *guspetti* for *spaghetti*.

☐ "Syllable collapses" may occur. Syllable collapses are not commonly reported in the literature, but we have found them to be a common characteristic. The client reduces and/or disrupts the number of syllables in motorically complex words or phrases. For example, a client might say *glost gers* for *Los Angeles Dodgers* or *be neers* for *Tampa Bay Buccaneers*. In both examples, the number of syllables is collapsed and the remaining syllables are inaccurately produced.

☐ Receptive language abilities are often, but not always, superior to expressive abilities. However, the language skills are separate from the apraxia.

☐ People with apraxia of speech are usually aware of their incorrect articulatory productions. Therefore, they may be able to identify many of their own correct and incorrect productions without feedback from the clinician.

☐ Apraxia of speech can occur in isolation or in combination with other communicative disorders such as dysarthria, delayed speech or language development, aphasia, and/or hearing loss.

☐ Oral apraxia and/or limb apraxia may or may not be present with verbal apraxia. In our experience, however, an individual with oral apraxia will also have verbal apraxia.

☐ Severity varies from client to client. We have seen clients who could not volitionally produce a target vowel such as /a/, and others whose speech was fine until they attempted to produce motorically challenging phrases such as *statistical analysis* or *theoretical implications*.

We have provided an "Identifying Apraxia of Speech" worksheet (Form 9–3) to help you confirm or rule out verbal apraxia. Use this worksheet in conjunction with the "Checklists for Limb, Oral, and Verbal Apraxia" for a thorough evaluation. Evaluate your client's speech during automatic speech, spontaneous speech, and oral reading. To obtain a sample of automatic speech, ask the client to count to 50, name the days of the week, name the months of the year, or perform a similar task. To obtain the spontaneous speech sample, ask the client to describe pictures, describe the plot of a movie, or talk about hobbies or other interests. To obtain the oral reading sample, have the patient read a section from a book, a popular magazine, or one or more of the reading passages from pages 122–124 of this manual.

Be sure to compare the errors found in different speech contexts. Clients with apraxia of speech usually exhibit multiple errors in spontaneous speech and oral reading, while fewer or no errors are exhibited during automatic speech. If the patient exhibits an excessive number of errors during automatic speech, dysarthria may be present.

Published tests for the diagnosis of apraxia of speech include:

- *Screening Test for Developmental Apraxia of Speech* (Blakeley, 1980)
- *Apraxia Battery for Adults* (Dabul, 1986)
- *Comprehensive Apraxia Test* (DiSimoni, 1989)

Several aphasia batteries also include subsections for identifying apraxia.

Form 9–2. Checklists for Limb, Oral, and Verbal Apraxia

Name: _____ Age: _____ Date: _____

Examiner: _____

Instructions: Select several items from each section and ask the client to complete the task or repeat the utterance. Many items are provided to offer a wide range of tasks; you do not need to complete each item. Score each presented item as correct (+ or ✔) or incorrect (– or ∅). Transcribe errors phonetically on the right-hand side. Also note accompanying behaviors such as delays with initiation, struggling, groping, or facial grimacing. The diagnosis of apraxia is made by evaluating the nature and accuracy of movement, as well as the type and severity of error patterns present.

Limb Apraxia   **Comments**

_____ wave hello or goodbye _____

_____ make a fist _____

_____ make the "thumbs up" sign _____

_____ make the "okay" sign _____

_____ pretend you're zipping your coat _____

_____ pretend you're combing your hair _____

_____ pretend you're petting a dog _____

_____ pretend you're turning a doorknob _____

_____ pretend you're hitting a baseball (or golf ball) _____

_____ pretend you're tieing a shoe _____

_____ pretend you're using scissors to cut a piece of paper _____

_____ pretend you're knocking on a door _____

_____ pretend you're writing _____

_____ pretend you're going to make a fire _____

_____ pretend you're going to make coffee _____

_____ pretend you're going to drive a car out of a driveway _____

Oral Apraxia   **Comments**

_____ smile _____

_____ open your mouth _____

Oral Apraxia   **Comments**

_____ blow _____

_____ whistle _____

_____ puff out your cheeks _____

_____ show me your teeth _____

_____ chatter your teeth as if you are cold _____

_____ pucker your lips _____

_____ bite your lower lip _____

_____ smack your lips _____

_____ lick your lips _____

_____ stick out your tongue _____

_____ touch your nose with the tip of your tongue _____

_____ move your tongue in and out _____

_____ wiggle your tongue from side to side _____

_____ click your tongue _____

_____ clear your throat _____

_____ cough _____

_____ alternately pucker and smile _____

Verbal Apraxia   **Comments or Transcription**

_____ love—loving—lovingly _____

_____ jab—jabber—jabbering _____

_____ zip—zipper—zippering _____

_____ soft—soften—softening _____

_____ hope—hopeful—hopefully _____

_____ hard—harden—hardening _____

_____ thick—thicken—thickening _____

_____ please—pleasing—pleasingly _____

_____ sit—city—citizen—citizenship _____

_____ cat—catnip—catapult—catastrophe _____

_____ strength—strengthen—strengthening _____

(continued)

Form 9–2. *(continued)*

Verbal Apraxia   **Comments or Transcription**

_____ door—doorknob—doorkeeper—dormitory _____

_____ tornado _____

_____ radiator _____

_____ artillery _____

_____ linoleum _____

_____ inevitable _____

_____ delegation _____

_____ probability _____

_____ cauliflower _____

_____ declaration _____

_____ refrigeration _____

_____ unequivocally _____

_____ thermometer _____

_____ parliamentarian _____

_____ catastrophically _____

_____ disenfranchised _____

_____ statistical analysis _____

_____ alternative opinion _____

_____ regulatory authority _____

_____ ruthlessly malicious _____

_____ barometric pressure _____

_____ indescribably delicious _____

_____ Mississippi River _____

_____ Tallahassee, Florida _____

_____ Kalamazoo, Michigan _____

_____ Boston, Massachusetts _____

_____ Sacramento, California _____

_____ Madison Square Garden _____

_____ Minneapolis, Minnesota _____

_____ Chattanooga, Tennessee _____

_____ Encyclopedia Britannica _____

_____ Saskatoon, Saskatchewan _____

_____ Philadelphia, Pennsylvania _____

_____ Oakland-Alameda Coliseum _____

_____ Vancouver, British Columbia _____

_____ Vancouver, British Columbia _____

_____ Nuclear Regulatory Commission_____

Form 9–3. Identifying Apraxia[1]

Name: _____ Age: _____ Date: _____

Examiner: _____

Instructions: Evaluate each behavior in automatic speech, spontaneous speech, and oral reading. Mark a plus (+) if the client has no difficulty. Use the severity scale if the client does exhibit problems with production. Add comments on the right-hand side as needed.

    1. = mild difficulties
    2. = moderate difficulties
    3. = severe difficulties

Oral Reading	Automatic Speech	Spontaneous Speech		Comments
_____	_____	_____	phonemic anticipatory errors (e.g., *kreen crayon* for *green crayon*)	_____
_____	_____	_____	phonemic perseveratory errors (e.g., *babyb* for *baby*)	_____
_____	_____	_____	phonemic transposition errors (e.g., *snapknack* for *knapsack*)	_____
_____	_____	_____	phonemic voicing errors (e.g., *Paul* for *green ball*)	_____
_____	_____	_____	phonemic vowel errors (e.g., *might* for *meet*)	_____
_____	_____	_____	visible or audible searching	_____
_____	_____	_____	numerous and varied off-target attempts	_____
_____	_____	_____	highly inconsistent errors	_____
_____	_____	_____	errors increase with phonemic complexity	_____
_____	_____	_____	fewer errors in automatic speech	_____
_____	_____	_____	marked difficulties initating speech	_____
_____	_____	_____	intrudes a schwa sound	_____
_____	_____	_____	abnormal prosodic features	_____
_____	_____	_____	aware of errors but difficult to correct	_____
_____	_____	_____	receptive-expressive language gap	_____

---

[1]Adapted from B. Dabul, *Apraxia Battery for Adults*. TX: PRO-ED. Copyright © 1979, 1986 and used by permission.

Developmental Apraxia of Speech

As already stated, apraxia results from damage to the central nervous system. The term *developmental apraxia of speech* (also called *childhood apraxia* or *developmental apraxia*) is sometimes used as a clinical diagnosis with children who exhibit the communicative symptoms associated with apraxia, even though they may not have a specifically identified central nervous system lesion. From a clinical standpoint there is little question that some children do exhibit the speech characteristics of verbal apraxia. Their speech is often delayed, with characteristics similar to apraxia, including struggling behaviors, metathesis, increase in errors in more complex tasks, variable sound productions, and so forth. Improvement in therapy is often very slow. For additional information, descriptions of developmental apraxia are found in works by Blakeley (1980), Haynes (1985), Love (1992), and Yoss and Darley (1974).

If you are completing a diagnostic evaluation on a child with a suspected apraxic disorder, use the same testing materials provided in this manual that you would use for assessing an adult (i.e., "Checklists for Limb, Oral, and Verbal Apraxia" and "Identifying Apraxia"). Of course, you will need to use age-appropriate stimulus items for collecting a reading sample and spontaneous speech sample (see "Reading Passages" on pp. 122–124 or "Conversation Starters for Eliciting a Speech-Language Sample" on pp. 98–99). Other published assessment materials can also be used.

ASSESSMENT OF APHASIA

Aphasia is defined as a loss of language function due to an injury to the brain in an area associated with the comprehension and production of language. Aphasia is most often caused by a stroke, or cerebral vascular accident (CVA). Other etiologies include accident, tumor, infection, and toxicity (Hegde, 1996). Aphasia can have multiple ramifications. Every client will be different depending on a variety of factors, including the site of the injury, the severity of the injury, and the uniqueness of the individual. The fact that clients may vary so dramatically from one another makes it challenging to clearly define aphasia in terms of a set of behaviors and deficits.

Experts have different opinions about how aphasia ought to be classified or whether classifications should exist at all. This difference of opinion is due to the fact that the brain functions to integrate all aspects of language, and an injury to a particular site typically affects all language modalities to one degree or another. Therefore, clear-cut symptoms following a brain injury simply do not exist. On the other hand, classification systems do help us clarify broad categories of language deficiencies based on the site of the injury even though there is a degree of variation from one client to another (Hegde, 1995a).

Table 9–3 summarizes several types of aphasia according to one of the most commonly used classification systems. The aphasia types are differentiated according to fluent and nonfluent characteristics. Keep in mind when using this type of classification system that aphasia is not always so easily simplified. In practice, you will typically not find "textbook cases" of the different types of aphasia. In reality, aphasia is manifest differently in every client, and the lines separating one type from another are not clearly defined.

Table 9–3. Types and Characteristics of Aphasia Categorized by Fluent and Nonfluent Characteristic

Type	Characteristics
Nonfluent Aphasias	
Broca's aphasia	Agrammatism
	Effortful speech
	Short, telegraphic phrases
	Presence of apraxia
	Marked naming problems
	Slow speech rate, lacking intonation
	Poor reading and writing ability
	Relatively good auditory comprehension
Transcortical motor aphasia	Intact repetition
	Lack of spontaneous speech
	Naming problems
	Short, telegraphic sentences
	Good articulation
	Agrammatism
	Paraphasias
Isolation aphasia	Marked naming difficulty
	Severely impaired comprehension
	Mild to moderately impaired repetition skills
Global aphasia	All language functions severly affected
	Severe deficits in comprehension and production
	Naming problems
	Difficulty with gestural skills
	Impaired reading and writing
Fluent Aphasias	
Wernicke's aphasia	Fluent but meaningless speech
	Severe auditory comprehension deficit
	Jargon, paraphasias, and neologisms
	Good articulation and intonation
	Naming difficulties
	Poor reading comprehension
	Writing deficits
Conduction aphasia	Marked difficulty repeating words and phrases
	Only minor comprehension problems

Fluent Aphasias

Conduction aphasia	Good articulation and prosody
	Naming problems
	Recognition of errors with attempts to self-correct
Transcortical sensory aphasia	Intact repetition
	Poor auditory comprehension
	Naming difficulties
	Paraphasias
Anomic aphasia	Marked naming problems
	Near-normal language
	Good comprehension
	Good repetition skills
	Relatively good auditory comprehension
	Good articulation
	Good grammatical structures

Adapted and summarized from Hegde (1996, 1995a).

Although there is variation from one aphasic client to the next, there are certain behaviors and deficits of communication that are characteristic of aphasia. These include:

- Impaired auditory comprehension.
- Impaired verbal expression.
- Presence of paraphasias.
- Perseveration.
- Agrammatism, or grammatical errors.
- Nonfluent speech or nonmeaningful fluent speech.
- Impaired prosodic features of speech.
- Difficulty repeating words, phrases, and/or sentences.
- Problems with naming and word finding (anomia).
- Impaired reading ability.
- Impaired writing ability (possibly confounded by loss of use of the dominant right hand due to hemiparesis).
- In bilingual clients, unequal impairment between the two languages.
- Pragmatic deficits.

- Difficulty using or understanding gestures (summarized from Brookshire [1992], Davis [1993], and Hegde [1994, 1996]).

When completing an evaluation of aphasia it is important to identify strengths and deficiencies within all these areas in order to make the most complete and realistic diagnosis and treatment plan for the client. Several formal tests are available for the assessment of aphasia. Some of the most commonly used published tests include:

- *Boston Assessment of Severe Aphasia* (Helm-Estabrooks, Ramsberger, Morgan, & Nicholas, 1989)
- *Boston Diagnostic Aphasia Examination* (Goodglass & Kaplan, 1983a)
- *Minnesota Test for Differential Diagnosis of Aphasia* (Schuell, 1965)
- *Porch Index of Communicative Ability* (Porch, 1981)
- *Western Aphasia Battery* (Kertesz, 1982).

Tasks for identifying skills and deficits of aphasic clients are found in Form 9–4 (pp. 305–319). These evaluation procedures are based on principles and tasks common to many examinations of aphasia. The materials in Form 9–4 allow you to assess a variety of receptive and expressive skills by using simple tasks that vary in difficulty. In the "Comments" sections make specific notes about the client's behaviors, such as delayed responses (include length of time), self-corrections, numbers and types of cues provided by the therapist, perseverations, visual neglect, response accuracy (e.g., incorrect response but correct response class), etc. Gain as much relevant information as possible for a complete assessment. "Evaluation of Aphasia" is not a standardized formal test but, in the hands of someone familiar with aphasia, it can be used for diagnostic purposes.

While failure to respond correctly to some items may be the result of aphasia, incorrect responses may also be the result of other disorders (e.g., language deficiencies secondary to severe hearing impairment, visual impairment, mental impairment, poor academic skills, schizophrenia, etc.). Be sure you know your client's medical history! Aphasia results from a neurological insult. The symptoms have a sudden onset (at the time of neurological insult), not a gradual onset as in the case of other disorders that have similar symptoms. To accurately assess aphasia, it is important to obtain as much information as possible about the nature of the disorder, including events surrounding its onset, communicative abilities prior to its onset, and results of any related neurological assessments (e.g., Magnetic Resonance Imaging [MRI], computerized tomographic [CT] scan, etc.).

The test items are not score-based or criterion-based. Rather, the tasks are designed to identify strengths and weaknesses. When administering the items, include tasks from each section. You can administer entire sections or sample from within each section. The tasks are arranged in an easy-to-difficult sequence, so be sure to sample some of the more difficult tasks before assuming your client does or does not have a deficit in that given area.

Form 9—4. Evaluation of Aphasia

Name: _____ Age: _____ Date: _____

Primary care physician: _____

Medical diagnosis: _____

Date of incident: _____

Condition prior to incident: _____

Date of CT scan/MRI_____Findings: _____

Relevant medical history: _____

_____

_____

Medications:_____

Examiner:_____

Instructions: Administer selected sections or all sections as appropriate for the client. Specific instructions are provided under each subheading.

Conversational speech

Use pictures or converse with the client to stimulate speech, noting specific difficulties the client exhibits.

Comments

agrammaticism_____

anomia _____

circumlocution _____

dysfluency _____

effortful speech _____

jargon _____

paraphasia _____

perseveration _____

telegraphic speech _____

other _____

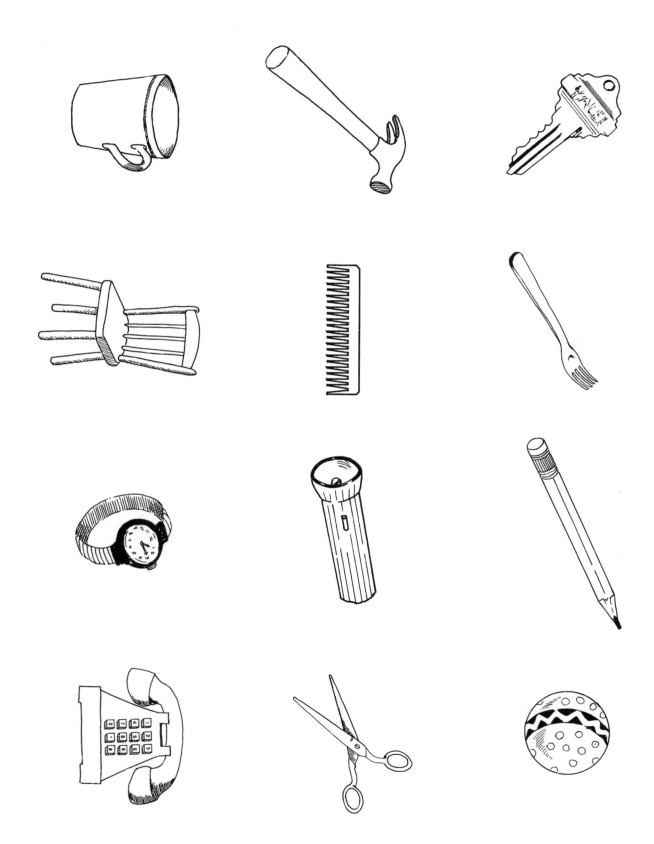

Checklist for Common Nouns and Functions

	Recognition of Word	Naming Word	Recognition of Functions
fork	_____	_____	_____
key	_____	_____	_____
ball	_____	_____	_____
flashlight	_____	_____	_____
chair	_____	_____	_____
hammer	_____	_____	_____
scissors	_____	_____	_____
watch	_____	_____	_____
pencil	_____	_____	_____
comb	_____	_____	_____
cup	_____	_____	_____
telephone	_____	_____	_____

Recognition of Common Nouns

Name each picture on the left-hand page one at a time and have the client point to the picture requested. If the client is unable to point, observe eye gaze. Record responses on the checklist on the right-hand side.

Naming Common Nouns

Use the same pictures and ask the client to name each item. Record responses on the checklist on the right-hand side.

Recognition of Common Functions

Use the same pictures and ask the client to identify the correct item for the following questions. Record responses on the checklist on the right-hand side.

What do you eat with?

What do you use to see at night?

What do you use to write something?

What do you use to talk to someone who is not in the room with you?

What do you use to hit a nail?

What do you use to cut paper?

What do you use to unlock the door?

What do you sit on?

What do you use on your hair?

What do you drink out of?

What do you use to play a game with?

What do you use to tell time?

Yes-No Questions

Ask the following questions to evaluate appropriateness of yes and no responses. Score a plus (+) or minus (−) for correct or incorrect responses.

Comments

_____Are you sitting on a chair? _____

_____Are we in Paris, France? _____

_____Is a book an animal? _____

_____Is a dog an animal? _____

_____Are you wearing a swimsuit? _____

_____Am I an adult? _____

Do you butter toast with a comb? _____

Do frogs swim? _____

Do cars fly? _____

Do trains carry people? _____

Following Commands

Ask the client to carry out each of the following commands. Make sure your client waits until you have finished the entire command before responding.

One-part Command   **Comments**

_____Touch your nose _____

_____Raise your hand_____

_____Look at the door _____

Two-part Command

_____Touch your head, then your mouth _____

_____Clap your hands, then touch your knees _____

_____Nod your head twice, then close your eyes _____

_____Touch your chair, then clap twice _____

Three-part Command　　　　　　　　　　　　　　　　**Comments**

_____Nod your head, clap your hands, then make a fist　_____

_____Look at the door, look at me, then close your eyes　_____

_____Touch your chin, then your nose, then raise your hand　_____

Repeating Phrases

Read each phrase and ask the client to repeat it. Syllabic complexity of each phrase increases as you read down the list (the number of syllables for each phrase is indicated in parentheses). Note the syllable length at which the client exhibits difficulty.

Comments

_____(1) Cap _____

_____(1) Boat_____

_____(2) Laughing _____

_____(2) Not now _____

_____(3) Piano _____

_____(3) Forty-two_____

_____(4) Geography _____

_____(4) It's time to go. _____

_____(5) Magnifying glass_____

_____(5) The car was dirty. _____

_____(6) Personal computer _____

_____(6) Put everything away. _____

_____(7) Revolutionary War _____

_____(7) She is not very happy. _____

_____(8) Mechanical engineering _____

_____(8) The letter arrived yesterday. _____

_____(9) Recreational motorcycle _____

_____(9) Put it in the microwave oven. _____

Logic Questions

Ask the following questions to evaluate logic and problem-solving skills. Suggested answers are provided below, but other responses may also be appropriate.

Comments

_____ Why do you store ice in the freezer? (so it won't melt) _____

_____

_____ Why do you brush your teeth? (so you don't get cavities, to clean them, etc.) _____

_____

_____ Why don't people swim outdoors in the winter? (it's too cold) _____

_____

_____ Why don't people eat house plants? (they aren't edible, they are for decoration, etc.)

_____

_____ What would you do if your car ran out of gas? (call someone for help, walk to a gas station, etc.)

_____

_____ What would you do if you couldn't find a friend's phone number? (look it up in a phone book, ask someone else, call information, etc.)

_____

_____ How could you learn about current news if you didn't have a newspaper? (listen to the radio, watch television, etc.)

_____

_____ How could you get downtown if you didn't have a car? (take a bus, walk, etc.) _____

_____

Sequencing

Ask the client to describe the steps necessary to complete the following tasks. Make a note of difficulties with thought organization or sequencing.

Comments

_____ make a sandwich _____

_____ wash a car _____

Sequencing   **Comments**

_____prepare a frozen dinner _____

_____change a light bulb   _____

_____write and send a letter _____

Definition of Terms

Ask the client to define each of the terms below. Note behaviors such as paraphasias and circumlocutions.

Comments

_____car _____

_____tree_____

_____window _____

_____bathe _____

_____shopping _____

_____cloudy _____

_____solo _____

_____tricky_____

_____northern _____

_____controversial _____

_____fleeting _____

_____content _____

_____opinion _____

6	3	8	one hundred and twenty-seven
11	29	49	two hundred and twelve
173	207	151	two thousand and forty-four
297	2,046	7,921	
one	six	four	
nine	seven	three	
thirteen	twenty-two	seventeen	
thirty-three	forty-one	ninety-one	

Number Recognition

Ask the client to identify each number on the left-hand page. Circle correct responses and mark a slash (/) through incorrect responses.

8	3
49	29
151	207
7,921	2,046

6
11
173
297

Numeric Word Recognition

Ask the client to read each number on the left-hand page. Circle correct responses and mark a slash (/) through incorrect responses.

four	six	one
three	seven	nine
seventeen	twenty-two	thirteen
ninety-one	forty-one	thirty-three

one hundred and twenty-seven

two hundred and twelve

two thousand and forty-four

baby

radio

ordinary

sometimes

Put it away.

Open the door.

They don't want any.

Peanut butter and honey

What happened to the flowers?

Send it to your friend before Thursday.

Writing Words and Sentences

Give the client a blank sheet of unlined paper and a pencil or pen. Ask him or her to write the following words and sentences. Observe ease of writing and make a note of paraphasic or spelling errors, incomplete sentences, and overall legibility.

Comments

car _____

tree _____

summer _____

I saw her. _____

We ate dinner. _____

They went outside. _____

The television set was broken. _____

He is saving his money for a rainy day. _____

It's too bad they can't come tomorrow. _____

I would rather have chicken than spaghetti. _____

Reading Words and Sentences Orally

Ask the client to read each word or sentence on the left-hand side of the page. Make a note of specific difficulties.

Comments

baby _____

radio _____

ordinary _____

sometimes _____

Put it away. _____

Open the door. _____

They don't want any. _____

Peanut butter and honey _____

What happened to the Bowers? _____

Send it to your friend before Thursday. _____

_____

$$
\begin{array}{r} 1 \\ +7 \\ \hline \end{array}
\qquad
\begin{array}{r} 9 \\ +3 \\ \hline \end{array}
\qquad
\begin{array}{r} 77 \\ +58 \\ \hline \end{array}
$$

$$
\begin{array}{r} 7 \\ +2 \\ \hline \end{array}
\qquad
\begin{array}{r} 13 \\ +4 \\ \hline \end{array}
\qquad
\begin{array}{r} 17 \\ +4 \\ \hline \end{array}
$$

$$
\begin{array}{r} 5 \\ +3 \\ \hline \end{array}
\qquad
\begin{array}{r} 12 \\ +7 \\ \hline \end{array}
\qquad
\begin{array}{r} 107 \\ +92 \\ \hline \end{array}
$$

$$
\begin{array}{r} 3 \\ -2 \\ \hline \end{array}
\qquad
\begin{array}{r} 17 \\ -7 \\ \hline \end{array}
\qquad
\begin{array}{r} 72 \\ -13 \\ \hline \end{array}
$$

$$
\begin{array}{r} 8 \\ -5 \\ \hline \end{array}
\qquad
\begin{array}{r} 16 \\ -12 \\ \hline \end{array}
\qquad
\begin{array}{r} 82 \\ -14 \\ \hline \end{array}
$$

$$
\begin{array}{r} 11 \\ -2 \\ \hline \end{array}
\qquad
\begin{array}{r} 56 \\ -9 \\ \hline \end{array}
\qquad
\begin{array}{r} 171 \\ -83 \\ \hline \end{array}
$$

Mathematic Calculations (Addition and Subtraction)

Ask the client to calculate the problems on the left-hand page. Circle correct responses and make a slash (/) through incorrect responses.

Subtraction

$$\begin{array}{r} 11 \\ -2 \\ \hline 9 \end{array} \qquad \begin{array}{r} 8 \\ -5 \\ \hline 3 \end{array} \qquad \begin{array}{r} 3 \\ -2 \\ \hline 1 \end{array}$$

$$\begin{array}{r} 56 \\ -9 \\ \hline 47 \end{array} \qquad \begin{array}{r} 16 \\ -12 \\ \hline 4 \end{array} \qquad \begin{array}{r} 17 \\ -7 \\ \hline 10 \end{array}$$

$$\begin{array}{r} 171 \\ -83 \\ \hline 88 \end{array} \qquad \begin{array}{r} 82 \\ -14 \\ \hline 68 \end{array} \qquad \begin{array}{r} 72 \\ -13 \\ \hline 59 \end{array}$$

Addition

$$\begin{array}{r} 5 \\ +3 \\ \hline 8 \end{array} \qquad \begin{array}{r} 7 \\ +2 \\ \hline 9 \end{array} \qquad \begin{array}{r} 1 \\ +7 \\ \hline 8 \end{array}$$

$$\begin{array}{r} 12 \\ +7 \\ \hline 19 \end{array} \qquad \begin{array}{r} 13 \\ +4 \\ \hline 17 \end{array} \qquad \begin{array}{r} 9 \\ +3 \\ \hline 12 \end{array}$$

$$\begin{array}{r} 107 \\ +92 \\ \hline 199 \end{array} \qquad \begin{array}{r} 17 \\ +4 \\ \hline 21 \end{array} \qquad \begin{array}{r} 77 \\ +58 \\ \hline 135 \end{array}$$

$$\begin{array}{r} 3 \\ \times 2 \\ \hline \end{array} \qquad \begin{array}{r} 7 \\ \times 1 \\ \hline \end{array} \qquad \begin{array}{r} 3 \\ \times 3 \\ \hline \end{array}$$

$$\begin{array}{r} 4 \\ \times 3 \\ \hline \end{array} \qquad \begin{array}{r} 5 \\ \times 5 \\ \hline \end{array} \qquad \begin{array}{r} 9 \\ \times 3 \\ \hline \end{array}$$

$$\begin{array}{r} 13 \\ \times 14 \\ \hline \end{array} \qquad \begin{array}{r} 23 \\ \times 17 \\ \hline \end{array} \qquad \begin{array}{r} 19 \\ \times 26 \\ \hline \end{array}$$

$$3\overline{)9} \qquad 9\overline{)27} \qquad 12\overline{)36}$$

$$2\overline{)4} \qquad 7\overline{)56} \qquad 6\overline{)126}$$

$$7\overline{)42} \qquad 9\overline{)81} \qquad 9\overline{)144}$$

Mathematic Calculations (Multiplication and Division)

Ask the client to calculate the problems on the left-hand page. Circle correct responses and make a slash (/) through incorrect responses.

Division

$$7\overline{)42} \quad \xrightarrow{6}$$

$$2\overline{)4} \quad \xrightarrow{2} \qquad 3\overline{)9} \quad \xrightarrow{3} \qquad \begin{array}{r} 3 \\ \times 3 \\ \hline 9 \end{array} \qquad \begin{array}{r} 7 \\ \times 1 \\ \hline 7 \end{array} \qquad \begin{array}{r} 3 \\ \times 2 \\ \hline 6 \end{array}$$

$$9\overline{)81} \quad \xrightarrow{9}$$

$$7\overline{)56} \quad \xrightarrow{8} \qquad 9\overline{)27} \quad \xrightarrow{3} \qquad \begin{array}{r} 9 \\ \times 3 \\ \hline 27 \end{array} \qquad \begin{array}{r} 5 \\ \times 5 \\ \hline 25 \end{array} \qquad \begin{array}{r} 4 \\ \times 3 \\ \hline 12 \end{array}$$

Multiplication

$$9\overline{)144} \quad \xrightarrow{16}$$

$$6\overline{)126} \quad \xrightarrow{21} \qquad 12\overline{)36} \quad \xrightarrow{3} \qquad \begin{array}{r} 19 \\ \times 26 \\ \hline 114 \\ +380 \\ \hline 494 \end{array} \qquad \begin{array}{r} 23 \\ \times 17 \\ \hline 161 \\ +230 \\ \hline 391 \end{array} \qquad \begin{array}{r} 13 \\ \times 14 \\ \hline 52 \\ +130 \\ \hline 182 \end{array}$$

RIGHT HEMISPHERE DYSFUNCTION

Traditionally, the left hemisphere of the brain is known as the hemisphere of language function. However, both cerebral hemispheres perform specific tasks that complement and are integrated with tasks that are specific to the opposite hemisphere. Simply stated, both hemispheres are vitally important for normal and functional communication. The left hemisphere is primarily responsible for basic language functions, such as phonology, syntax, and simple-level semantics. The right hemisphere is primarily responsible for complex linguistic processing and the nonverbal, emotional aspects of communication (Burns, 1985).

Injury to the right hemisphere of the brain results in a unique set of deficits that can significantly affect a person's ability to communicate and function appropriately in his or her environment. As with other neurologically based disorders, outcomes from right hemisphere damage can vary significantly from one client to another. However, there are specific impairments that are characteristic of right hemisphere damage. These are summarized from Brookshire (1992) and Tompkins (1995) and fall into four categories:

Perceptual and Attentional Deficits

- Neglect of the left visual field.
- Difficulty with facial recognition (prosopagnosia).
- Difficulty with constructional tasks.
- Impulsivity, distractibility, and poor attention to tasks.
- Excessive attention to irrelevant information.
- Denial of deficits (anosognosia).

Affective Deficits

- Difficulty expressing emotions.
- Difficulty recognizing emotions of others.
- Depression.
- Apparent lack of motivation.

Communicative Deficits

- Difficulty with word retrieval.
- Impaired auditory comprehension.
- Reading and writing deficits.
- Impaired prosodic features of speech.
- Difficulty with pragmatics.
- Dysarthria.

Cognitive Deficits

- Disorientation.
- Impaired attention.
- Difficulty with memory.
- Poor integration of information.
- Difficulty with logic, reasoning, planning, and problem solving.
- Impaired comprehension of inferred meanings.
- Difficulty understanding humor.

Many of the characteristics of right hemisphere dysfunction are similar to those of aphasia, resulting from left hemisphere damage. To assist in the differential diagnosis of these two disorders, see Table 9–4.

Table 9–4. Differential Characteristics of Right Hemisphere Dysfunction and Aphasia

Right Hemisphere Syndrome	Aphasia
Only mild problems in naming, fluency, auditory comprehension, reading, and writing	Significant or dominant problems in naming, fluency, auditory comprehension, reading and writing.
Left-sided neglect	No left-sided neglect
Denial of illness	No denial of illness
Speech is often irrelevant, excessive, rambling	Speech is generally relevant
Often lack of affect	Generally normal affect
Possibly, impaired recognition of familiar faces	Intact recognition of familiar faces
Rotation and left-sided neglect	Simplification of drawings
More prominent prosodic defect	Less prominent prosodic defect
Inappropriate humor	Appropriate humor
May retell only nonessential, isolated details (no integration)	May retell the essence of a story
Understands only literal meanings	May understand implied meanings
Pragmatic impairments more striking (eye contact, topic maintenance, etc.)	Pragmatic impairments less striking
Though possessing good language skills, communication is very poor	Though limited in language skills, communication is often good
Pure linguistic deficits are not dominant	Pure linguistic deficits are dominant

Source: From M. N. Hegde, *PocketGuide to Assessment in Speech-Language Pathology* (pp. 350–351). San Diego, CA: Singular Publishing Group. Copyright © 1996 and used by permission.

We have provided an informal assessment tool for evaluating clients with right hemisphere damage. The "Cognitive-Linguistic Evaluation" (Form 9–5) is a nonstandardized assessment designed to identify specific problem areas that may be present in a client with a right cerebral hemisphere injury. There are also a variety of other assessment materials included in this book that you may find helpful. These include:

- *Evaluation of Aphasia* (Form 9–4). Selected subsections may be used to assess memory, logic, reasoning, problem solving, auditory processing, thought organization, reading, and writing.

- *Assessment of Pragmatic Skills* (Form 6–4). This worksheet may be useful for assessing a variety of pragmatic responses.

- *Informal Assessment of Traumatic Brain Injury* (Form 9–5). Selected questions in this behavioral profile may be helpful for gathering specific information from family members or other caregivers.

- *Reading Passages* (pp. 122–124). These may be useful for assessing reading ability and visual function.

- *Narratives with Pictures* (pp. 104–111). These may be useful for assessing memory and thought organization.

Several commercially available sources for assessment are listed below. Keep in mind that many of them were not developed for evaluating right hemisphere dysfunction specifically. However, administered in their entirety or in selected subsections, they can be adapted for such use.

- *Boston Diagnostic Aphasia Examination* (Goodglass & Kaplan, 1983a)

- *Communicative Abilities in Daily Living (CADL)* (Holland, 1980)

- *Discourse Comprehension Test* (Brookshire & Nicholas, 1993)

- *Mini Inventory of Right Brain Injury (MIRBI)* (Pimental & Kingsbury, 1989)

- *Rehabilitation Institute of Chicago (RIC) Evaluation of Communication Problems in Right Hemisphere Dysfunction-2 (RICE-2)* (Burns, Halper, & Mogil, 1985)

- *Revised Token Test (RTT)* (McNeil & Prescott, 1978)

- *Right Hemisphere Language Battery (RHLB)* (Bryan, 1989)

- *Ross Information Processing Assessment-2* (Ross-Swain, 1996)

- *Ross Information Processing Assessment—Geriatric* (Ross-Swain & Fogle, 1996)

- *Test of Visual Neglect* (Albert, 1973)

- *Wechsler Memory Scale—Revised* (Wechsler, 1987)

- *Western Aphasia Battery* (Kertesz, 1982).

Form 9–5. Cognitive Linguistic Evaluation

Name: _____ Age: _____ Date: _____

Primary care physician: _____

Medical diagnosis: _____

Date of incident: _____

Condition prior to incident: _____

Date of CT scan/MRI_____Findings: _____

Relevant medical history: _____

_____

_____

Medications: _____

Examiner: _____

Instructions: Administer selected sections or all sections as appropriate for the client. Specific instructions are provided under each subheading. Make additional observations in the right-hand column. The client will need a pen or pencil to complete the writing portion of the evaluation.

Orientation and Awareness

Ask the client the following questions. Score a plus (+) or minus (−) for correct or incorrect responses.

Comments

____What day is it? _____

____What month is it? _____

____What year is it? _____

____What season is it? _____

____Approximately what time do you think it is?_____

____What state are we in? _____

____What city are we in? _____

____What county are we in? _____

____Where do you live?_____

____What is the name of this building?_____

____Why are you in the hospital? _____

____How long have you been here? _____

____When did you have your accident?_____

____What kinds of problems do you have because of your accident? _____

Orientation and Awareness

Comments

____What is my name? _____

____What is my profession? _____

____Who is your doctor? _____

____About how much time has passed since we started talking together today? _____

Memory

Immediate Memory. Ask the client to repeat the following sequences or sentences. Score a plus (+) or minus (−) for correct or incorrect responses.

Comments

____0, 8, 4, 6 _____

____8, 6, 0, 1, 3 _____

____2, 9, 1, 4, 6, 5 _____

____car, duck, ring, shoe _____

____rain, desk, ladder, horse, cake _____

____The keys were found under the table. _____

____He always reads the newspaper before he has breakfast. _____

____After their victory, the baseball team had pizza and watched a movie. _____

Ask the client to retell this story:

____Helen had a birthday party at the petting zoo. Ten of her friends came.

All the children laughed when a goat was found eating the cake and ice cream.

Recent Memory. Ask the client the following questions. Score a plus (+) or minus (−) for correct or incorrect responses.

Comments

____What did you have for breakfast? _____

____What did you do after dinner last night? _____

____What did you do after breakfast this morning? _____

____What else have you done today? _____

____Have you had any visitors today or yesterday? _____

____What other therapies do you receive? _____

(continued)

Form 9–5. *(continued)*

____Who is your doctor? _____

____How long have you been a resident here? _____

Long-Term Memory. Ask the client the following questions. Score a plus (+) or minus (−) for correct or incorrect responses.

Comments

____Where were you born? _____

____When is your birthday? _____

____What is your husband's/wife's name? _____

____How many children do you have? _____

____How many grandchildren do you have? _____

____Where did you used to work? _____

____How much school did you complete? _____

____Where did you grow up? _____

____How many brothers and sisters do you have? _____

Auditory Processing and Comprehension

Ask the client the following questions. Score a plus (+) or minus (−) for correct or incorrect responses.

Comments

____Is your last name Williams? _____

____Is my name Jim? _____

____Are you wearing glasses? _____

____Do you live on the moon? _____

____Have you had dinner yet? _____

____Do cows eat grass? _____

____Do fish swim? _____

____Do four quarters equal one dollar? _____

____Are there forty-eight hours in a day? _____

____Is Alaska part of the United States? _____

Problem Solving

Ask the client the following questions. Score a plus (+) or minus (−) for correct or incorrect responses.

Comments

____What would you do if you locked your keys in your house? _____

_____What would you do if your newspaper did not get delivered? _____

_____What would you do if you could not find your doctor's phone number? _____

_____What would you do if your TV stopped working? _____

_____What would you do if you forgot to put the milk away when you got home from the grocery store?

_____

Logic, Reasoning, Inference

Ask the client what is wrong with these sentences? Score a plus (+) or minus (−) for correct or incorrect responses.

Comments

_____He put salt and pepper in his coffee._____

_____Six plus one is eight. _____

_____I put my socks on over my shoes._____

_____Hang up when the phone rings._____

_____The dog had four kittens. _____

Ask the client what these expressions mean? Score a plus (+) or minus (−) for correct or incorrect responses.

Comments

_____Haste makes waste. _____

_____An apple a day keeps the doctor away._____

_____When it rains it pours. _____

_____He's a chip off the old block. _____

_____Beauty is only skin deep. _____

Ask the client the following questions. Score a plus (+) or minus (−) for correct or incorrect responses.

Comments

_____What is worn on your feet, knit, and used to keep you warm? _____

_____What has a bushy tail, climbs trees, and stores nuts? _____

_____What is thin and lightweight, used to wipe tears, used during a cold? _____

_____How are a sweater, pants, and a blouse alike?_____

_____How are orange juice, soda, and milk alike? _____

Thought Organization

Ask the client to answer the following questions or tasks. Score a plus (+) or minus (−) for correct or incorrect responses.

(continued)

Form 9–5. *(continued)*

Thought Organization

                                                       Comments

____What does the word "affectionate" mean?   _____

____What does the word "deliver" mean?   _____

____What are the steps you follow to wash your hair?   _____

____What are the steps you follow to make your bed?   _____

____How would you plan a meal for two dinner guests?   _____

Calculation

Ask the client to answer the following questions. Score a plus (+) or minus (−) for correct or incorrect responses.

                                                       Comments

____If you went to the mall and spent $8.00 in one store and $7.50

     in another store, how much did you spend? _____

____If tomatoes cost $1.50 per pound and you bought 2 pounds,

     how much did you spend on tomatoes?   _____

____If you went to the store with $3.00 and returned home with

     $1.75, how much did you spend? _____

____If toothbrushes cost $3.00 each and you have $10.00, how

     many toothbrushes can you buy? _____

____If you have a doctor's appointment at 10:30 and it takes you

     30 minutes to get there, what time should you leave? _____

Reading and Visual Processing

Ask the client to read the six words in each row and cross out the one that does not belong. Score a plus (+) or minus (−) for correct or incorrect responses.

__ Cow   Apple   Carrot   Cheese   Banana   Oatmeal

__ Desk   Chair   Blue   Bed   Couch   Table

Ask the client to read the following sentences and do what they say. Score a plus (+) or minus (−) for correct or incorrect responses.

Comments

__ Look at the ceiling. _____

__ Point to the door, then blink your eyes. _____

__ Sing Happy Birthday. _____

Ask the client to read the following paragraph out loud and answer the questions about it. Score a plus (+) or minus (−) for correct or incorrect responses.

Mark and Rick are brothers. They both entered a tennis tournament, hoping to win the $100 grand prize. Mark won his first two matches, but was eliminated after losing the third match. Rick made it all the way to the semi-finals. He lost, but was awarded a can of tennis balls as a consolation prize.

Comments

___Are Mark and Rick cousins?_____

___What sport did they play?_____

___What was the grand prize? _____

___Did one of them win the grand prize? _____

___Which one did the best in the tournament? _____

Show the client these two clocks and ask what time the clocks say? Score a plus (+) or minus (−) for correct or incorrect responses.

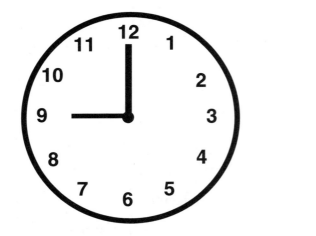
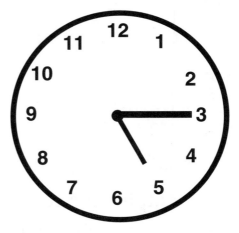

Now ask the client to copy the clocks below. Note accuracy of construction.

Ask the client to put an x through all the circles on this page. Note the client's attention to the left half of the page.

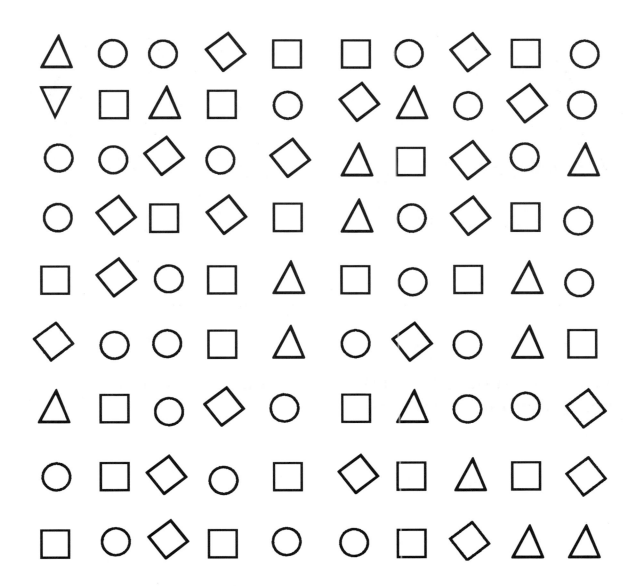

Write your name.

Write today's date.

Write a short description of what you have done today in speech therapy.

Writing

Ask the client to complete the writing tasks presented on the opposite page. Observe accuracy of response, completeness and organization of response, legibility, and observance of left visual field. Make comments in the right margin.

Comments

Write your name. _____

Write today's date. _____

Write a short description of what you have done today in speech therapy. _____

_____

Pragmatics and Affect

Check all behaviors observed during your assessment.

Comments

____Inappropriate physical proximity _____

____Inappropriate physical contacts_____

____Left visual field neglect_____

____Poor eye contact _____

____Lack of facial expression _____

____Gestures (inappropriate, absent) _____

____Lack of prosodic features of speech (intensity, pitch, rhythm)_____

____Poor topic maintenance_____

____Lack of appropriate turn taking_____

____Perseveration _____

____Presupposition (too much, too little)_____

____Inappropriately verbose_____

____Lack of initiation _____

____Easily distracted _____

____Frequent interruptions _____

____Impulsive _____

____Poor organization _____

____Incompleteness _____

ASSESSMENT OF TRAUMATIC BRAIN INJURY

A traumatic brain injury (TBI) is the result of an acute assault on the brain. Causes of TBI include motor vehicle accidents, sports injuries, falls, home- or work-related accidents, gunshot wounds, and other mishaps (Naugle, 1990). There are two subcategories of TBIs: penetrating injuries and closed-head injuries. Penetrating injuries occur when an object, such as a bullet or a knife, penetrates the skull and rips through the soft brain tissue, damaging nerve fibers and nerve cells. The neurological damage is focal (localized) and the resulting behaviors vary, depending on the severity and location of the injury. Closed-head injuries are incurred from the collision of the head with an object or surface that does not penetrate the skull. Even though the skull remains intact, the brain can be severely damaged. Upon impact, the soft, fragile brain is thrust to and fro against the hard, rough surface of the cranium (skull), becoming damaged, twisted, and bruised in the process. The damage is diffuse (nonlocalized), and the resulting behaviors vary depending on the severity and location(s) of the injury. Other than in a war zone environment, closed-head injuries are the most common type of TBI (National Institutes of Health, 1984).

Considering the varying nature of a TBI, one can understand why there is no such thing as a typical brain injury. Also, a brain injury can occur at any age. These factors pose a unique challenge to the clinician attempting to assess the communicative skills of a client who has suffered a head injury. A uniform set of symptoms characteristic of all TBIs simply does not exist. However, some commonly seen consequences of brain injury include:

Cognitive Deficits:

- Attention deficits
- Memory disorders
- Language impairments
- Impaired abstraction and judgment capabilities (inflexibility)
- Decreased speed, accuracy, and consistency
- Defective reasoning processes
- Susceptibility to internal and external stressors

Perceptual Deficits:

- Decreased acuity or increased sensitivity in vision, hearing, or touch
- Vestibular deficits
- Spatial disorientation
- Disorders of smell and taste

Physical Deficits:

- Disorders such as ataxia, spasticity, and tremors
- Musculoskeletal disorders

Behavioral and Emotional Deficits:

- Irritability
- Impatience
- Poor frustration tolerance
- Dependence
- Denial of disability (Hamlin, 1987, p. 59)

These sequelae will vary in severity across clients. This requires the clinician to identify the individual assessment needs of each client, and use assessment instruments that are appropriate for the client's age and abilities.

Before beginning the direct assessment, obtain as much information as possible about the nature of the brain injury. Research the type and severity of the injury, the date of onset, and the cerebral areas affected. Investigate the client's medical history and pretrauma personality so you can predict behavior patterns (Ylvisaker & Holland, 1985). Obtain evaluation dates and assessment results from CT scans or MRIs. Also, identify the client's cognitive status. The Rancho Los Amigos Levels of Cognitive Functioning (Malkus, Booth, & Kodimer, 1980) is a frequently used scale for describing cognitive status in clients with recent onset, severe head injuries. Each level is identified with a Roman numeral:

I. No response to stimuli
II. Generalized response to stimuli
III. Localized response to stimuli
IV. Confused—agitated
V. Confused, inappropriate—nonagitated
VI. Confused—appropriate
VII. Automatic—appropriate
VIII. Purposeful and appropriate

All of these factors influence the client's behaviors and will prepare you to administer the most appropriate assessment.

Specific neuropsychological and communicative factors you may identify or observe during the assessment will vary depending on:

- The type of TBI (penetrating or closed-head injury),
- The cerebral systems involved,
- The extent and severity of the injury, and
- The presence of additional neuromedical variables (extended coma, cerebral hemorrhage, etc.) (Cullum, Kuck, & Ruff, 1990).

In many cases, speech and language characteristics resulting from TBI resemble aspects of aphasia, but not closely enough to label the disorder an aphasic syndrome in all clients. The most prominent aphasia-like symptoms include anomie, circumlocution, paraphasia, and perseveration. Dysarthria, especially spastic dysarthria, and/or dysphagia are also reported in some cases of TBI (Helm-Estabrooks, 1991; Marquardt, Stoll, & Sussman, 1990). The primary objection to making a diagnosis of aphasia for all TBI clients is that the pragmatic and language behaviors associated with a true aphasia differ from those associated with TBI. In most cases, clients with aphasia resulting from a CVA exhibit mild to severe deficits across all language modalities, yet they maintain intact social and pragmatic skills. In contrast, clients with TBI often have relatively normal receptive and expressive language skills, but they are unable to communicate effectively because of their deficits (Marquardt et al., 1990). To complete a thorough assessment, it is important to obtain a good sampling of pragmatic and communicative functions. Cullum et al. (1990) identify eight areas of cognitive functioning that should be assessed:

1. General cognitive/intellectual abilities
2. Language functions
3. Visuospatial, visuomotor, and visuoconstructional abilities
4. Attention/Concentration
5. A. Learning ability
    a. Verbal modality
    b. Nonverbal modality
   B. Memory ability
    a. Verbal modality
    b. Nonverbal modality
6. Motor functioning
7. Higher cognitive functioning
8. Emotional functioning (pp. 141–153)

Ylvisaker and Holland (1985) report that the predominant language disturbance associated with TBI is a cognitive impairment. TBI clients often exhibit problems attending, processing, reasoning, and executing normal functions. The assessment process frequently includes complete neuropsychological test batteries (typically administered by a neuropsychologist) and language test batteries. Two of the more commonly used neuropsychological batteries are:

- *Halstead-Reitan Neuropsychological Test Battery* (Reitan & Davison, 1974)
- *Luria-Nebraska Neuropsychological Battery* (Golden, Hammeke, & Purisch, 1980)

Several formal speech and language assessment instruments that are appropriate for assessing the communicative effects of TBI include:

- *Assessment of Intelligibility of Dysarthric Speech* (Yorkston et al., 1984)
- *Boston Diagnostic Aphasia Examination* (Goodglass & Kaplan, 1983a)
- *Boston Naming Test* (Goodglass & Kaplan, 1983b)
- *Brief Test of Head Injury* (Helm-Estabrooks & Hotz, 1991)
- *Detroit Tests of Learning Aptitude-2* (Hammill, 1985)

- *Expressive One-Word Picture Vocabulary Test* (Gardner, 1979)
- *Illinois Test of Psycholinguistic Abilities* (Kirk, McCarthy, & Kirk, 1968)
- "Logical Memory" subtest of *Wechsler Memory Scale—Revised* (Wechsler, 1987)
- *Minnesota Test for the Differential Diagnosis of Aphasia* (Schnell, 1972)
- *Peabody Picture Vocabulary Test—Revised* (Dunn & Dunn, 1981)
- *Ross Information Processing Assessment—Revised* (Ross-Swain, 1996)
- *Scales of Cognitive Ability for Traumatic Brain Injury* (Adamovich & Henderson, 1991)
- *The Word Test* (Jorgenson, Barrett, Huisingh, & Zachman, 1981)
- *Token Test—Revised* (McNeil & Prescott, 1978)
- *Wechsler Adult Intelligence Scale—Revised* (Wechsler, 1981)
- *Western Aphasia Battery* (Kertesz, 1982)
- *Woodcock-Johnson Psychoeducational Battery* (Woodcock & Johnson, 1977)

The specific tests you administer should be selected according to the behaviors and assessment needs of the client. In the absence of formal tests, you can administer a variety of assessment materials included in this manual. For example, selected sections of the "Evaluation of Aphasia" (Form 9–4) are appropriate for assessing memory, logic, reasoning, semantic concepts, problem solving, and language skills; the "Assessment of Pragmatic Skills" worksheet (Form 6–4) is appropriate for assessing a variety of pragmatic responses; the "Reading Passages" (pp. 122–124) or "Narratives With Pictures" (pp. 104–111) can be used to assess memory and language organization; selected sections of the "Cognitive-Linguistic Evaluation" (Form 9–5) are appropriate for assessing memory, orientation, auditory processing and comprehension, problem solving, reasoning, thought organization, visual processing, and graphic expression; and a speech-language sample is appropriate for assessing conversational competence. Since these materials (and most formal, commercially available tools) are not designed specifically for assessing the effects of TBI, you will need to be creative in selecting and administering stimulus items. Keep in mind the behaviors you want to assess and adapt your assessment materials as needed to achieve your goal.

Cullum, Kuck, and Ruff (1990) and Ylvisaker and Holland (1985) stress the importance of supplementing formal evaluative measures with informal measures. In many cases, the clinician is able to identify functional deficits affecting the client's academic, social, and vocational adjustment only through informal assessment. Form 9–6 is a worksheet for informally observing behaviors of clients with a TBI. Ylvisaker and Holland identify the client's family members as key informants for this important information, as they witness functional problems in everyday environments that cannot be detected during formal assessment sessions. Family members are also most able to describe subtle or blatant changes in the client's behaviors since the onset of the TBI. Ideally, the form is designed to be completed over an extended period of time (preferably several hours or even 1–2 days) by someone who spends a lot of time with the client. Some less impaired clients may be able to answer the questions themselves. If a family member or care provider is not available to complete the form, a nurse or other care provider may be able to provide the most complete and accurate information about the client's abilities and deficits. If another person is not available to complete the form, the clinician may need to adapt stimulus materials (e.g., sections of assessment batteries, informal assessment tasks) to construct situations for direct-

Form 9–6. Informal Assessment of Traumatic Brain Injury

Name: _____ Age: _____ Date: _____

Primary care physician: _____

Medical diagnosis: _____

Date of incident: _____

Condition prior to incident: _____

Date of CT scan/MRI_____Findings: _____

Relevant medical history: _____

_____

_____

Medications:_____

Examiner:_____

Instructions: Ask a family member or care provider to observe the client over an extended period of time and then answer each question. If another person is not available to complete the form, adapt stimulus materials to directly observe and evaluate the behaviors described. If possible, ask the client, family members, and/or care providers those questions not answered by observation. Provide clarifying comments in the space provided.

Is the client aware of personal orientation? (e.g., time, place)

Does the client attend to stimuli?

How long can the client attend to a task? (in seconds or minutes)

What distracts the client the most? (e.g., someone entering the room, noise from a TV or radio, too much visual stimulation, etc.)

Is the client able to shift attention from one activity to another?

Is the client able to attend to more than one activity at a time? (e.g., converse while preparing a meal)

Does the client attend to certain activities better than others?

What are the most difficult activities?

What are the easiest activities?

Is the client able to follow immediate directions?

Is the client able to follow complex directions?

(continued)

Form 9–6 *(continued)*

Is the client able to remember things that happened earlier that day?

Is the client able to remember things that happened earlier that month or year?

Is the client able to recall events that happened many years ago?

Is the client able to remember future activities? (e.g., take the garbage out this afternoon, or take the roast out of the oven in 1 hour)

Is the client able to shift from one activity to another without difficulty?

Is the client able to follow a conversation that shifts from one topic to another?

Is the client able to change the topic appropriately during a conversation?

What strategies does the client use to complete tasks?

Is the client aware of the strategies used? How does the client respond to the question, "How did you do that?"

How does the client respond to problem-solving situations?

What are some things the client is able to problem-solve?

What are some things the client is unable to problem-solve?

How does the client respond to stressful situations?

What kinds of everyday tasks does the client have difficulties with?

What are some things that the client needs to do on a daily basis?

Is the client having difficulty with any of these things? (if yes, identify)

(continued)

Form 9–6 *(continued)*

Is the client about to convey thoughts in writing?

Is the client able to use good judgment during everyday tasks?

Does the client seem to have good safety awareness?

What is the client's behavior like at home? (passive, aggressive, compulsive, etc.)

Please add additional comments about the client's behaviors and abilities.

ly observing the client. If possible, the clinician may also directly ask the client, family members, and/or care providers certain questions during a formal or informal interview to complete as much of the form as possible.

ASSESSMENT OF DEMENTIA

As our population ages, speech-language pathologists will become more and more involved in the assessment and treatment of clients with dementia. Dementia is characterized by progressive deterioration of memory, orientation, intellectual ability, and behavioral appropriateness. It generally progresses from a very mild to a very severe cognitive impairment over the course of months or even years. This section on the assessment of dementia focuses on irreversible dementias, but there are forms of dementia that are reversible. For example, certain medications can cause symptoms of dementia. Depression can manifest in dementia-like behaviors. Also, certain medical conditions such as tumors or infections may result in dementia (Ripich, 1995). These reversible forms of dementia are generally treated by other health care professionals, yet it is still important for the speech-language pathologist to be knowledgeable about nonreversible dementias and conditions related to reversible dementia.

The most common form of progressive, irreversible dementia is Alzheimer's disease (also called dementia of the Alzheimer's type, or DAT). Other dementias include multi-infarct dementia (MID), Pick's disease, Parkinson's disease (PD), Huntington's disease (HD), Wilson's disease, supranuclear palsy, Creutzfeldt-Jakob disease, and Korsakoff's syndrome. Most dementias follow a general pattern of progression. We have divided this pattern into three stages, although variability may vary significantly from one client to another and from one dementia type to another. The stages below are primarily related to dementia of the Alzheimer's type, however several other forms of dementia have similar patterns of progression. The information below is based on Hegde (1996), Kempler (1995), Overman and Geoffrey (1987), Ripich (1991), and Reisberg, Feris, DeLeon, and Crook (1982). Consult these sources and others for further information on the progression of dementia and differentiating characteristics of specific dementia types.

Stage I: Early Dementia

- Slow, insidious onset
- Some memory loss
- Word finding problems
- Poor attention span
- Disorientation
- Reasoning and judgment problems
- Difficulty with abstract concepts
- Empty speech at times
- Intact automatic speech
- Intact articulation and phonological skills

- Intact syntactic skills
- Mechanics of writing and reading intact, although meaning may be obscured
- Possible anxiety, depression, agitation, and/or apathy
- Attitude of indifference toward deficits

Stage 2: Intermediate Dementia

- Increasing memory loss. Client may forget names of loved ones, although usually remembers his or her own name
- Increasing word-finding deficits
- Decreasing orientation
- Empty speech
- Poor topic maintenance
- Intact automatic speech
- Intact articulation and phonological skills
- Intact syntactic skills
- Mechanics of writing and reading still intact, although meaning is more obscured
- Wandering
- Unable to take care of own needs
- Inability to perform complex tasks
- Perseveratory behaviors such as chewing or lip smacking
- Withdrawal from challenging situations
- Personality and emotional changes such as delusional behaviors, obsessive behaviors, anxiety, agitation, and/or previously nonexistent violent behaviors

Stage 3: Advanced Dementia

- Severely impaired memory
- Profound intellectual deterioration
- Severely impaired verbal abilities. Speech is meaningless or absent
- Unable to participate in social interaction
- Physical debilitation
- Aimless wandering
- Restlessness and agitation
- Possible violent outbursts
- Client requires assistance for all activities of daily living.

During the speech-language evaluation, the case history questions will be especially important for determining the etiology and prognosis of a client's dementia. As many of the client's primary caregivers and family members as possible need to be consulted to offer details related to the onset and progression of the client's condition. In addition to traditional case history questions, you may also want to ask:

- What behaviors were first noticed and when?
- How have the behaviors changed over time?
- Was the onset sudden? or gradual?
- What other events were occurring in the client's life at the time of onset?
- What is the client's psychiatric history?
- What kinds of problems is the client having, taking care of his or her daily needs?
- How has the client attempted to compensate for his or her deficits?
- How do you and others currently communicate with the client?

One frequently used dementia assessment tool is the *Mini-Mental State Examination (MMSE)* (Folstein, Folstein, & McHugh, 1975). It is often used as an initial test for a possible diagnosis of dementia. The examination is quick to administer, only taking about 10 minutes, and the outcome can provide direction for further assessment. The examination measures memory, orientation, and cognitive abilities. We have adapted it and reprinted it in Form 9–7.

Form 9–7. The Mini-Mental State Examination[1]

Name: _____ Age: _____ Date: _____

Primary care physician: _____

Medical diagnosis: _____

Relevant medical history: _____

_____

_____

Medications:_____

Examiner:_____

To administer this examination, you will need a wrist watch, a pencil, and some blank paper.

1. Ask the client to answer the following questions. Score 1 point for each correct answer:
    ___What is today's date?
    ___What is the day?
    ___What is the month?
    ___What is the year?
    ___What is the season?
    ___Total (maximum of 5 points)

2. Ask the client to answer the following questions. Score 1 point for each correct answer :
    ___What is the name of this building/hospital/or clinic?
    ___What is the name of the street it is on?
    ___Which floor are we on?
    ___What is the name of this city?
    ___What is the name of this state?
    ___Total (maximum of 5 points)

3. Slowly name three unrelated objects (e.g., dog, rose, bicycle). Ask the client to repeat them. Score one point for each correctly remembered object. The first attempt determines the score, but repeat the test up to six trials if the client is not successful.
    ___Total (maximum of 3 points)

(continued)

[1]Adapted from M. F. Folstein, S. E. Folstein, and P. R. McHugh (1975). Mini-Mental State: A Practical Method for Grading the Mental State of Patients for the Clinician. *Journal of Psychiatric Research, 12,* 189–198.

Form 9–7 *(continued)*

4. Ask the client to count backwards from 100 in 7s. Stop after five answers (93, 86, 79, 72, 65). Score 1 point for each correct answer. If the client is unable to perform this task, ask him or her to spell "world" backward, scoring 1 point for the number of letters in the correct order.
___Total (maximum of 5 points)

5. Ask the client to name the three objects you named earlier in question 3. Score 1 point for each correct response.
___Total (maximum of 3 points)

6.   a. Show the client a wrist watch and ask what it is. Score 1 point for a correct answer.
    b. Show the client a pencil and ask what it is. Score 1 point for a correct answer.
___Total (maximum of 2 points)

7. Ask the client to repeat this sentence: "No ifs, ands, or buts." Score 1 point if the client repeats it correctly on the first trial.
___Total (maximum of 1 point)

8. Hand the client a piece of paper and ask him or her to follow this three-step directive: "Take the paper in your right hand, fold it in half, and put it on the floor." Score 1 point for each part of the command correctly followed.
___Total (maximum of 3 points)

9. Show the client the sentence "Close your eyes" on the next page. Ask the client to read it and do what it says. Score 1 point for a correct response.
___Total (maximum of 1 point)

10. Give the client a blank piece of paper and ask him or her to write a sentence for you. It must contain a noun and a verb and make sense to score 1 point. Correct grammar and punctuation are not necessary.
___Total (maximum of 1 point)

11. Show the client the drawing of two pentagons on the next page. Ask the client to copy the drawing exactly as it is. All ten angles must be present and two angles must intersect to score 1 point. Tremor or paper rotation can be ignored.
___Total (maximum of 1 point)

___Total Score

Interpretation: The highest possible score is 30. Consider additional cognitive testing for a score of 23 or under.

CLOSE YOUR EYES

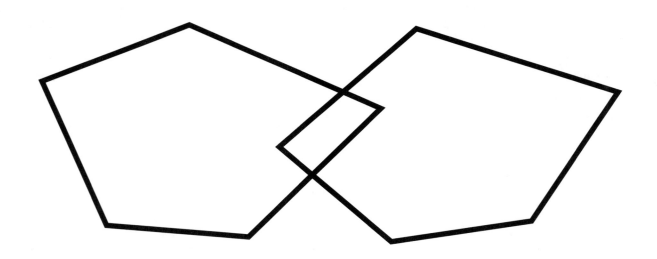

If you administer the MMSE and the outcome indicates a need for further evaluation, there are several commercially available assessment tools for dementia that are available. Take care to select testing materials that are appropriate for the client's level of cognition and awareness, as assessment tools vary widely in their focus, length, and application. Some evaluative tools you may wish to consider include:

- *Arizona Battery for Communication Disorders of Dementia (ABCD)* (Bayles & Tomoeda, 1993)

- *Boston Naming Test* (Kaplan, Goodglass, & Weintraub, 1983)

- *Communicative Abilities in Daily Living* (Holland, 1980)

- *Clinical Dementia Rating Scale (CDR)* (Hughes, 1982)

- *Global Deterioration Scale* (Reisberg et. al., 1982)

- *Rating Scale of Communication in Cognitive Decline* (Bollinger & Hardiman, 1990)

- *Severe Impairment Battery* (Saxton, McGonigle, Swihart, & Boller, 1993). Appropriate for a client who scores less than 8 on the MMSE.

- *Wechsler Memory Scale—Revised* (Wechsler, 1987)

- Selected portions of the *Boston Diagnostic Aphasia Examination* (Goodglass & Kaplan, 1983a) and/or the *Western Aphasia Battery* (Kertesz, 1982).

- Selected portions of the *Ross Information Processing Assessment-2* (Ross-Swain, 1996).

There are also assessment materials in this book that can be adapted for evaluating a client with a dementia disorder. For example, subsections of the "Cognitive Linguistic Evaluation" (Form 9–5) are appropriate for assessing orientation, memory, auditory processing and comprehension, thought organization, and pragmatics. The "Evaluation of Aphasia" (Appendix 9–A) is useful for assessing memory, semantic concepts, and language skills. The "Assessment of Pragmatic Skills" (Form 6–4) can be adapted for the assessment of a variety of pragmatic skills. The Reading Passages (pp. 122–124) can be adapted for the assessment of reading comprehension and/or memory of written material. The "Pictures" (pp. 100–103) can be used to evaluate thought organization, confrontational naming, and language skills. Finally, the "Narratives with Pictures" (pp. 104–111) can be used to assess auditory comprehension and memory.

CONCLUDING COMMENTS

The basic principles and methods for the assessment of six neurologically based disorders have been addressed in the preceding sections. Each disorder presents a different pattern of symptoms and communicative behaviors. Even though each neurologically based disorder is a distinct clinical entity, many clients are affected by several disorders simultaneously.

This requires the clinician to carefully evaluate a variety of communicative skills and abilities. The clinician must determine a hierarchy of clinical importance for each disorder diagnosed. It is important to view the "whole picture" and prioritize immediate and less-immediate needs for making appropriate diagnostic and treatment decisions.

SOURCES OF ADDITIONAL INFORMATION

Aphasia

Boone, D. R., & Plante, E. (1993). *Human communication and its disorders* (2nd ed.). Englewood Cliffs, NJ: Prentice-Hall.

Brookshire, R. H. (1992). *An introduction to neurogenic communication disorders* (4th ed.). St. Louis: Mosby-Year Book.

Code, C., & Muller, D. J. (1991). *Aphasia therapy* (2nd ed.). San Diego: Singular Publishing Group.

Collins, M. (1991). *Diagnosis and treatment of global aphasia*. San Diego: Singular Publishing Group.

Haynes, W. O., Pindzola, R. H., & Emerick, L. L. (1992). *Diagnosis and evaluation in speech pathology* (4th ed.). Englewood Cliffs, NJ: Prentice-Hall.

Hegde, M. N. (1991). *Introduction to communicative disorders*. Austin, TX: PRO-ED.

Helm-Estabrooks, N., & Albert, M. L. (1991). *Manual of aphasia therapy*. Austin, TX: PRO-ED.

Johns, D. F. (Ed.). (1985). *Clinical management of neurogenic communicative disorders* (2nd ed.). Boston: Little, Brown and Co.

LaPointe, L. L. (1990). *Aphasia and related neurogenic language disorders*. New York: Thieme Medical Publishers Inc.

Payne, J. C. (1997). *Adult neurogenic language disorders: Assessment and treatment*. San Diego, CA: Singular Publishing Group.

Peterson, H. A., & Marquardt, T. P. (1990). *Appraisal and diagnosis of speech and language disorders* (2nd ed.). Englewood Cliffs, NJ: Prentice-Hall.

Rosenbek, J. C., LaPointe, L. L., & Wertz, W. T. (1989). *Aphasia: A clinical approach*. Austin, TX: PRO-ED.

Dementia

Bayles, K., Kaszniak, A.W., & Tomoeda, C. (1987). *Communication and cognition in normal aging and dementia*. Austin, TX: PRO-ED.

Cummings, J. L., & Benson, D. F. (1983). *Dementia: A clinical approach*. Boston: Butterworths.

Lubinski, R. (Ed.). (1995). *Dementia and communication*. San Diego, CA: Singular.

Payne, J. C. (1997). *Adult neurogenic language disorders: Assessment and treatment*. San Diego, CA: Singular.

Ripich, D. N. (Ed.). (1991). *Handbook of geriatric communication disorders*. Austin, TX: PRO-ED.

Ripich, D. N., & Wykle, M. L. (1996). *Alzheimer's disease and communication guide*. Tucson, AZ: Communication Skill Builders.

Shadden, B. B., & Toner, M. A. (1997). *Aging and communication*. Austin, TX: PRO-ED.

Shekim, L. O. (1990). Dementia. In L. L. LaPointe (Ed.), *Aphasia and related neurogenic language disorders* (pp. 210–220). New York: Thieme Medical Publishers.

Stokes, G., & Goudie, F. (1995). *Working with dementia*. Bicester, Oxton, United Kingdom: Winslow.

Dysarthria and Apraxia

Brookshire, R. H. (1992). *An introduction to neurogenic communication disorders* (4th ed.). St. Louis: Mosby-Year Book.

Darley, F. L., Aronson, A. E., & Brown, J. R. (1975). *Motor speech disorders*. Philadelphia: W. B. Saunders Co.

Duffy, J. R. (1995). *Motor speech disorders: Substrates, differential diagnosis and management*. St. Louis: Moseby.

Dworkin, J. P. (1991). *Motor speech disorders: A treatment guide*. St. Louis: Mosby-Year Book.

Johns, D. F. (Ed.). (1985). *Clinical management of neurogenic communicative disorders* (2nd ed.). Boston: Little, Brown and Co.

Love, R. J. (1992). *Childhood motor speech disability*. Columbus, OH: Merrill/Macmillan.

Perkins, W. H. (Ed.). (1983). *Dysarthria and apraxia*. New York: Thieme-Stratton.

Wertz, R. T., LaPointe, L. L., & Rosenbek, J. C. (1991). *Apraxia of speech in adults: The disorder and its management*. San Diego: Singular Publishing Group.

Yorkston, K, Beukelman, D., & Bell, K (1988). *Clinical management of dysarthric speakers*. Austin, TX: PRO-ED.

Right Hemisphere Dysfunction

Brookshire, R. H. (1992). *An introduction to neurogenic communication disorders* (4th ed.). St. Louis: Mosby-Year Book.

Joanette, Y., & Brownell, H. H. (Eds.). (1990). *Discourse ability and brain damage: Theoretical and empirical perspectives*. New York: Springer-Verlag.

Joanette, Y., & Goulet, P., & Hannequin, D. (1990). *Right hemisphere and verbal communication*. New York: Springer-Verlag.

LaPointe, L. L. (Ed.). (1990). *Aphasia and related neurogenic language disorders*. New York: Thieme Medical Publishers.

Myers, P. S. (1994). Communication disorders associated with right-hemisphere brain damage. In R. Chapey (Ed.), *Language intervention strategies in adult aphasia* (3rd ed., pp. 514–534). Baltimore: Williams & Wilkins.

Payne, J. C. (1997). *Adult neurogenic language disorders: Assessment and treatment*. San Diego, CA: Singular Publishing Group.

Tompkins, C. A. (1995). *Right hemisphere communication disorders: Theory and management*. San Diego, CA: Singular Publishing Group.

Traumatic Brain Injury

Adamovich, B. B., Henderson, J. A., & Auerbach, S. (1985). *Cognitive rehabilitation of closed head injured patients: A dynamic approach*. Boston: Little, Brown and Co.

Beukelman, D. R., & Yorkston, K. M. (Eds.). (1991). *Communication disorders following traumatic brain injury*. Austin, TX: PRO-ED.

Bigler, E. D. (Ed.). (1990). *Traumatic brain injury*. Austin, TX: PRO-ED.

Helm-Estabrooks, N., & Albert, M. L. (1991). *Manual of aphasia therapy*. Austin, TX: PRO-ED.

National Institutes of Health. (1984). *Head injury: Hope through research*. Bethesda, MD: Author.

Payne, J. C. (1997). *Adult neurogenic language disorders: Assessment and treatment*. San Diego: Singular Publishing Group.

Sohlberg, M. M., & Mateer, C. A. (1989). *Introduction to cognitive rehabilitation: Theory and practice*. New York: The Guilford Press.

Ylvisaker, M. S., & Holland, A. L. (1985). Coaching, self-coaching, and rehabilitation of head injury. In D. F. Johns (Ed.), *Clinical management of neurogenic communicative disorders* (pp. 243–257). Boston: Little, Brown and Co.

Internet Sources

Alzheimer's Association
　http://www.alz.org

Institute of Neurotoxicology and Neurological Disorders
　http://www.innd.org

Listservers of Interest to Communication Disorders Folks
　http://www.shc.uiowa.edu/wjshc/iiscdl.html

National Aphasia Association
　http://www.aphasia.org

National Parkinson Foundation
　http://www.parkinson.org

☐ CHAPTER 10 ☐

Assessment of Dysphagia

Many of the muscles used for speech production are also used for chewing and swallowing. Because speech-language pathologists are knowledgeable about oral and pharyngeal anatomy and physiology, we frequently participate in the evaluation and treatment of dysphagia (chewing and/or swallowing dysfunction), even when a client does not have a communicative disorder. This chapter describes the normal swallow function and procedures for evaluating a client with a possible swallowing impairment. Assessment procedures unique to tracheostomized clients are also included.

It is critical that you exercise caution when completing any evaluation with a client with suspected dysphagia; it is a life-threatening disorder. For example, aspiration pneumonia, which can be caused by food or liquid in the lungs, can lead to death. Speech-language pathologists will need to work closely with physicians, nurses, and other medically related personnel to provide safe client care.

OVERVIEW OF ASSESSMENT

History of the Client

    Procedures

        Written Case History
        Information-getting Interview
        Information from Other Professionals

    Contributing Factors

        Medical Diagnosis
        Pharmacological Factors
        Age
        Intelligence, Motivation, and Levels of Concern

Oral-facial Examination

Assessment of Dysphagia

    Procedures

        Screening
        Bedside Evaluation
        Radiographic Study
        Blue-dye Test

    Analysis

        Type of Dysphagia
        Severity of Risk for Aspiration

Cognitive Assessment

Speech Assessment

Language Assessment

Hearing Assessment

Determining the Diagnosis

Providing Information (written report, interview, etc.)

OVERVIEW OF A NORMAL SWALLOW

Before you evaluate a client for a swallowing disorder, it is important to understand the dynamics of a functional swallow. The normal swallow occurs in four phases, each described below. The client with dysphagia will exhibit difficulties within one or more of these phases.

☐ *Oral Preparatory Phase.* The food or liquid is manipulated in the oral cavity, chewed (if necessary), and made into a bolus, which is sealed with the tongue against the hard palate.

☐ *Oral Phase.* The tongue moves the food or liquid toward the back of the mouth (toward the anterior faucial pillars). To achieve this, the tongue presses the bolus against the hard palate and squeezes the bolus posteriorly. The oral-preparatory and oral phases are voluntary, not reflexive, actions.

☐ *Pharyngeal Phase.* During this phase, the swallow reflex is triggered and the bolus is carried through the pharynx, while these simultaneous actions occur: (a) the velopharyngeal port closes; (b) the bolus is squeezed to the top of the esophagus (cricopharyngeal sphincter); (c) the larynx elevates as the epiglottis, false vocal folds, and true vocal folds close to seal the airway; and (d) the cricopharyngeal sphincter relaxes to allow the bolus to enter the esophagus.

☐ *Esophageal Phase.* During this fourth and final phase, the bolus is transported through the esophagus into the stomach (Logemann, 1983).

The first three phases are of most interest for the speech-language pathologist's treatment. The fourth phase (esophageal phase) is not amenable to direct therapy and normally is treated medically.

BEDSIDE ASSESSMENT OF DYSPHAGIA

Form 10–1 will help you complete a bedside assessment for dysphagia. The form is divided into two segments. The first involves information gathering and an oral-facial evaluation specific to dysphagia. The second involves presentation of foods and/or liquids.[1] It is not necessary to administer both segments with all dysphagic clients. If your client is not alert or if you know which type of dysphagia is present, you can complete the evaluation without presenting food or liquids. If you do administer food or liquid orally, and the client exhibits

---

[1]**Caution:** Do not administer the feeding portion of the evaluation without some prior training and experience or without the direct supervision of a trained and knowledgeable professional.

signs of aspiration after swallowing (i.e., choking, coughing, wet voice quality), discontinue the evaluation. Then notify the physician to modify or discontinue oral feeding. You can proceed with therapy or refer the client for a radiographic examination to diagnose the disorder more specifically. Be aware that *silent* aspiration can occur. In this case, the client does not exhibit the outward signs of aspiration. If you suspect your client is aspirating silently, a radiographic study will be necessary to confirm or rule out dysphagia.

Administration and Interpretation[2]

Before you begin the direct assessment, gather as much information about the client's current status as you can. The best way to obtain this information is to consult with the client's physician or nurse or review the client's medical records. Sometimes a family member or the client can provide this information. Specifically:

☐ Identify the client's neurological and medical status. For example, was there a recent stroke? Does the client have Parkinsonism? Are there any neurological indicators? Does the client have a history of aspiration pneumonia? Does the client wear dentures?

☐ Identify the client's feeding status. For example, is the client on a regular diet? Puree diet? Fed via a nasogastric tube? Has the client been losing weight or refusing to eat? Has the client been experiencing backflow, reflux, or vomiting after meals? Is the client fed by someone else? Who will feed the client after discharge from a hospital?

☐ Be aware of dietary limitations. For example, does the client have food allergies? Is the client diabetic? Obtain this information so you do not present foods or liquids that could be detrimental to the client.

☐ Identify the client's cognitive status. For example, is the client alert? Is the client able to follow commands? Is there dementia? Will the client be able to cooperate in therapy if treatment is indicated?

Once you have gathered this preliminary information, assess the integrity of the oral mechanism. This assessment is similar to the oral-facial evaluation administered as a standard procedure for most communicative disorders, but for a dysphagic client you also need to make special note of behaviors or deficits that may alter the person's ability to safely chew and swallow.

☐ Poor oral control may be a result of weak lips, tongue, and/or jaw, or poor oral sensitivity. Oral sensitivity may be compromised, and the client may have difficulty keeping the food in the mouth. If the weakness is unilateral, the food typically leaks from the weaker side.

---

[2]The information in this section is based on Cherney, Cantieri, and Pannell (1986); Logemann (1983); Perlman and Schulze-Delrieu (1997); and our own clinical experiences.

☐ Chewing difficulties may be caused by incoordination or weakness of the jaw. Also, normal food textures may not be appropriate for a client if teeth are absent or if the client's dentures do not fit properly.

☐ Poor oral control may result from a weak, uncoordinated, or insensitive tongue. The client may have difficulty forming a bolus and manipulating the food for chewing or propelling the food back for swallowing.

☐ Nasal regurgitation may occur if velopharyngeal movement is impaired.

☐ Penetration of the bolus into the airway or complete aspiration may result from weak or uncoordinated laryngeal musculature. If the larynx does not have normal range of motion or if the laryngeal reflex is slow or delayed, the airway is at risk of being obstructed during swallowing. Also, the client may not be able to productively clear food out of the airway if aspiration does occur.

For the second segment of the bedside dysphagia evaluation, present small bites of different textures of food or liquids in order from the easiest to manage (puree) to the most difficult to manage (liquid). A puree texture (e.g., mashed potatoes or applesauce) easily forms into a cohesive bolus and does not need to be chewed. Soft texture foods (e.g., chopped meat with gravy or cooked beans) require some chewing, but are easier to manage than regular textures. Regular texture foods (e.g., toast or chunks of meat) are the most difficult foods to chew and prepare into a bolus. Liquids are the most difficult to manipulate because swallowing liquids involves the least voluntary and reflexive control. Assess the client's ability to manage liquids presented from a spoon, a straw, and a cup. Do not present liquids at all to a client who has difficulty with puree textures.

Part II of the bedside evaluation form lists behaviors you may observe during the presentation of foods or liquids. The behaviors are grouped according to the applicable phase of the normal swallow. Suspect dysphagia if the client is having difficulty with one or several of these behaviors:

Oral Preparatory Phase:

☐ Food or liquid spills out of the mouth because of poor labial seal. Normally it leaks from the weaker side of the mouth if unilateral paresis is present.

☐ Food is not chewed adequately because of reduced mandibular strength, reduced lingual strength and range of motion, or reduced oral sensitivity.

☐ A proper bolus is not formed because of reduced lingual strength and range of motion or reduced oral sensitivity.

☐ Residual food is pocketed between the cheeks and tongue (lateral sulcus) after the swallow due to reduced buccal tension.

☐ Residual food is pocketed under the tongue after the swallow due to reduced lingual strength.

Oral Phase:

☐ Food or liquid spills out of the mouth due to poor labial and lingual seal. Normally, leakage occurs from the weaker side of the mouth if unilateral paresis is present.

☐ Food or liquid falls over the base of the tongue and may be aspirated because of reduced tongue strength and/or range of motion, or reduced oral sensitivity.

☐ Residual food is pocketed between the cheeks and tongue (lateral sulcus) after the swallow due to reduced buccal tension.

☐ Residual food is pocketed under the tongue after the swallow due to reduced lingual strength.

☐ Residual food is present on the hard palate after the swallow because of reduced lingual elevation.

☐ Food is spit out of the oral cavity from tongue thrusting.

☐ The time taken to move the bolus posteriorly is abnormally slow.

☐ Excessive tongue movement is noted during the swallow due to lingual incoordination, or as a compensatory strategy due to a delayed or absent swallow reflex.

Pharyngeal Phase:

☐ Coughing, choking, or a wet voice quality occurs when food or liquid enters the airway because of a delayed or absent swallow reflex, reduced laryngeal elevation, reduced laryngeal closure, reduced pharyngeal peristalsis (squeezing), or cricopharyngeal dysfunction. With some clients, these outward symptoms do not occur even when aspiration has taken place.

☐ Nasal regurgitation occurs due to inadequate velopharyngeal closure.

☐ Excessive saliva and mucous are present due to aspiration and the body's attempt to clear away the foreign material.

Esophogeal Phase:

☐ Coughing, choking, or a wet voice quality occurs when food or liquid enters the esophagus, is partially regurgitated, and then enters the airway because of cricopharyngeal dysfunction.

☐ Regurgitation occurs due to cricopharyngeal dysfunction.

Form 10–1. Adult Dysphagia Bedside Evaluation

Name: _____   Age: _____   Date: _____

Examiner:_____

Part I

Current medical/neurological status: _____

Current feeding status: _____

Dietary limitations: _____

Cognitive status:_____

Ask the client to do the following. Model as necessary. Make a check (✔) on the left-hand column and circle any observations.

Jaw:

_____ open and close mouth: normal/incomplete/deviates right/deviates left

_____ open and close mouth against mild pressure: normal/weak

Is the client groping?

Look at the client's dentition. Make a note of abnormal occlusion or missing teeth.

Does the client wear dentures or partials? If yes, do they fit properly?

(continued)

Form 10–1. *(continued)*

Lips:

_____ pucker the lips: normal/reduced excursion

_____ smile: normal/droops right/droops left/droops bilaterally

_____ protrude tongue: normal/droops right/droops left/droops bilaterally

_____ say "ma ma ma": normal/poor labial seal

_____ hold air in the cheeks: normal/poor labial seal/nasal emission

Is the client drooling? If yes, from which side?

Brush the lips lightly with hot, cold, sweet, and lemon-flavored cotton-tip swabs. How does the client respond to the different stimuli?

Tongue:

_____ lick lips: normal/incomplete excursion

_____ protrude tongue: normal/deviates right/deviates left

_____ elevate tongue, normal/incomplete excursion

_____ say "la, la, la": normal/slow/poor alveolar contact

_____ say "ga, ga, ga": normal/slow/poor velar contact

Is the client's articulation normal? Is dysarthria present?

Brush the tongue lightly with hot, cold, sweet, and lemon-flavored cotton-tip swabs. How does the client respond to the different stimuli?

Pharynx:

_____ sustain "ah" (observe velopharyngeal movement): normal/absent/weak on right/weak on left/hypernasality

Is a gag reflex present? If yes, is it abnormal? Describe the reflex (e.g., hypoactive, hyperactive, delayed, etc.).

Larynx:

_____ say "ah" for 5 seconds: normal/unable to sustain

_____ clear your throat: normal/weak/absent

_____ cough: normal/weak/absent

_____ swallow (feel laryngeal area): larynx elevates normally/reduced excursion

_____ change pitch upward: normal/reduced range

_____ say "ah" and get louder: normal/no intensity change

_____ say "ah" (note voice quality): normal/wet/breathy/hoarse

PART II[1]

Check the behaviors the client exhibits for each texture presented. Also note whether the client is aware of difficulties and is able to compensate appropriately.

	puree	chopped	regular	liquid
food falls out of mouth (indicate side)	_____	_____	_____	_____
food is pushed out of mouth	_____	_____	_____	_____
struggle while chewing	_____	_____	_____	_____
unable to form bolus	_____	_____	_____	_____
unable to move bolus side-to-side	_____	_____	_____	_____
unable to move bolus back to pharynx	_____	_____	_____	_____
pocketing of food (indicate location)	_____	_____	_____	_____

(continued)

_____

[1]**Caution:** Do not administer the feeding portion of this evaluation without some prior training and experience, or without the direct supervision of a trained and knowledgeable professional.

Form 10–1. *(continued)*

	puree	chopped	regular	liquid
multiple attempts to swallow	_____	_____	_____	_____
residual food on tongue	_____	_____	_____	_____
residual food on hard palate	_____	_____	_____	_____
unable to suck liquid through a straw	_____	_____	_____	_____
difficulty grasping cup with lips	_____	_____	_____	_____
difficulty holding straw with lips	_____	_____	_____	_____
nasal regurgitation	_____	_____	_____	_____
swallow too rapid	_____	_____	_____	_____
swallow delayed (indicate seconds)	_____	_____	_____	_____
laryngeal elevation absent	_____	_____	_____	_____
laryngeal elevation delayed (indicate seconds)	_____	_____	_____	_____
laryngeal elevation incomplete	_____	_____	_____	_____
coughing after swallow	_____	_____	_____	_____
throat clearing after swallow	_____	_____	_____	_____
wet voice quality after swallow	_____	_____	_____	_____
excessive saliva and mucus present	_____	_____	_____	_____
oral regurgitation	_____	_____	_____	_____

Was the client aware of difficulties?

What did the client do to compensate for chewing or swallowing problems?

RADIOGRAPHIC ASSESSMENT OF DYSPHAGIA

A radiographic examination provides a motion x-ray of the swallow. There are several titles for this procedure, including videofluroscopy, modified barium swallow (MBS), and oral pharyngeal motility study (OPMS). During the assessment, the client is presented with barium of varying consistencies (e.g., thin liquid, thick, pudding) and sometimes foods coated with barium (e.g., cracker, banana). The client swallows the barium while being x-rayed as the examiner observes the progression of the barium through the oral and pharygeal cavities and into the esophogus. The test provides valuable diagnostic information by allowing the clinician to determine whether a client is aspirating or penetrating the airway, and if he or she is, specifically identifying the site of aspiration or penetration, its cause, and strategies that will maximize swallowing safety for the client (e.g., body and head positioning, food texture, and amount and rate of food presentation). Although the examination is administered by a radiologist, the speech-language pathologist should make explicit requests about positioning, food consistencies, and compensatory strategies (e.g., modify head position, amount of food, etc.) that need to be assessed by the study. If possible, the clinician should be present during the examination to maximize its diagnostic benefits.

BEDSIDE ASSESSMENT OF THE TRACHEOSTOMIZED CLIENT

When evaluating a tracheostomized client, the swallowing evaluation is modified somewhat. The presence of a tracheostomy changes the pharyngeal pressures that contribute to a functional swallow. Also, the actual hardware can obscure a client's ability to swallow normally and safely (Dikeman & Kazandjian, 1995). Due to complicating factors related to the tracheostomy, it is critical that the client's physician and respiratory therapist be consulted prior to administering the swallowing assessment. The client's physician can provide valuable information about the client's history and current medical status, and the respiratory therapist can provide information about the client's respiratory status. If possible, it is a good idea to have the respiratory therapist present during portions of the evaluation. He or she can monitor the client's ventilation status, assist with cuff deflation and inflation, and suction as needed.

The first portion of the evaluation is the case history. Review medical records, communicate with other caregivers, and talk to the client to gather as much relevant information as possible. In addition to more traditional case history queries, you will also want to ask:

☐ Why is the person tracheostomized?

☐ How long has the tracheostomy been in place?

☐ What kind of tracheostomy tube is present? Is it cuffed? Is it fenestrated?

☐ What stage, if any, of weaning is the client in?

☐ What is the client's medical status?

Next, complete the oral-motor assessment. Apply traditional evaluation techniques for determining lip, tongue, and jaw integrity. Occlude the opening of the tracheostomy briefly and ask the client to say "ah" to see if the client can phonate. If the tracheostomy is cuffed, it will need to be deflated to continue the assessment. It is vitally important that the client's physician authorize cuff deflation. Due to other health issues, cuff deflation may be life threatening. If this is the case, postpone further laryngeal evaluation and presentation of food or liquid until the client is more medically stable. If the client can tolerate cuff deflation, deflate the cuff and continue the assessment of laryngeal function.

The Blue-dye Test

The blue-dye test is a useful diagnostic tool for determining whether a client is aspirating. Ideally, a blue-dye test is administered over several sessions and days with only one texture introduced per day. This allows the most accurate assessment of the client's abilities to manage varying textures (Dikeman & Kazandjian, 1995). Before introducing foods or liquids, ask the respiratory therapist to suction the mouth, the tracheostomy region, and the lungs. If the cuff is still inflated, deflate it now (with physician approval). Once completed, begin the blue-dye test. Add blue food coloring to food or liquid, preferably testing only one texture at a time. Present small amounts of the blue-dyed food or liquid to the client and occlude the tracheostomy tube during every swallow. The client is then suctioned and monitored for the presence of blue dye in the tracheal region. Suctioning is repeated every 15 minutes for the next hour, and the tracheal area is continously monitored for the next 24 hours. Any positive identification of blue food coloring in the tracheal region indicates some degree of aspiration has occurred. It is important to let other caregivers know that a blue-dye test is in progress so that they can continue to watch for blue coloring in your absence.

The blue-dye test can also be used to assess a client's management of his or her saliva even if no food or liquid is introduced. Dab a small amount of blue food coloring on the client's tongue and monitor the tracheal region as you would if food or liquid had been introduced. The blue-dye test is a helpful assessment tool but we must offer this word of caution concerning its reliability: the *presence* of blue dye in the tracheal region will positively identify aspiration; however, the *absence* of blue dye does not necessarily mean the absence of aspiration. Aspiration can be missed (Dikeman & Kazandjian, 1995).

CONCLUDING COMMENTS

Although dysphagia is not a disorder of communication, its evaluation and treatment is frequently under the domain of the speech-language pathologist. It is a potentially life-threatening disorder and should be evaluated with caution and a thorough understanding of dysphagia. It is important to communicate regularly with a client's physician and other health care professionals so the client's health and safety are not jeopardized. A bedside evaluation is often adequate for making diagnostic conclusions about a client with suspected dysphagia; however, there are cases when a radiographic study is necessary for completing a thorough examination.

There are diagnostic procedures unique to tracheostomized clients that are followed when completing a dysphagia evaluation. The client's physician and respiratory therapist are invaluable sources of assistance and information. It is especially important to discuss the assessment protocol with the physician prior to completing the evaluation so you know whether the client is medically stable enough to tolerate the assessment. The blue-dye test can be administered to detect aspiration in a tracheostomized client.

SOURCES OF ADDITIONAL INFORMATION

Dikeman, K. J., & Kazandjian, M. S. (1995). *Communication and swallowing management of tracheostomized and ventilator-dependent adults*. San Diego, CA: Singular Publishing Group.

Gilardeau, C., Kazandjian, M. S., Bach, J. R., Dikeman, K. J., Willig, T. N., & Tucker, L. M. (1995). The evaluation and management of dysphagia. *Seminars in Neurology, 15*(1), 46–51.

Groher, M. (Ed.). (1992). *Dysphagia: Diagnosis and management* (2nd ed.). Stoneham, MA: Butterworth-Heinemann.

Hendrix, T. (1993). Art and science of history taking in the patient with difficulty swallowing. *Dysphagia, 8*, 69–73.

Logemann, J. (1983). *Evaluation and treatment of swallowing disorders*. Austin, TX: PRO-ED.

Logemann, J. A. (1990). Dysphagia. *Seminars in Speech and Language, 2*, 157–164.

Perlman, A. L., & Schulze-Delrieu, K. S. (Eds.). (1997). *Deglutition and its disorders*. San Diego, CA: Singular Publishing Group.

Internet Sources

American Speech-Language-Hearing Association
http://www.asha.org/

Dysphagia Resource Center
http://www.dysphagia.com/

□ CHAPTER 11 □

Assessment of Three Special Populations

In some clinical environments, speech-language pathologists work with clients who have uncommon communicative disabilities. In such cases, the assessment procedure needs to be tailored to evaluate the client's unique communicative skills and deficits. This chapter presents basic diagnostic procedures for assessing three such populations: clients who may benefit from an augmentative or alternative communication (AAC) system, laryngectomized clients, and clients with cleft lip and/or palate.

If your experience with these client populations is limited, we recommend you consult a speech-language pathologist who has experience in these areas. This resource manual is intended to summarize basic assessment procedures. The evaluation process for these special populations is sometimes complex, with many factors to consider. An experienced clinician can offer valuable insight into the administration and interpretation of assessment data. The *Sources of Additional Information* listed at the end of this chapter can also provide additional guidance.

OVERVIEW OF ASSESSMENT

History of the Client

> Procedures

>> Written Case History
>> Information-getting Interview
>> Information from Other Professionals

> Contributing Factors

>> Medical Diagnosis
>> Pharmacological Factors
>> Age
>> Intelligence, Motivation, and Levels of Concern

Assessment for Augmentative or Alternative Communication (AAC)

> Procedures

>> Screening
>> Consultation with Caregivers and Client
>> Formal Testing
>> Structured Observations

> Analysis

>> Current Needs
>> Sensory Skills
>> Motor Skills
>> Cognitive Abilities
>> Language Abilities
>> Appropriate AAC Options

Assessment of Laryngectomees

    Procedures

        Pre-operative Consultation
        Informal Testing
        Speech and Language Sampling
        Post-operative Consultation

    Analysis

    Current Needs
    Cognitive-Linguistic Abilities
    Client Preferences for Alaryngeal Communication
    Most Appropriate Alaryngeal Communication Method

Assessment of Clients with Cleft Lip and/or Palate

    Procedures

        Screening
        Speech Sampling
        Formal Testing
        Use of Instrumentation
        Stimulability

    Analysis

        Type of Cleft
        Velopharyngeal Integrity
        Resonance
        Expressive/Receptive Abilities
        Cognitive-linguistic Abilities
        Intelligibility

Oral-facial Examination

Hearing Assessment

Determining the Diagnosis

Providing Information (written report, interview, etc.)

Ongoing Assessment

ASSESSMENT FOR AUGMENTATIVE OR ALTERNATIVE COMMUNICATION (AAC)

Some individuals are severely limited in their ability to communicate verbally due to cognitive disabilities or physical impairments. These clients are often candidates for augmentative or alternative communication (AAC). AAC is a communication system that compensates for impairments and disabilities of clients with severe expressive communication disorders (American Speech-Language Hearing Association, 1989). There are a variety of AAC systems available, ranging from inexpensive, low-technology options such as sign language or communication boards, to costly, high-technology communication devices utilizing synthesized speech output. An AAC system may be needed temporarily or permanently, depending on the client's individual abilities and prognosis.

A speech-language evaluation can determine whether AAC will be beneficial and what type of AAC system will be most appropriate for a client. When completing an evaluation of clients with a severe expressive impairment, the evaluation process needs to be modified to accommodate the client's language and physical limitations. The evaluation typically involves consulting a team of professionals, such as physicians, therapists, psychologists, social workers, and teachers, who can provide valuable information to help you make the most appropriate assessment decisions. The assessment of clients for AAC generally includes four broad areas. They are:

- ☐ Determining the clients communicative needs.
- ☐ Assessing the client's sensory and motor abilities.
- ☐ Assessing the client's language and cognitive abilities.
- ☐ Predicting the most suitable AAC system.

When determining the client's communicative needs, you will need to consider the client's current communication system, how effective that system is, what kind of success or failure the client has experienced with other systems, and what communicative situations and messages are typical for the client. This information can be gathered by interviewing the client as well as other caregivers who interact with the client regularly, especially parents and teachers. The assessment environment needs to be as natural as possible, mimicking what the client experiences during routine day-to-day activity. Glennen and DeCoste (1997) have devised an assessment worksheet that is helpful for evaluating a nonverbal client's communicative needs. We have adapted it and reprinted it in Form 11–1.

Form 11–1. Augmentative and Alternative Communication Information and Needs Assessment[1]

Name: _____ Age:_____ Date:_____

Examiner: _____

Informants: Relationship to Client:

_____   _____

_____   _____

_____   _____

I. **Current Methods of Communication.** For each modality ask the informant (1) whether the modality is used, and if it is to describe the client's current use of the modality, (2) to indicate the size of the client's vocabulary using the modality, and (3) to indicate how well the client is understood when using the modality. Use the spaces provided to record notes.

Modality	Description	Vocabulary Size	Intelligibility
Speech			
Vocalizations			
Sign language			

(continued)

Form 11-1 *(continued)*

Gesture/pointing

Head nods

Eye gaze

Facial expressions

AAC device

Other

II. **Past AAC Experience.** Ask the informant the following questions. Record notes in the spaces provided.

Has this individual ever used a picture or letter-based AAC device in the past? If yes describe the system.

Name of device:_____ Length of time used:_____

Number of symbols:_____ Size of symbols:_____

Symbol system used:_____ Organization of symbols:_____

Access method:_____

What were the strengths and limitations of the AAC system described above?

(continued)

Form 11–1 *(continued)*

III. **Communication Environments**. Ask the informant to describe how the AAC will be used and with whom. Also determine barriers to using the AAC. Take notes in the spaces provided.

Environment	Description	Interaction Partner
Home		
School		
Work		
Community		
Other		

What barriers to AAC implementation exist in any of the environments listed above?

IV. **Mobility and Access**. Ask the informant to describe the client's mobility and access regarding use of an AAC system. Also determine specific mobility, seating, or positioning concerns.

Mobility	Description	Environment Used
Fully ambulatory		
Ambulatory with assistance		
Manual wheelchair		
Power wheelchair		
Other		

Are there any mobility, seating, or positioning concerns that will affect the implementation of an AAC system? If yes, describe.

(continued)

Form 11–1 *(continued)*

Functional Access	Description	Access Limitations
Left arm/hand		
Right arm/hand		
Head		
Left leg/foot		
Right leg/foot		
Eye gaze		
Other		

V. **Other Technologies**. Ask the informant what other technologies will need to be integrated with an AAC system. Record notes in the spaces provided.

Technology	Description	Environment Used
Wheelchair		
Computer		
Environmental controls		
Switch toys		
Other		

VI. **AAC Expectations**. Ask the informant the following questions. Record notes in the space provided.

What goals could be achieved if the client had access to an AAC system?

Assessing Sensory and Motor Capabilities

A client with limited verbal skills may have severe sensory and/or motor impairments that will need to be identified in order to make the most appropriate assessment decisions and AAC recommendations. It is important to modify test administrations to accommodate certain deficits, and to carefully consider the client's abilities and disabilities when selecting an AAC system. The specific sensory and motor abilities that you will need to consider are: positioning, hearing, visual tracking and scanning, and motor dexterity.

During the assessment, position the client so that success in completing evaluative tasks is maximized. Pillows, wedges, foam rolls, or other support structures are sometimes helpful for achieving optimal positioning. Consider whether the client can position him- or herself or if restraints are needed for maintaining the most desirable posture. Also note whether the client is able to walk or is confined to a wheelchair. Various AAC systems accommodate a variety of user postures and positions.

The client's visual tracking and scanning abilities will also need to be considered. Visual tracking refers to the ability to watch an object or person move through more than one visual plane, and visual scanning refers to the ability to look for and locate an object among several other objects (Baumgart, Johnson, & Helmstetter, 1990). Both skills will have an impact on assessment administration and recommendations for AAC. Evaluate the client's ability to visually track vertically, horizontally, and diagonally in two directions. Evaluate the client's ability to visually scan words, objects, and/or symbols that may be used for utilizing an AAC system. Use a variety of stimulus items and include repeated trials. Also determine:

- Whether the client can visually focus on an object;
- If the eyes move in a smooth, continuous motion;
- If nystagmus (oscillating movement of the eyeball) is present;
- Whether there are areas of visual neglect;
- If the eyes move together;
- At what rate the client tracks or scans (e.g, slowly, quickly, inconsistently);
- The distance from the face the item needs to be to successfully view it;
- Where the client begins tracking or searching for objects (e.g., at midline, to the right, to the left, up, down);
- Whether there is an identifiable pattern of scanning; and
- The number of items the client is able to scan.

Form 11–2, "Visual Scanning and Tracking Checklist," is provided to help you evaluate a client's visual skills for the assessment for AAC.

Form 11–2. Visual Scanning and Tracking Checklist

Name: _____ Age:_____ Date:_____

Examiner: _____

Instructions: Make the following observations. Mark a check (✓) if a statement describes the client. Record additional comments in the right-hand column.

Comments

Client is able to track from:

_____ left to right _____

_____ right to left _____

_____ up and down _____

_____ down and up _____

_____ diagonally up and down, left to right _____

_____ diagonally up and down, right to left _____

_____ diagonally down and up, left to right _____

_____ diagonally down and up, right to left _____

Client is able to:

_____ read words (indicate size of print) _____

_____ read phrases (indicate size of print) _____

_____ recognize pictures or objects _____

_____ recognize symbols_____

Client is able to:

_____ visually focus on stimuli _____

_____ scan stimuli for desired word/picture/symbol (circle one and indicate number of stimulus items in

field) _____

_____ identify desired stimulus quickly/slowly (circle one and indicate seconds) _____

_____ identify desired stimulus consistently _____

_____ identify desired stimulus with cues (indicate type) _____

(continued)

Form 11–2 *(continued)*

Client demonstrates:

_____ visual neglect (indicate areas) _____

_____ nystagmus (oscillating movement of the eyeball) _____

_____ strabismus (eyes turn in or out) _____

_____ poor ability to move eyes together _____

_____ difficulty seeing stimuli more than 12 inches away from face _____

Note any identifiable patterns of scanning, including where the client begins visually searching (e.g., at midline, top left, top right, etc.) _____

_____

_____

Hearing acuity becomes particularly important if visual skills are deficient, as many AAC devices have auditory scan features which clients with adequate hearing can access. Assessment of hearing is usually straightforward, and an audiologist with or without AAC experience can evaluate hearing abilities (Beukelman & Mirenda, 1992).

The evaluation process also includes a determination of the client's motor abilities and deficits and how they will impact the usefulness of various AAC systems. Specific considerations include:

- The primary medical diagnosis,
- The presence of abnormal reflexes associated with spasticity,
- The presence of tremor, and
- How easily and how much the client fatigues (Silverman, 1995).

To use certain AAC systems, a client must be able to use some part of the body, preferably a hand, to produce voluntary, controlled, and consistent movements. If physical disability precludes the use of either hand, the head and chin, feet, knees, elbows, or other body part could possibly be used. Even controlled eye blinks or movements of the tongue have been used to access AAC devices (Buekelman, Yorkston, & Dowden, 1985).

Assessing Language and Cognitive Skills

The assessment of language and cognitive skills are important for determining current levels of expressive and receptive abilities, understanding how the client perceives the world, and accurately predicting the most suitable AAC system to maximize the client's communication. To determine cognitive levels, make observations about the client's abilities and deficits in the following areas:

☐ *Alertness.* Note whether the client is aware of his or her surroundings and if the client is oriented to time and space. The Rancho Los Amigos Levels of Cognitive Functioning (Malkus, Booth, & Kodimer, 1980) (described on p. 335 of this book) are often used to assign or describe general levels of alertness.

☐ *Fatigue level.*

☐ *Attention span.* Determine how long the client can attend to an activity or conversation.

☐ *Knowledge of "cause and effect."* Note whether the client understands the concept that one behavior causes another, such as activating a switch causes a tape recorder to play music.

☐ *Symbolic representation skills.* Note whether the client recognizes symbols, such as pictures of common objects, and is able to correlate pictures with real objects. Also determine the client's reading and writing skills.

☐ *Memory skills.*

Knowledge of a client's cognitive status will help you make appropriate judgments and recommendations regarding the most appropriate AAC system. Also important is knowledge of the client's receptive and expressive language abilities. Clearly, the method of assessing language will have to be modified to accommodate physical and verbal disabilities. For example, you may need to allow the client to use eye gaze in place of pointing when administering certain tests. You may also need to create client-specific stimulus activities to elicit desired responses. For example, to assess the client's ability to follow simple or complex commands, present directives that you know the client is motorically capable of doing. Note whether comprehension occurs with verbal direction only or with verbal direction accompanied by gesture.

The Nonspeech Test for Receptive/Expressive Language (Huer, 1983) is an assessment tool designed specifically for evaluating expressive and receptive language skills of nonverbal clients. Other commercially available tests that are not designed for this population but can be modified for such use include:

- *Boehm Test of Basic Concepts* (Boehm, 1986)
- *Peabody Picture Vocabulary Test*—Revised (Dunn & Dunn, 1981)
- *Preschool Language Scale III.* Auditory Comprehension Scale (Zimmerman, Steiner, & Evatt-Pond, 1991)
- *Receptive One-Word Picture Vocabulary Test* (Gardner, 1985)
- *Test for Auditory Comprehension of Language—Revised* (Carrow-Woolfolk, 1985)
- Selected subtests of *Clinical Evaluations of Language Functions—3* (Wiig & Semel, 1995) and *Clinical Evaluation of Language Functions—Preschool* (Wiig, Secord, & Semel, 1992)
- Selected subtests of *Peabody Individual Achievement Test—Revised* (Markwardt, 1989).

You can also adapt certain assessment materials presented in Chapter 4, *Assessment Procedures Common to Most Communicative Disorders*, and Chapter 6, *Assessment of Language*, in this resource manual.

The client's ability to identify objects and pictures will need to be known prior to administering certain language assessments. This will help you determine whether incorrect responses are truly language based or simply due to physical limitations. You can then proceed with more complex communicative tasks that will help you select an appropriate AAC system based on the client's language, cognition, sensory skills, and motor skills. During the assessment, determine whether the client can associate icons with real objects and concepts, use multiple icons to convey a message (e.g., "I want" "to eat" "some cereal"), and recognize categories of icons, pictures, or objects. Also assess the client's ability to read and write. Take note of the size and position of the stimulus materials presented. This will be important to consider when selecting an appropriate AAC system.

Determining the Most Appropriate AAC System

Once the assessment information is gathered and evaluated, a recommendation is made regarding the type of AAC system most appropriate to meet the client's needs. This is a complex decision, and the recommendation should be made by an individual—or team of individuals—with knowledge and experience with the various types of AAC systems and devices available. Often, several options can be presented. Even with the most carefully considered decision, field testing is necessary. Judgments should be made concerning:

- The appropriateness of the AAC system,
- The client's proficiency in accessing the AAC system,
- The client's progress in developing communication skills, and
- The proficiency of the client's communication partners in utilizing the AAC system.

In some cases, assessment results may indicate the client is a poor candidate for AAC. Glennen and DeCoste (1997) recommend that the client be given an opportunity to try AAC anyway. Their rule of thumb is "never say never." Initial assessment results may not consider all the factors that night make an AAC system beneficial.

The selection of the most beneficial AAC system for a client is an ongoing process and is usually not completed during a single evaluation. There are many factors to consider, including the client's proficiency at utilizing a particular system, the client's willingness to use it, and changes in the client's disability, needs, and maturation over time. Commercially available tests that are useful for initial evaluation and subsequent ongoing assessment include:

- *INteraction CHecklist for Augmentative Communication (INCH) (Revised)* (Bolton & Dashiell, 1991)
- *Lifespace Access Profile: Assistive Technology Assessment and Planning for Individuals with Severe or Multiple Disabilities* (Williams et al., 1993)
- *Non-Oral Communication Assessment* (Fell, Linn, & Morrison, 1984)

Probably the ultimate consideration in selecting AAC is the client's desire and willingness to use it. A recommended device may be seen as the answer to a client's communicative needs and have the enthusiastic support of the clinician, the client's family, teachers, and other communicative partners. However, if the client resists or rejects a device, it will serve as nothing more than a futile (and perhaps expensive) undertaking. Counseling, ongoing assessment, and alternative means of communication may be offered until an accepted system is found.

ASSESSMENT OF LARYNGECTOMEES

Laryngectomy is the surgical removal of all or part of the larynx. Most commonly laryngectomy is performed to remove cancerous tumors or, in the case of traumatic injury, to remove a larynx that is severely damaged and not repairable. A person whose larynx has been removed is called a laryngectomee. Obvious and immediate changes occur to the physiology of the speech mechanism as a result of laryngectomy. Illustration 11–1 shows the anatomical changes, and the major respiratory and vocal changes are summarized in Table 11–1.

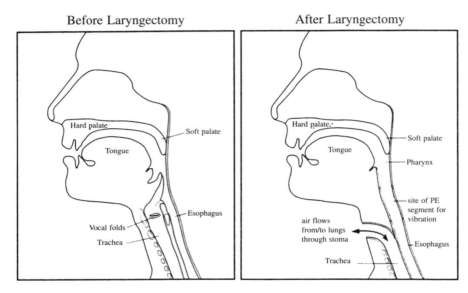

Illustration 11–1. Preoperative and postoperative anatomy of the head and neck related to laryngectomy. (From J. K. Casper and R. H. Colton (1993), *Clinical Manual for Laryngectomy and Head/Neck Cancer Rehabilitation* (p. 66). San Diego, CA: Singular. Reprinted with permission.)

Table 11–1. Pre- and Post-Operative Changes in Respiratory Structures and Behaviors

Pre-Operative	Post-Operative
Inhalation and exhalation are possible through the nose or the mouth or both.	Inhalation and exhalation occur only through a stoma in the neck.
Air taken in through the nose is warmed, moistened, and filtered before entering the lungs.	Air taken in through a stoma passes much more quickly and directly into the lungs without passing through the upper respiratory tract.
Continuity exists from the lungs through the bronchi, trachea, and larynx to the pharynx, mouth, and nose.	No continuity exists between the mouth, nose, and lungs. The stoma is the end point of the tracheal stump.
Voice is produced by airflow through the larynx during exhalation.	Loss of voice. The larynx is removed, and air from the lungs is exhaled directly through the stoma.

Source: Adapted from M. L. Andrews, *Manual of Voice Treatment: Pediatrics through Geriatrics*, p. 316. San Diego, CA: Singular. Copyright © 1995 and used by permission.

Because the vocal mechanism is gone completely or partially, oral communication is profoundly impaired following laryngectomy. A primary responsibility of the speech-language pathologist is to maximize a client's opportunity to establish an adequate post-operative means of communication as soon as possible (Morrison et al., 1994; Stemple, Glaze, & Gerdeman, 1995). The assessment procedure involves pre-operative and post-operative consultations. Prior to the pre-operative visit, it is important to consult the client's physician and review all relevant medical records to learn as much information as possible about the surgery. This will prepare you to answer questions and determine the most feasible post-operative communication strategies. You may use Form 11–3, "Case History for Pre- and Post-Operative Laryngectomee," to help with the collection of this information.

Form 11–3. Case History for Pre- and Post-Operative Laryngectomee[1]

Name: _____ Age:_____ Date:_____

Examiner: _____

Medical History

Surgery: _____

Date of surgery:_____Primary TEF[*]? yes/no   Planned TEF? yes/no

Surgeon: _____

History of present problems: _____

Previous treatment of problem:_____

General health: _____

Medications: _____

Previous surgeries: _____

Radiation treatment pre-op: yes/no   If yes, number of visits_____

Radiation treatment post-op: yes/no   If yes, number of visits_____

Social/Occupational History

Occupation: _____

Will client return to work?: _____

With whom does the client live?: _____

Family/friends adjustment?: _____

---

[1]Adapted from J. K. Casper & R. H. Colton, (1993), *Clinical Manual for Laryngectomy and Head/Neck Cancer Rehabilitation* (Appendix D). San Diego, CA: Singular. Copyright 1993 and used by permission.

[*]tracheoesophogeal fistulization

Current Status

Hearing:_____

Vision: _____Dental: _____

Swallowing: _____

Chewing:_____Taste: _____Smell: _____

Tongue: if resectioned, how much? _____

   range of motion: _____

   reconstruction or prosthesis: _____

Cognitive status: _____

Emotional status: _____

Prognosis for acquisition of:

Electronic/mechanical speech: _____

Esophageal speech: _____

Tracheoesophageal speech: _____

Recommendations: _____

_____

_____

The pre-operative consultation provides an opportunity to describe the effects of surgery on communication and discuss post-surgery communication options. Other objectives, summarized from Casper and Colton (1993) and Hegde (1996), are listed below. During this initial visit, be sensitive to just how much information the client is prepared to receive. Some of the information may need to be repeated or deferred until the post-operative consultation.

- [ ] Determine what the client already knows.
- [ ] Be positive about post-surgery outcomes.
- [ ] Instruct the client to be patient with him- or herself as a new mode of communication is learned.
- [ ] Correct misunderstandings, reinforce correct information, and provide new information.
- [ ] Provide information about support groups.
- [ ] Encourage family involvement.
- [ ] If the client is amenable, have a rehabilitated laryngectomee visit the client and/or family.
- [ ] Discuss communication options.
- [ ] Provide printed information about laryngectomy, postoperative care, and alaryngeal communication options.
- [ ] Informally assess cognition and speech and language skills, including writing.

After surgery, a post-operative consultation is completed. This visit focuses on a more detailed discussion and demonstration of alaryngeal communication options. During this session, review the information presented during the initial visit and include more detailed information to help the client make educated decisions. Provide demonstrations and encourage the client to try a variety of options. When providing information, consider the client's needs and personal situation. Some alaryngeal communication options are not suitable for certain laryngectomees. Therefore, make recommendations that are client-appropriate.

Alaryngeal Communication Options

There are three primary communication modes available to laryngectomees. They are:

- [ ] Electromechanical devices (pneumatic devices and electric larynxes).
- [ ] Esophageal speech.
- [ ] Tracheoesophageal speech resulting from surgical prosthesis.

Electromechanical devices enable sound to be generated outside of the body as speech is shaped by the articulators. Electromechanical devices include pneumatic devices and electric larynxes. A pneumatic device contains a reed that vibrates with exhalation. The device covers the stoma and utilizes tubing to carry the vibrations to the mouth for the production of speech. Pneumatic devices are sometimes the best option immediately after surgery because they typically are easy to use and do not interfere with post-surgical healing. Electric larynxes utilize a mechanical vibrator to create a sound source. Hand-held neck devices direct sound through the skin, and intraoral electronic devices direct sound into the mouth via tubing for the production of speech. All electromechanical devices produce an external source of sound.

Esophageal speech relies on a client's remaining anatomical structures to produce an internal source of sound. Air in the nose and mouth is injected or inhaled into the esophagus and then expelled. The expelled air vibrates the cricopharyngeus muscle of the upper esophagus and the middle and inferior pharyngeal constrictor muscles. These structures are collectively referred to as the pharyngo-esophageal, or PE, segment. The client then articulates normally, utilizing this compensatory sound source to produce speech (Stemple, Glaze, & Gerdeman, 1995).

Esophageal speech is difficult to learn, with some clients unable to learn it even with much practice and instruction. Berlin (1963) described four skills a client should demonstrate that help predict a client's ability to proficiently use esophageal speech. The skills and methods by which they are assessed are:

1. *Ability to phonate reliably on demand.* The client should be able to vocalize /a/ for .4 seconds or longer over 20 repeated trials.

2. *A short latency between inflation of the esophagus and vocalization.* The client should be able to phonate within .2 to .6 seconds after inflating the esophagus over 10 repeated trials.

3. *Adequate duration of phonation.* The client should be able to sustain /a/ for 2.2 seconds over 10 repeated trials.

4. *Ability to sustain phonation during articulation.* The client should be able to articulate the syllable /dɑ/ 8 to 10 times on one injection or inhalation over 5 repeated trials.

Berlin's four skills are meant to predict success with esophageal speech. They are a guideline only. A client who appears to be a poor candidate based on Berlin's criteria should still be given an opportunity to learn esophageal speech if he or she is motivated and has no other contraindicators.

Tracheoesophageal speech relies on a voice prosthesis surgically placed in the tracheoesophageal wall. The surgery is referred to as a tracheoesophageal puncture or fistula (TEP or TEF), and it creates a small hole in the common wall shared by the trachea and esophagus. This hole is fitted for a prosthetic device. When the stoma is occluded, the prosthesis shunts air directly from the lungs into the esophagus, which vibrates the PE segment to create an internal sound source for the production of speech. A tracheostoma valve is sometimes used to eliminate the need to manually occlude the stoma.

All three alaryngeal communication modes have advantages and disadvantages that need to be considered during the evaluation process. These advantages and disadvantages are summarized in Table 11–2. Also, there may be certain contraindicators that would rule out the use of a particular alaryngeal communication option. Candidacy for each mode of post-surgical communication is based on the following criteria (summarized from Casper & Colton, 1993; Duguay & Feudo, 1988; Hegde, 1996; Stemple et al., 1995):

Electromechanical Devices

- Appropriate for almost all laryngectomees.
- Heavy post-surgical scar tissue may preclude the use of a neck device, in which case an intraoral device would be indicated.
- Client must demonstrate adequate manual dexterity to be able to handle and manipulate the unit.
- Articulation must be precise for good intelligibility.
- A variety of units from various manufacturers should be tried to select the most appropriate option for the client.
- Client must express a desire to use the device on a temporary or permanent basis.

Esophageal Speech

- Extensive surgical alteration may preclude the use of the pharyngo-esophageal (PE) segment as a source of vibration for phonation.
- Client should have good hearing acuity.
- Tongue strength and mobility must be adequate for air injection and articulatory production.
- The esophagus must be functionally and structurally sound.
- Radiation damage to oral or pharyngeal tissue may make esophageal speech production more difficult.
- Client must express a desire and willingness to learn esophageal speech.

Tracheoesophageal Speech

- Client must be healed from previous surgery, be disease-free, and exhibit no evidence of cancer recurrence.
- The tracheoesophageal wall must be healthy.
- The stoma should be at least 1.5 cm and located at the manubrium, above the jugular notch.
- Manual dexterity, visual acuity, alertness, and hygienic habits must be adequate for properly maintaining the prosthetic device.
- Pharyngoesophageal spasm, identified through insufflation testing is a contraindicator.[1]
- Client must express a desire to use tracheoesophageal speech and a willingness to maintain the prosthetic device over time.

---

[1]Insufflation testing is done by inserting a rubber catheter through the nasal passage into the esophagus. Air is introduced into the esophagus through the catheter and the client is instructed to use that air to phonate. A Blom-Singer insufflation test kit is commonly used to conduct this test.

Table 11–2. Advantages and Disadvantages of the Three Primary Alaryngeal Communication Options

Electromechanical Devices	Advantages:	Easy to use
		Speech is generally intelligible
		Pneumatic varieties are relatively inexpensive to purchase and operate
		Electronic larynxes are compact and have volume and pitch controls
		Pneumatic devices are suitable for use immediately after surgery in most cases
		Can be an interim source of communication
	Disadvantages:	Mechanical, "robot-like" vocal quality
		Electric larynxes are moderately expensive to purchase and maintain
		Intraoral devices may be initially awkward to use
		Require good articulation skills
Esophageal Speech	Advantages:	Does not require reliance upon a mechanical device
		Both hands are free while speaking
		Vocal productions are the client's "own voice"
		More natural sounding than electromechanical devices
	Disadvantages:	Difficult to learn
		Requires extensive therapy and practice to learn proficiently (approximately 4 to 6 months is typical)
		Approximately one-third of laryngectomees are unable to learn esophageal speech
		Client may need to learn to habitually speak in shorter phrases

(continued)

Table 11–2. *(continued)*

		Vocal intensity is sometimes insufficient
		Client may have a hoarse voice quality
		Potential articulatory errors, excessive stoma noise, "klunking," and facial grimacing need to be overcome during the learning process
Tracheoesophageal Speech	Advantages:	Most natural voice quality of all alaryngeal communication options
		Greater pitch and intensity range than esophageal speech
		Easier and faster to learn than esophageal speech
		Clients can effectively produce sentences of normal length
	Disadvantages:	Requires additional surgery
		Maintenance of the prosthesis is required
		Manual occlusion of the stoma is required if a tracheostoma valve is not used
		Client must have good breath control to use a tracheostoma valve
		Coughing or excessive moisture may interfere with tracheostoma valve function
		Some risk of aspiration of the prosthesis

Source: Summarized from Andrews (1995), Casper and Colton (1993), Martin (1994), and Stemple, Glaze, and Gerdeman (1995).

The selection of one alaryngeal communication method does not preclude the use of another. In some cases, one method is used initially and another is used later. For example, an electromechanical device may be used temporarily while a client learns esophageal speech. Consider initial selections tentative, because the assessment process is ongoing and should be continually modified to achieve the best communication possible for the client.

ASSESSMENT OF CLIENTS WITH CLEFT LIP AND/OR PALATE

Speech-language pathologists are concerned with clefts of the lip and/or palate because of their potential negative impact on normal speech development. Clefts vary in size, extent, and severity from one client to another. Currently, there is no universally accepted system of classifying clefts, although one frequently used classification is Olin's (1960) system which classifies clefts on the basis of three major groups:

- Cleft of the lip only,
- Cleft of the palate only, and
- Cleft of the lip and palate.

Olin's classification is broad, and within each classification there are a variety of potential cleft types. For example, a cleft of the lip can be bilateral, unilateral, at the midline, partial, complete, or a combination of these features. Identifying types of clefts will help in the assessment process, as different locations of clefts affect different aspects of speech production.

The management of a child with a cleft usually involves an interdisciplinary team of specialists, including a physician, dentist, and speech-language pathologist. Each professional offers valuable information regarding the client's immediate and long-term needs. The speech-language evaluation of a client with a cleft follows traditional protocols for evaluating many aspects of speech, language, and voice, but also considers issues specific to clefting. For example, the oral-facial examination is a procedure common to most communicative disorders. We have provided a description of this procedure and an evaluation form on pages 88–94 of this book. In addition to the traditional oral-facial examination, there are several other factors you should consider when evaluating a client with a cleft. These include:

- ☐ Type of cleft. The cleft should be classified and described. If the cleft is repaired, make a judgment about the adequacy of the repair.
- ☐ Presence of other facial abnormalities.
- ☐ Presence of a submucosal cleft. This is often indicated by a bifid uvula, reduced or asymmetrical palatal movement, translucency or thinning of musculature at the velum midline, and/or a palpable notch on the posterior edge of the hard palate.
- ☐ Labial pits in the lower lip.
- ☐ Labiodental, alveolar, palatal, and/or velar fistulas (holes).
- ☐ Velar elevation pattern (e.g., symmetrical, asymmetrical, extent).

☐ Perceived length of the velum.

☐ Perceived depth of the nasopharynx.

☐ Shape of the alveolar ridge (e.g., notched, cleft, wide, collapsed).

Voice is another area that may require special consideration when evaluating a client with a cleft. Deficient vocal resonance is a primary characteristic of cleft palate speech. The issue of vocal resonance and velopharyngeal integrity will be discussed in greater detail on the following pages. However, it is also important to note that children with clefts are also at an increased risk for the development of laryngeal voice disorders, including abnormal voice quality and vocal nodules. This is typically due to the client's effort to:

- produce intelligible speech,
- achieve normal pitch change and loudness,
- compensate for velopharyngeal incompetence by using the glottis to produce plosives and fricatives, and/or
- mask hypernasality and nasal emission (D'Antonio & Scherer, 1995).

Chapter 8, *Assessment of Voice and Resonance*, contains a variety of worksheets you may use to assess the client's voice.

Language assessment is also part of the evaluation process. Procedures for the assessment of language are generally the same for children with or without clefts. Language disorders are not necessarily associated with clefts, as many children in this population develop language normally. However, children with clefts sometimes have language disorders due to cleft-related hearing loss, negative social and emotional factors, and/or cognitive delay, especially if the cleft co-exists with other conditions (McWilliams, Morris, & Shelton, 1990). Use the information in Chapter 6, *Assessment of Language*, for procedures and protocols for the assessment of receptive and expressive language skills.

Assessing Speech and Resonance

Clefts potentially have the most significant negative impact on the development of speech and resonance. However, children with clefts do not always develop speech or resonance disorders, especially when there has been early surgical intervention. Surgical closure of a cleft before single-word development begins (approximately age 1) may preclude the development of cleft-related speech and resonance problems (Trost-Cardamone & Bernthal, 1993).

Many of the assessment guidelines for evaluating the speech and resonance of children with clefts are the same as those for evaluating children without clefts. Chapter 5, *Assessment of Articulation and Phonological Processes*, and Chapter 8, *Assessment of Voice and Resonance*, contain assessment procedures and protocols that can be used when evaluating children with clefts. There are, however, certain characteristics of speech and resonance that are related to clefts, and these need to be considered when completing a speech-language evaluation.

Cleft-related speech impairments primarily include disorders of resonance, poor production of pressure consonants, and the presence of compensatory articulation strategies

(Moller & Starr, 1993). Resonance problems include hypernasality, hyponasality, cul-de-sac resonance, and nasal emission. Specific assessment procedures for evaluating nasal resonance are described on pages 275–277 of this book. Clients with cleft palates may be particularly hypernasal during the production of vowels, glides, and liquids. Nasal emission may be especially evident during the production of pressure consonants. Note if hypernasality is consistent, as this is an indicator of possible velopharyngeal incompetence, or if hypernasality is inconsistent or phoneme-specific, which suggests a behavioral issue rather than a physiologic issue.

Poor production of pressure consonants is an indication of inadequate velopharyngeal closure. As a result, the client is unable to produce sufficient intra-oral pressure for the production of certain consonants. The pressure consonants, along with words and phrases for assessing velopharyngeal function, are presented on pages 277–278. These are useful for assessing a client's ability to produce high-pressure phonemes in a variety of contexts (e.g., syllables, words, phrases).

Other methods for assessing velopharyngeal integrity are also available. The modified tongue anchor procedure (described on p. 279) is one helpful assessment tool. You can also use a mirror or nasal listening tube to assess velopharyngeal integrity (Shipley, 1990). When a mirror is placed below the nares, emitted air during speech causes temporary cloudiness on the mirror. To use a nasal listening tube, place a small nasal bulb in the client's nostrils with an attached tube directed into the clinician's ear. The clinician can identify nasal emission when sound through the tube intensifies. When using the mirror or nasal listening tube, ask the client to produce non-nasal sounds, words, and phrases to determine if there is oral or nasal resonance.

Keep in mind that these procedures may not identify borderline velopharyngeal incompetence. Instruments that directly view the velopharyngeal mechanism during speech production, such as multi-view videofluoroscopy, ultrasonography, tomography, and fiberoptic endoscopy, may need to be used in such cases (Witzel & Stringer, 1990).

Compensatory articulation strategies are learned behaviors that clients with clefts sometimes use in an effort to compensate for velopharyngeal incompetence. These speech patterns may persist even after surgical intervention has resolved the physiologic defect (Morris, 1990). Several specific patterns have been identified and are described below. The phonetic symbols used to notate these productions during phonetic transcription are provided in parentheses.

☐ *Glottal stops* (/ʔ/). The vocal folds are used in an effort to produce plosive consonants. This strategy is frequently detected in cleft palate speech.

☐ *Pharyngeal stops* /ʖ/, unvoiced; /ʖ/ voiced). Produced by lingual contact with the posterior pharyngeal wall.

☐ *Mid-dorsum palatal stops* (/ɞ/, unvoiced; /ɟ/ voiced). The mid-dorsum of the tongue makes contact with the mid-palate.

☐ *Pharyngeal fricatives* (/ʕ/, unvoiced; /ʕ/ voiced). Produced by narrowing the pharyngeal airway through linguapharyngeal constriction. These are attempted substitutes for sibilant fricatives.

☐ *Velar fricatives* (/X/, unvoiced; /ɣ/ voiced). Fricatives are produced in the approximate place where /k/ and /g/ are normally produced.

☐ *Nasal fricatives.* Excessive nasal emission is used as a substitute for consonants. These are also referred to as "nasal snorts," "nasal rustles," or "nasal friction."

☐ *Posterior nasal fricatives* (/Δ/). Produced when the velum or uvula approximates the posterior pharyngeal wall of the nasopharynx. The back of the tongue may elevate in an attempt to assist in velopharyngeal closure.

☐ *Nasal grimaces.* A narrowing of the nostrils produced in an attempt to control nasal emission and inefficient use of the air source (Bzoch, 1989; Trost, 1981; Trost-Cardamone & Bernthal, 1993).

Morley (1970) identified several other patterns of articulation that are common in clients with clefts. These are not compensatory strategies, yet they are important to consider during the evaluative process. They include:

☐ Substitution of /t/ for /k/ and /d/ for /g/, or vice versa.

☐ Substitution of /n/ for /t/ and /d/.

☐ Substitution of /m/ for /p/ and /b/.

☐ Substitution of /n/ for /ŋ/, or vice versa.

☐ Phonemes /k/ and /g/ may be produced by contact of the back of the tongue and the posterior pharyngeal wall, or by substitution of /h/ for /k/ and /g/.

☐ Labiodental and interdental phonemes may be produced bilabially.

☐ Phonemes /t/ and /d/ may be produced interdentally.

We have provided an assessment worksheet, Form 11–4 "Checklist for the Assessment of Clients with Clefts," to help you summarize information gathered during the speech-language evaluation. The worksheet is intended to help you focus on areas of speech and voice that may be deficient in clients with clefts. In addition to this worksheet, there are other assessment instruments that are helpful for evaluating clients with clefts. These include:

• *Great Ormand Street Speech Assessment* (Sell, Harding, & Grunwell, 1994)
• *Iowa Pressure Articulation Test*, a subtest of the *Templin-Darley Tests of Articulation* (Templin & Darley, 1969)
• Several assessment protocols in *Communicative Disorders Related to Cleft Lip and Palate* (3rd ed.) (Bzoch, 1989)

Form 11–4. Checklist for the Assessment of Clients with Clefts

Name: _____ Age:_____ Date:_____

Primary care physician: _____

Type of cleft: _____

Date of surgery:_____

Other conditions and medical history: _____

_____

_____

Examiner: _____

Oral-Facial Examination

Instructions: Administer a standard oral-facial examination (you may wish to use Form 4–1 in this book). Additionally, make observations about the following oral-facial features. Check and circle each item noted. Include descriptive comments in the right-hand margin.

Comments

_____ Type of cleft: lip/palate/lip and palate (describe) _____

_____ Adequacy of cleft repair: good/fair/poor _____

_____ Other facial abnormalities: absent/present (describe) _____

_____ Submucosal cleft: absent/present _____

_____ Labial pits in lower lip: absent/present _____

_____ Labiodental fistulas: absent/present _____

_____ Alveolar fistulas: absent/present_____

_____ Palatal fistulas: absent/present _____

_____ Velar fistulas: absent/present _____

_____ Perceived length of velum: normal/short/long _____

_____ Perceived depth of nasopharynx: normal/shallow/deep_____

_____ Shape of the alveolar ridge: notched/cleft/wide/collapsed_____

_____ Notes from standard oral-facial examination_____

_____

_____

(continued)

Form 11–4 *(continued)*

Assessment of Voice

Instructions: Evaluate the client's voice, paying particular attention to possible cleft-related problems. Check deficits that are present and indicate severity. Record additional notes in the right-hand margin. (You may also use Form 8–2, Vocal Characteristics Checklist, for a more detailed analysis.)

    1 = mild
    2 = moderate
    3 = severe

Comments

_____ Pitch variation is reduced _____

_____ Vocal intensity is reduced _____

_____ Vocal quality is hoarse/harsh/breathy (circle) _____

_____ Vocal quality is strangled _____

_____ Client produces glottal stops in place of plosives and fricatives _____

_____ Client attempts to mask hypernasality and nasal emission _____

_____ Client strains voice to achieve adequate pitch change and loudness_____

_____ Client strains voice in attempt to increase speech intelligibility _____

Assessment of Resonance and Velopharyngeal Integrity

Instructions: Evaluate the client's voice, listening for the following qualities of resonance. Check each characteristic the client exhibits and indicate severity. Record additional notes in the right-hand margin.

    1 = mild
    2 = moderate
    3 = severe

Comments

_____ Hypernasality _____

_____ Nasal emission _____

_____ Cul-de-sac resonance _____

_____ Hyponasality _____

Instructions: Use the administration guidelines for the modified tongue anchor procedure described on page 279 of this book. Check your observation below:

_____ Velopharyngeal function is adequate (no nasal emission)

_____ Velopharyngeal function is inadequate (nasal emission present)

_____ Further testing using objective instrumentation is necessary

Instructions: Ask the client to produce the pressure consonants /p/, /b/, /k/, /g/, /t/, /d/, /f/, /v/, /s/, /z/, /ʃ/, /ʒ/, /tʃ/, /θ/, and /ð/ (see pp. 277–278 for suggested stimulus words and phrases), and listen for hypernasality and nasal emissions. Check the appropriate observations below.

_____ Velopharyngeal function is adequate (no nasal emissions or hypernasality)

_____ Velopharyngeal function is inadequate (nasal emissions or hypernasality present)

_____ Further testing using objective instrumentation is necessary

_____ Nasal emissions and hypernasality are consistent

_____ Nasal emissions and hypernasality are inconsistent

Assessment of Articulation and Phonology

Instructions: Listen to the client's articulatory accuracy. Pay particular attention to the client's production of stop-plosives, fricatives, and affricates, which are most likely to be negatively affected by a cleft. Indicate severity and make additional comments in the right-hand margin.

    1 = mild
    2 = moderate
    3 = severe

Comments

_____ Stop-plosive errors _____

_____ Fricative errors _____

_____ Affricate errors _____

_____ Glide errors _____

_____ Liquid errors _____

_____ Nasal errors_____

_____ Vowel errors _____

_____ Error patterns are consistent _____

_____ Error patterns are inconsistent _____

_____ Further assessment is recommended _____

Instructions: Check the following compensatory strategies the client uses during speech production and indicate severity. Make additional comments in the right-hand margin.

    1 = mild
    2 = moderate
    3 = severe

(continued)

Form 11–4 *(continued)*

Comments

_____ Glottal stops _____

_____ Pharyngeal stops_____

_____ Mid-dorsum palatal stops _____

_____ Pharyngeal fricatives _____

_____ Velar fricatives _____

_____ Nasal fricatives _____

_____ Posterior nasal fricatives_____

_____ Nasal grimaces _____

Summary

Instructions: Check areas that require further assessment. Make additional comments in the right-hand margin.

Comments

_____ Articulation — Cleft-related _____

_____ Articulation — Non–cleft-related _____

_____ Cognition_____

_____ Hearing _____

_____ Language_____

_____ Velopharyngeal integrity_____

_____ Voice _____

CONCLUDING COMMENTS

Basic assessment procedures for three special populations were presented in this chapter—specifically, assessment for AAC, assessment of laryngectomees, and assessment of clients with cleft lip and/or palate. Each population presents a unique pattern of symptoms and communicative behaviors. The assessment processes are typically ongoing, requiring multiple visits to modify the recommended treatment program and meet the client's changing communicative needs. If you do not have experience in the assessment of these special populations, we encourage you to seek guidance from a clinician who does. An experienced clinician can offer insight into nuances and unique situations that a resource manual of this nature is not intended to present. We also encourage you to consult the resources listed below for further information on these three special populations.

SOURCES OF ADDITIONAL INFORMATION

Augmentative and Alternative Communication

Baumgart, D., Johnson, J., & Helmstetter, E. (1990). *Augmentative and alternative communication systems for persons with moderate and severe disabilities*. Baltimore: Paul H. Brookes.

Beukelman, D. R., & Mirenda, P. (1992). *Augmentative and alternative communication: Management of severe communication disorders in children and adults*. Baltimore: Paul H. Brookes.

Blackstone, S. W., & Bruskin, D. M. (1986). *Augmentative communication: An introduction*. Rockville, MD: ASHA.

Church, G., & Glennen, S. (1991). *The handbook of assistive technology*. San Diego, CA: Singular Publishing Group.

Glennen, S. L., & DeCoste, D. C. (1997). Handbook of augmentative and alternative communication. San Diego, CA: Singular Publishing Group.

Silverman, F. H. (1995). *Communication for the speechless* (3rd ed.). Boston: Allyn & Bacon.

Laryngectomy

Andrews, M. L. (1995). *Manual of voice treatment: Pediatrics through geriatrics*. San Diego, CA: Singular Publishing Group.

Casper, J. K., & Colton, R. H. (1993). *Clinical manual for laryngectomy and head/neck cancer rehabilitation*. San Diego, CA: Singular Publishing Group.

Doyle, P. C. (1994). *Foundations of voice and speech rehabilitations following laryngeal cancer*. San Diego, CA: Singular Publishing Group.

Keith, R. L., & Darley, F. L. (1994). *Laryngectomee rehabilitation* (3rd ed.). Austin, TX: PRO-ED.

Stemple, J. C., Glaze, L. E., & Gerdeman, B. K. (1995). *Clinical voice pathology: Theory and management*. San Diego, CA: Singular Publishing Group.

Cleft Lip and Palate

American Cleft Palate-Craniofacial Association. (1993). Parameters for evaluation and treatment of patients with cleft lip/palate or other craniofacial anomalies. *Cleft Palate-Craniofacial Journal, 30*, (Supplement).

Bardach, J., & Morris, H. L. (1990). *Multidisciplinary management of cleft lip and palate*. Philadelphia: W. B. Saunders Co.

Berkowitz, S. (1996). *Cleft lip and palate: Perspectives in management*. San Diego: CA: Singular Publishing Group.

Bzoch, K. R. (Ed.). (1989). *Communicative disorders related to cleft lip and palate*. Austin, TX: PRO-ED.

McWilliams, B. J., Morris, H. L., & Shelton, R. L. (1990). *Cleft palate speech* (2nd ed.). Philadelphia: B. C. Decker, Inc.

Moller, K. T., & Starr, C. D. (1993). *Cleft palate: Interdisciplinary issues and treatment*. Austin, TX: PRO-ED.

Shprintzen, R. J., & Bardach, J. (Eds.) (1995). *Cleft palate speech management: A multidisciplinary approach*. St. Louis: Mosby.

Internet Sources

American Cleft Palate-Craniofacial Association (ACPA) and Cleft Palate Foundation (CPF)
http://www.cleft.com

An Introduction to Alaryngeal Speech
http://www.ahs.uwo.ca/orcn/asha/phil.html

The United States Society for Augmentative and Alternative Communication
http://kaddath.mt.cs.cmu.edu/scs/93-7.html

The Voice Center at Eastern Virginia Medical School
http://www.voice-center.com/laryngectomy.html

□ CHAPTER 12 □

Assessment of Hearing

The assessment of hearing is within the professional province of the audiologist, not the speech-language pathologist. However, the speech-language clinician is interested in clients' hearing abilities since hearing loss directly affects the development or maintenance of optimal communicative skills. Specifically, we are interested in the effects of hearing impairment:

- On the assessment of communicative development and abilities,
- On the development or maintenance of a communication disorder,
- On treatment recommendations and the selection of appropriate treatment procedures and target behaviors, and
- On academic, social, or vocational development.

Speech-language pathologists are limited to screening their clients' hearing, but it is vitally important for the speech-language pathologist to understand hearing loss, audiological assessment procedures, interpretation of findings, and implications of hearing loss on speech and language development.

TYPES OF HEARING LOSS

Conductive Hearing Loss

A conductive hearing loss occurs when the transmission of sound is interrupted. This occurs in the outer ear or, more frequently, in the middle ear. In children, the most common cause of middle ear dysfunction is otitis media, or middle ear infection. (See "Medical Conditions Associated with Communicative Disorders" on page 49 and the Glossary for descriptions of otitis media.) In adults, the most common cause of conductive hearing impairment is otosclerosis, a disease of the middle ear ossicles which may cause the footplate of the stapes to attach to the oval window. The most common cause of conductive hearing impairment among the geriatric population is ear canal collapse. Other less common causes of conductive hearing loss are aural atresia (closed external auditory canal), stenosis (narrow external auditory canal), and external otitis (infected and swollen external auditory canal; also known as "swimmer's ear").

Sensorineural Hearing Loss

A sensorineural hearing loss occurs when the hair cells of the cochlea or the acoustic nerve (CN VIII) are damaged. The impairment is associated with the loss of hearing through bone conduction, and it is considered a permanent impairment. Causes of sensorineural hearing loss include:

- Ototoxicity, or damage from drugs (including certain antibiotics);
- Infections, such as meningitis or maternal rubella;

- Genetic factors, such as certain birth defects that result in partially developed or missing parts of the cochlea or auditory nerve;
- Syphilis or anoxia contracted during the birth delivery;
- Presbycusis associated with the effects of aging;
- Ménière's disease, a unilateral disease that is characterized by vertigo (dizziness) and tinnitus (noise in the ear).

Mixed Hearing Loss

Mixed hearing losses involve a combination of a conductive and sensorineural loss. Both air and bone conduction pathways are involved so the hearing loss is partially conductive and partially sensorineural, but the hearing by bone conduction is typically the better of the two (Bess & Humes, 1995). The sensorineural component of a mixed hearing loss determines the amount of speech sound distortion that is present. Thus, bone conduction audiograms are the best indicators of the degree of difficulty a client will have recognizing and discriminating speech, even if it has been amplified (Martin, 1990).

Central Auditory Disorder

Central auditory disorders stem from problems within the central auditory system, caused by damage that occurs somewhere along the auditory nerve or within the cochlear nuclei. Clients with central auditory disorders may have difficulties localizing sound, understanding (versus hearing) speech, or understanding speech in noise. Tinnitus may also be present.

Retrocochlear Pathology

Retrocochlear pathology involves damage to the nerve fibers along the ascending auditory pathways from the internal auditory meatus to the cortex. This damage is often, but not always, the result of a tumor (Bess & Humes, 1995). Depending on the pathology, a hearing loss may or may not be detected when hearing is tested with pure tones. However, many clients with retrocochlear pathology perform poorly on speech-recognition tasks, particularly when the speech signal is altered by filtering, adding noise, and so forth. Several speech-recognition tests as well as auditory brainstem response (ABR) tests and other auditory evoked potentials help identify the presence of retrocochlear pathology. Such testing is clearly beyond the province of the speech-language pathologist and, depending on their training and the equipment available to them, some audiologists as well.

STANDARD CLASSIFICATION OF HEARING LOSS AND THE EFFECTS ON COMMUNICATIVE DEVELOPMENT

Hearing losses vary in severity from individual to individual. A frequently used standard classification system for describing severity levels of hearing loss is presented in Table 12–1. The classifications described are related to average hearing levels obtained during pure tone audiometry. As hearing losses vary immensely, their influence on speech and language development also varies. Logically, the greater the severity of the hearing loss, the greater its potential negative impact on speech and language. You can easily see this relationship in Table 12–2, which presents the rehabilitative and communicative effects of hearing loss at different severity levels. Keep in mind that Boone and Plante's (1993) guidelines (in Table 12–2) are general. Hearing loss affects individuals differently, regardless of severity, and specific intervention is dependent on such factors as:

- The type of loss;
- The dB levels and frequencies affected;
- Age of onset;
- The client's age when the loss was diagnosed;
- Previous intervention (e.g., therapy or educational placement, type of intervention, communication mode);
- Medical intervention (e.g, ongoing, sporadic, etc.);
- The client's intelligence;
- The client's motivation;
- The client's general health;
- Care and stimulation provided by caregivers. For example, caregivers may provide speech and language stimulation in the home, learn sign language, learn how to "trouble shoot" hearing aid problems, include the client in family activities, etc.

Table 12–1. Description of Hearing Loss Severity by Decibel Levels

Average Hearing Level (in dB)	Severity of Hearing Loss
−10 to 15	Normal hearing
16 to 25	Slight hearing loss
26 to 40	Mild hearing loss
41 to 55	Moderate hearing loss
56 to 70	Moderately severe hearing loss
71 to 90	Severe hearing loss
91+	Profound hearing loss

Source: From J. G. Clark (1981), "Uses and abuses of hearing loss classification," *Asha, 23,* 493–500. Used by permission of the American Speech-Language-Hearing Association.

Table 12–2. Effects of Hearing Loss on Communication and Types of Habilitative Intervention with Children

Hearing Loss (500, IK, 2K)	Communication Effects	Habilitation Intervention
25–40 dB	Misses hearing many consonants	Possible surgical correction
	Difficulty in auditory learning	
	Mild speech-language problem	Fit with hearing aids
		Auditory training
		Needs speech-language therapy
40–65 dB	Speech-language retardation	Speech-language placement
	Learning disability	Special education placement
	Hears no speech at normal loudness levels	Fit with hearing aid
65–95 dB	Voice pathology (cul-de-sac resonance and pitch changes)	Voice therapy added to speech therapy
	Aural-oral language seriously compromised	Hearing aid, with total communication
	Severe learning problems	Classroom for the hearing-impaired
90 dB+	Profound hearing loss (deaf)	Hearing aid and total communication
	Voice-speech sound like deaf	Voice and speech therapy
	Severe problems in academic learning	Classroom (or school) for profoundly impaired

Source: From Daniel R. Boone & Elena Plante, *Human Communication and Its Disorders*, 2nd ed., © 1993, p. 183. Reprinted by permission of Prentice-Hall, Englewood Cliffs, NJ.

SCREENING

Speech-language pathologists often provide a hearing screen as part of the complete diagnostic evaluation to identify a potential peripheral hearing loss that may affect a client's communicative development or abilities. When a client fails a screen, he or she should be referred to an audiologist for further evaluation.

Screens are typically administered at 20 or 25 dB for the frequencies 1000, 2000, and 4000 Hz. For some clients, particularly children, you may wish to use more conservative criteria—15 dB at 500, 1000, 2000, 4000, and 8000 Hz—to reduce the risk of missing someone with a mild hearing loss. Form 12–1, the "Hearing Screening Form" is useful for recording your findings.

Form 12–1. Hearing Screening Form

Name: _____ Date: _____

Address/School: _____

DOB: _____ Age: _____

Patient History   **Comments**

_____ Family history of hearing loss _____

_____ Ear infections _____

_____ Earaches _____

_____ Tinnitus _____

_____ Surgery _____

_____ Hearing aid _____

_____ Medications _____

_____ Diseases associated with hearing loss _____

_____ Exposure to noise _____

_____ Other relevant information _____

Previous Hearing Evaluations (date, place, findings): _____

_____

Evaluation

X or ✔ = Responded appropriately
O or – = Did not respond
CTN = Could not test (specify reason)

dB level _____

	500 Hz	1000 Hz	2000 Hz	4000 Hz	8000 Hz
Right:	_____	_____	_____	_____	_____
Left:	_____	_____	_____	_____	_____

Conclusions

_____ Passed screen
_____ Failed Screen

Recommendations

INTERPRETING AUDIOGRAMS AND TYMPANOGRAMS

The audiologist is responsible for the complete evaluation and diagnosis of hearing impairment. However, the speech-language pathologist needs to understand hearing, how it is tested, how to interpret assessment results, and how the results apply to individual clients. The reference materials in this section are designed to help you more thoroughly understand your client's hearing impairment and its impact on the communicative disorder, diagnosis, treatment program, and referral process.

Audiograms are used to record the results of audiological testing. The most common symbols used on an audiogram are listed in Table 12–3.

Table 12–3. Symbols Commonly Found on Audiograms

Recommended set of symbols for those cases when thresholds are measured.

Response

MODALITY	EAR		
	LEFT	UNSPECIFIED	RIGHT
AIR CONDUCTION—EARPHONES			
UNMASKED	✗	⟨	◯
MASKED	☐		◁
BONE CONDUCTION—MASTOID			
UNMASKED	^	<	⌄
MASKED	⊓		⊔
BONE CONDUCTION—FOREHEAD			
UNMASKED			
MASKED	⌐	>	⌐
AIR CONDUCTION—SOUND FIELD	✶	S	∅
ACOUSTIC—REFLEX THRESHOLD			
CONTRALATERAL	⌐		Ч
IPSILATERAL	⊥		⊤

Recommended set of symbols for those cases when no responses are elicited.

No Response

MODALITY	EAR		
	LEFT	UNSPECIFIED	RIGHT
AIR CONDUCTION—EARPHONES			
UNMASKED	✗↘	←|	◯↙
MASKED	☐↘		◁↙
BONE CONDUCTION—MASTOID			
UNMASKED	↖	←|	↗
MASKED	⌐↗		⌐↖
BONE CONDUCTION—FOREHEAD			
UNMASKED			
MASKED	⌐↙	|→	⌐↘
AIR CONDUCTION—SOUND FIELD	✶↘	S→	∅↙
ACOUSTIC—REFLEX THRESHOLD			
CONTRALATERAL	⌐↗		Ч↙
IPSILATERAL	⊥↗		⊤↖

Source: From "Guidelines for Audiometric Symbols, *Asha* (April 1991, Supplement No. 2), 32(4), 25–30. Used by permission of American Speech-Language-Hearing Association.

Audiograms

The audiograms in Figures 12–1 through 12–7 illustrate several basic patterns of hearing loss. Exact configurations vary across individuals and according to the type, frequencies, and decibel levels of the loss. The hearing losses in these examples are bilateral (involving both ears), although unilateral hearing losses are also common.

The Three Basic Patterns (Conductive, Sensorineural, and Mixed Losses)

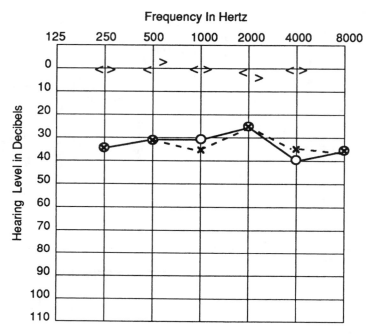

Figure 12–1. Audiogram of a conductive hearing loss. (Note the airbone gap.)

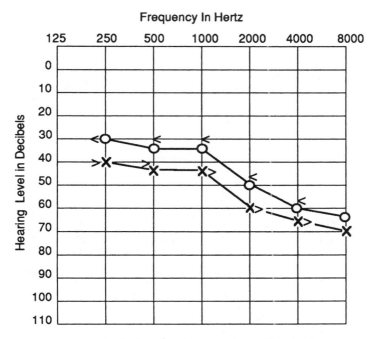

Figure 12–2. Audiogram of a sensorineural hearing loss.

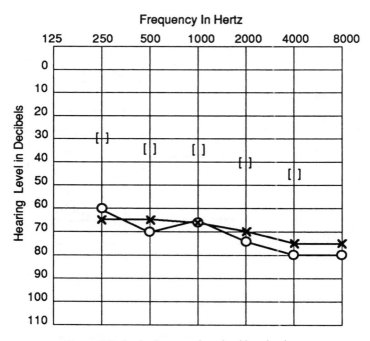

Figure 12–3. Audiogram of a mixed hearing loss.

Various Patterns of Hearing Losses

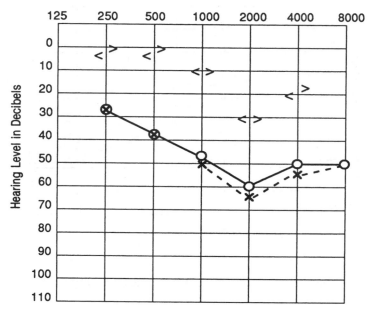

Figure 12–4. Audiogram of a conductive hearing loss caused by otosclerosis. (Note the Carhart notch in bone conduction.)

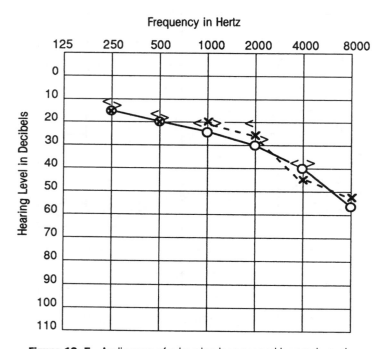

Figure 12–5. Audiogram of a hearing loss caused by presbycusis.

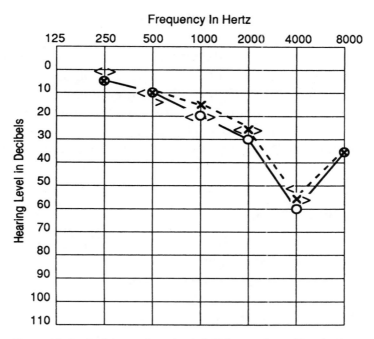

Figure 12–6. Audiogram of a noise-induced sensorineural hearing loss.

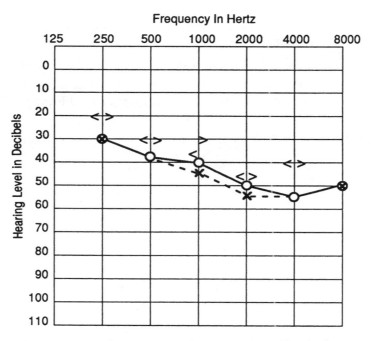

Figure 12–7. Audiogram of a moderate sensorineural hearing loss.

Tympanograms

The purpose of tympanometry is to determine the point and magnitude of greatest compliance (mobility) of the tympanic membrane. A tympanogram is a graph that illustrates the compliance on the y axis (left-hand side) and pressure (in mm H_2O) on the x axis (across the bottom). The results provide important information about middle ear function, and help diagnosticians detect different conditions and diseases of the middle ear. Tympanograms can be interpreted according to the peak pressure point, peak amplitude, and shape (Feldman, 1975). Based on dimensions of the tympanogram, several classifications and possible etiologies are:

Pressure (shown by location of peak)

Normal peak:	otosclerosis, ossicular chain discontinuity, tympanoclerosis, cholesteotoma in the attic space
No peak/Flat:	perforated tympanic membrane

Compliance (shown by height of peak)

increased amplitude:	eardrum abnormality, ossicular chain discontinuity
Reduced amplitude:	otosclerosis, tympanosclerosis, tumors, serous otitis media
Normal amplitude:	eustachian tube blockage, early acute otitis media

Shape (shown by slope)

Reduced slope:	otosclerosis, ossicular chain fixation, otitis media with effusion, tumor
Increased slope:	eardrum abnormality, ossicular chain discontinuity
Not smooth:	vascular tumors, patulous eustachian tube, ossicular chain discontinuity, eardrum abnormality (Feldman, 1975, 1976)

Figures 12–8 through 12–12 illustrate the five common patterns of tympanograms that clinicians encounter.

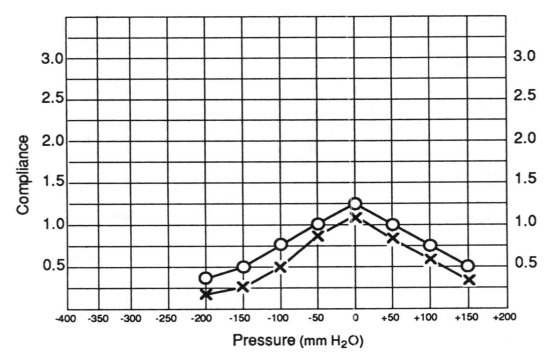

Figure 12–8. Type A tympanogram—Normal pressure and compliance functions.

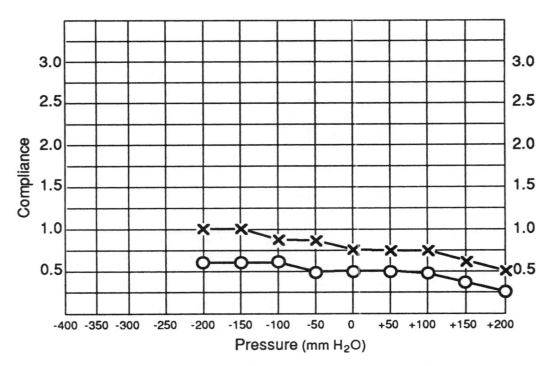

Figure 12–9. Type B tympanogram—Fluid in the middle ear (flat). This may indicate otitis media.

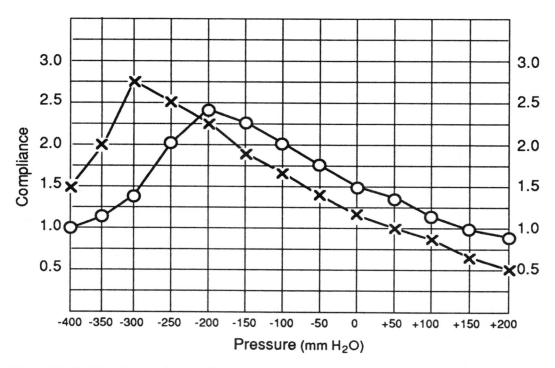

Figure 12–10. Type C tympanogram—Retracted tympanic membranes (shift to negative side). This may indicate eustachian tube blockage or otitis media.

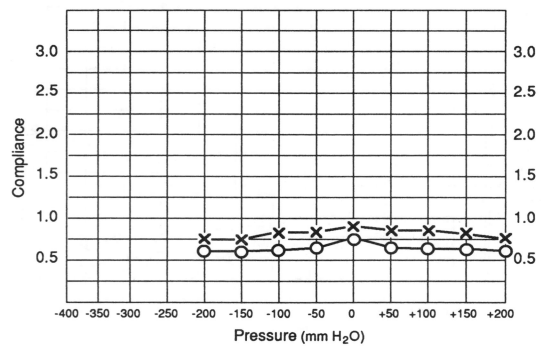

Figure 12–11. Type A_s tympanogram—Shallow. This may indicate otosclerosis or tympanosclerosis.

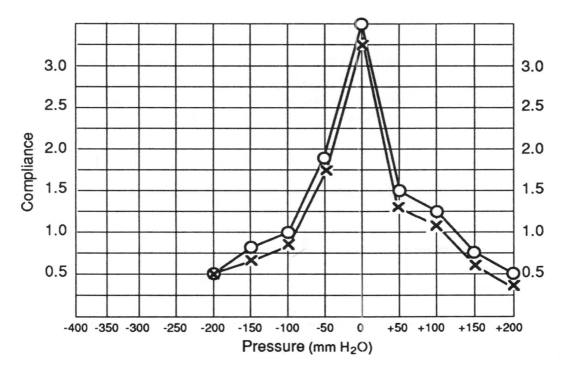

Figure 12–12. Type A$_D$—Deep. This may indicate ossicular chain discontinuity or flaccid tympanic membrane.

SPEECH AUDIOMETRY

Speech audiometry evaluates a client's ability to hear and understand speech. It can also be useful for assessing the effects of amplification. Two important speech audiometric findings are *Speech Reception Threshold* (SRT) and *Speech Recognition* scores. An SRT indicates the lowest decibel level at which a client can correctly identify a standard list of two syllable words (called *spondees*) 50% of the time. *Cupcake, baseball,* and *hotdog* are examples of spondee words. A normal SRT is within plus-or-minus 6 dB from the pure tone average (average of pure tone thresholds at 500 Hz, 1000 Hz, and 2000 Hz).

The speech recognition score reveals the client's ability to recognize words. The test is administered at a comfortable decibel level above the SRT. The client is asked to select the correct word from similar-sounding pairs (*cat-bat, beach-peach*, etc.), or repeat back single words (*day, cap*, etc.). A normal score is 90–100% correct.

THE ACOUSTIC-PHONETIC AUDIOGRAM

An acoustic-phonetic audiogram provides a pictorial representation of the typical acoustic properties of many environmental and speech sounds. It is useful for interpreting how losses at different intensities and frequencies affect the hearing and production of sounds in the English language. An acoustic-phonetic audiogram is shown in Figure 12–13.

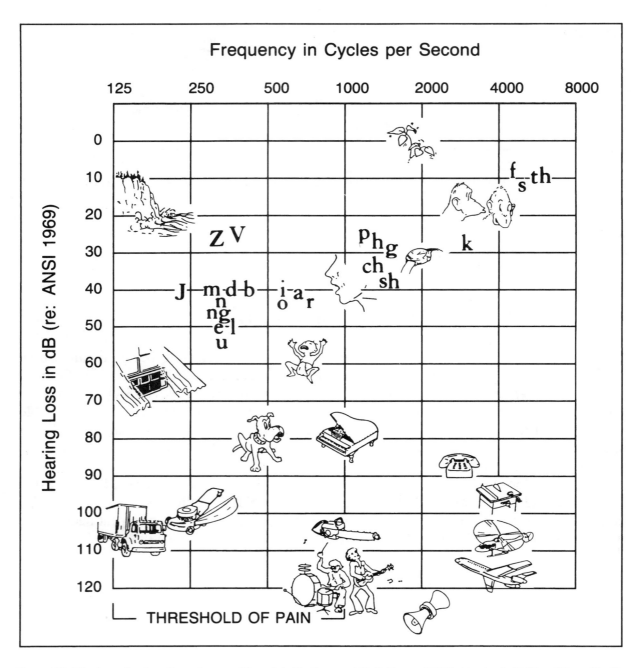

Figure 12–13. Acoustic-phonetic audiogram. (From J. L. Northern and M. P. Downs [1991], *Hearing in Children* [4th ea.] [p. 7]. Baltimore: Williams & Wilkins. Used by permission.)

ENVIRONMENTAL NOISE LEVELS

Table 12–4 contains select environmental noises that occur at different decibel levels. This information is useful for counseling clients or their caregivers about hearing loss and its effect on communication.

Table 12–4. Environmental Noise Levels

dB Level	Environmental Noise	dB Level	Environmental Noise
0 dB	Barely audible sound	80 dB	Muffled snowmobile Loud music
10 dB	Soft rustle of leaves Normal breathing		Niagara Falls Dog barking in the same room
20 dB	Average whisper 4 feet away Watch ticking	90 dB	Cocktail party Truck at 16 feet away A pneumatic drill 10 feet away
30 dB	Average residence Soft whisper at 16 feet away		Telephone ringing on work desk
40 dB	Birds chirping out the window Suburban street (no trafffic) Night noises in a city	100 dB	Loud auto horn 23 feet away Typical rock concert A riveter 35 feet away Outboard motor
50 dB	Moderate restaurant clatter Inside of a typical urban home A quiet automobile 10 feet away		Person shouting 3 feet away
		110 dB	Chain saw Jet engine at 800 feet
60 dB	Average busy street Normal conversational speech (50–70 dB) Department store	120 dB	Amplified rock band Thunderclap Jackhammer at 3 feet
		130 dB	Limit of ear's endurance Jet engine noise at 100 feet
70 dB	Bus Noisy restaurant Busy traffic Babies crying over 10 feet away	140 dB	Jet engine at take-off

Sources: Adapted from Boone (1978), Kuntz and Finkel (1987), Martin (1986), Martin and Noble (1994), Palmer and Yantis (1990), and Van Riper and Emerick (1996).

HEARING AIDS

There are five styles of hearing aids that audiologists and hearing aid dispensers supply to hearing-impaired clients. In descending order of popularity these are: in-the-ear aids, behind-the-ear aids, in-the-canal aids, eyeglass aids, and body aids. In-the-ear aids are most commonly used by adults, and behind-the-ear aids are most commonly used by children.

Before you begin a diagnostic evaluation of a client with a hearing impairment, do a quick listening check of his or her hearing aid(s). This is important! Imagine making a diagnosis of *moderate articulation disorder* or *mild receptive language impairment* only to discover that the client's malfunctioning hearing aid was impeding his or her typical communication. Do not allow a broken hearing aid to skew your diagnostic conclusions and recommendations. Complete a quick listening check by following these six steps. Attach the aid to a stethoscope or your own earmold for steps 2 through 5.

1. Check the battery. Is it missing? Is it weak?
2. Alternate the on-off switch. Do you hear distortions? Crackling noises? Other unusual sounds? No sound at all?
3. Turn the hearing aid to low volume and gradually increase to maximum volume. Is the transition smooth? Distorted?
4. Produce the sounds /a/, /i/, /u/, /ʃ/, and /s/. Are they audible? Clear?
5. Tap on the case. Do you hear changes in the sound?
6. Check for feedback. Is there a crack somewhere?

Troubleshooting Hearing Aid Problems

Depending on your work setting, you may see clients who are having trouble with their hearing aids. In some cases, the problem will have to be addressed by a trained hearing aid specialist (i.e., audiologist, hearing aid dispenser, hearing aid manufacturer). In other cases, you will be able to identify the problem and possibly correct it. For example, your client may report that the hearing aid is not amplifying anything. On inspection, you may discover that the tubing is twisted, the battery is dead, or the T (telecoil) switch is on. These problems are easily resolved on the spot by untwisting the tubing, replacing the battery, or turning the T switch off. When you are unable to resolve the problem, refer the client to the hearing aid dispenser or manufacturer if the aid is broken, or to a physician if the trouble is caused by impacted ear wax.

Table 12–5 is a troubleshooting guide for basic hearing aid problems. Refer to this table when you encounter a client with hearing aid trouble.

Table 12–5. Troubleshooting Hearing Aid Problems

Problem	Cause
Hearing Aid Dead	• bad battery • battery in backward • battery is wrong size • dirty cord contacts • broken cord • loose cord plug • tubing twisted • earmold plugged with cerumen • ear canal plugged with cerumen • receiver plugged with cerumen • switch turned to telecoil (T)
Hearing Aid Weak	• bad battery • earmold partially plugged with cerumen • microphone opening plugged with dirt or foreign object • moisture in the earmold • cracks in the earmold • ear canal plugged with cerumen • receiver plugged with cerumen
Intermittency	• dirty cord contacts • broken cord • loose cord plug • plastic tube collapsed • sweat in the hearing aid • dirty controls • telecoil switch is on
Acoustic Feedback	• earmold not inserted properly • child has outgrown earmold • earmold loose from receiver nubbin • microphone too close to receiver • volume control too high • microphone housing loose • crack or leak in earmold, plastic tubing, earhook, or opening to earhook • ear canal blocked with cerumen
Distorted or Muffled Sound	• weak battery • earmold partially plugged with cerumen • amplifier no longer working correctly • dirty microphone • ear canal plugged with cerumen
Noise in the Sound	• dirty or frayed cord • loose receiver cap • loose microphone housing • volume control worn • moisture in the aid • dirty microphone • poor battery contacts • telecoil switch is on • earmold blocked with cerumen • receiver plugged with cerumen

Source: Adapted in part from K. W. Berger and J. P. Millin, "Amplification/assistive devices for the hearing impaired." In R. L. Schow and M. A. Nerbonne (Eds.), *Introduction to Aural Rehabilitation* (2nd ed., p. 66). Austin, TX: PRO-ED. Copyright © 1989 and adapted by permission of Allyn and Bacon, current copyright holder.

COCHLEAR IMPLANTS

Cochlear implants have emerged in recent years as an alternative to conventional amplification. There are several types of these implants. Each implant serves to bypass the damaged cochlea by directly stimulating the auditory nerve (CN VIII). Martin and Noble (1994) describes cochlear implants as follows:

> Cochlear implants consist of an array of electrodes that is surgically placed into the cochlea of the inner ear. The electrodes are attached to an internal receiver, which is implanted in the bone behind the external ear. The acoustic signal is received by an externally worn microphone, which leads to a speech processor. The processor, in turn, amplifies and filters the signals and sends the electrical impulses to a transmitter. The implanted device may receive its electrical stimulation by a direct plug-in system through the skin, by magnetic induction, which converts the electric signals to magnetic impulses, or by frequency modulation (FM) transmission. When the cochlea is severely damaged, the cochlear implant can provide electrical stimulation to the auditory nerve for transmission to the brain. (p. 428)

Cochlear implants are still being refined. At the time of this publication, some of the best results have been for clients with profound sensorineural hearing loss who have acquired the loss after the development of speech and language. There is also increasing implant work with young nonhearing children (see Owens & Kessler, 1989). These implants do not create or restore normal hearing but, minimally, provide awareness of sound to the once-silent world of the deafened client (Bess & Humes, 1995). A cochlear implant is presently an alternative for only a small percentage of the hearing-impaired population—while research and refinement of the procedure continues. Candidates are very carefully selected, and extensive pre- and postoperative counseling and habilitation/rehabilitation for clients and their families is necessary (Martin, 1994; Martin & Noble, 1994).

VIBROTACTILE AIDS

Vibrotactile aids are sometimes used by clients with profound hearing losses. Essentially, the vibration of sound is felt through the skin. These vibratory aids are worn on the hand, wrist, stomach, back, arm, or thigh. Depending on the hearing loss, vibrotactile aids may be used together with more traditional amplification or used alone. One primary benefit of vibrotactile stimulation is its capacity to aid the client increase speechreading abilities (Bess & Humes, 1995; Martin, 1990).

CONCLUDING COMMENTS

Hearing is an extremely important factor in the development and maintenance of communicative abilities. A hearing loss can contribute to or even be the single cause of many communicative disorders. The audiologist is responsible for evaluating and diagnosing hearing loss. The speech-language pathologist is responsible for understanding the audiological assessment results and their impact on a client's speech and language. A client's best interests are clearly served when audiologists and speech-language pathologists pool their knowledge, abilities, and clinical skills on the client's behalf.

SOURCES OF ADDITIONAL INFORMATION

Bess, F. H. (Ed.) (1988). *Hearing impairment in children*. Parkton, MD: York Press.

Bess, F. H., & Hall, J. W., III (Eds.). (1992). *Screening children for auditory function*. Nashville, TN: Bill Wilkerson Center.

Bess, F. H., & Humes, L. E. (1990). *Audiology: The fundamentals*. Baltimore: Williams & Wilkins.

Cooper, H. (Ed.). (1991). *A practical guide to cochlear implants*. London: Whurr.

Hannley, M. (1986). *Basic principles of audiologic assessment*. Boston: Little, Brown and Co.

Hegde, M. N. (1995). *Introduction to communicative disorders* (2nd ed.). Austin, TX: PRO-ED.

Jerger, S., & Jerger, J. (1981). *Auditory disorders: A manual for clinical evaluation*. Boston: Little, Brown and Co.

Martin, F. N., & Noble, B. (1990). Hearing and hearing disorders. In G. H. Shames, E. H. Wiig, & W. A. Secord (Eds.), *Human communication and its disorders: An Introduction* (4th ed., pp. 388–436). New York: Macmillan.

Martin, F. N. (1991). *Introduction to audiology* (5th ed.). Englewood Cliffs, NJ: Prentice-Hall.

Northern, J. L. (Ed.). (1996). *Hearing disorders* (3rd ed.). Needham Heights, MA: Allyn & Bacon.

Northern, J. L., & Downs, M. (1991). *Hearing in children* (4th ed.). Baltimore: Williams & Wilkins.

Oller, D. K., & Eilers, R. E. (Eds.). (1988). Tactile artificial hearing for the deaf. In F. H. Bess (Ed.), *Hearing impairment in children* (pp. 310–328). Parkton, MD: York Press.

Owens, E., & Kessler, D. K. (Eds.). (1989). *Cochlear implants in young deaf children*. Boston: College-Hill Press.

Roeser, R. J. (1986). *Diagnostic audiology: The PRO-ED studies in communicative disorders*. Austin, TX: PRO-ED.

Roeser, R. J., & Downs, M. P. (Eds.). (1995). *Auditory disorders in school children: The law, identification, remediation* (3rd ed.). New York: Thieme Medical.

Sanders, D. A. (1993). *Management of hearing handicap: Infants to elderly* (3rd ed.). Englewood Cliffs, NJ: Prentice-Hall.

Internet Sources

League for the Hard of Hearing
    http://www.lhh.org
Listservers of Interest to Communication Disorders Folks
    http://www.shc.uiowa.edu/wjshc/iiscdl.html
National Institute on Deafness and Other Communication Disorders
    http://www.nih.gov/nidcd
Self Help for Hard of Hearing People, Inc.
    http://www.shhh.org

☐ APPENDIX A ☐

Dialectical and Bilingual/Multicultural Considerations

Owens (1991, 1995) has presented a series of concise tables illustrating some of the major differences between Standard American English and the three major ethnic dialects spoken in the United States—Black English, Hispanic English, and Asian English (Tables A–1 through A–6). He appropriately cautions that the terms Hispanic English and Asian English are probably misnomers. Actually, Hispanic English is more of a composite term which fails to account for factors such as the different Spanish dialects spoken, whether Spanish is spoken as a first or second language, the generation of the speaker, and the geographical location of the speaker.

The same factors are true for Asian English, but there is another very important distinction between Standard American English and Asian English. There are actually many Asian languages. Cheng (1991), Mattes and Omark (1991), and other sources contain detailed information about the various Asian languages. For example, Cheng notes that there are more than 80 languages and hundreds of dialects spoken in China alone. The two primary Chinese dialects spoken in the United States are Cantonese and Mandarin. There are several Indonesian languages, including the Vietnamese, Cambodian, and Laotian languages. In addition, there are many Asian groups such as the Filipinos, Koreans, Japanese, Hawaiians, Guamanians, and Micronesians (Cheng 1991; Owens, 1995). The languages spoken by these groups differ in many ways.

These introductory comments are intended to alert you to use the information in this appendix carefully. General patterns are described, but a good understanding of the complexity of each language is necessary when applying the information to individuals from specific cultural and linguistic backgrounds.

Table A–1. Phonemic Contrasts Between Black English and Standard American English

SAE Phoneme	Position in Word		
	Initial	**Medial**	**Final**†
/p/		Unaspirated /p/	Unaspirated /p/
/n/			Reliance on preceding nasalized vowel
/w/	Omitted in specific words (*I' as, too!*)		
/b/		Unreleased /b/	Unreleased /b/
/g/		Unreleased /g/	Unreleased /g/
/k/		Unaspirated /k/	Unaspirated /k/
/d/	Omitted in specific words (*I 'on't know*)	Unreleased /d/	Unreleased /d/
/ŋ/		/n/	/n/
/t/		Unaspirated /t/	Unaspirated /t/
/l/		Omitted before labial consonants (*help—hep*)	"uh" following a vowel (*Bill—Biuh*)
/r/		Omitted or /ə/	Omitted or prolonged vowel or glide
/θ/	Unaspirated /t/ or /f/	Unaspirated /t/ or /f/ between vowels	Unaspirated /t/ or /f/ (*bath—baf*)
/v/	Sometimes /b/	/b/ before /m/ and /n/	Sometimes /b/
/ð/	/d/	/d/ or /v/ between vowels	/d/, /v/, /f/
/z/		Omitted or replaced by /d/ before nasal sound (*wasn't—wud'n*)	

Blends

/str/ becomes /skr/
/ʃr/ becomes /str/
/θr/ becomes /θ/
/pr/ becomes /p/
/br/ becomes /b/
/kr/ becomes /k/
/gr/ becomes /g/

(continued)

Table A–1. *(continued)*

SAE Phoneme	Position in Word		
	Initial	**Medial**	**Final**[†]

Final Consonant Clusters (second consonant omitted when these clusters occur near the end of a word)

/sk/	/nd/	/sp/
/ft/	/ld/	/dʒd/
/st/	/sd/	/nt/

[†]Note weakening of final consonants.
[*Sources*: Data drawn from Fasold & Wolfram (1970), Labov (1972), Weiner & Lewnau (1979), and Williams & Wofram (1977)].

Source: From *Language Disorders: A Functional Approach to Assessment and Intervention* by Robert E. Owens, Jr. Copyright © 1991 by Macmillan Publishing Company. (p. 330). Reprinted with permission.

Table A–2. Grammatical Contrasts Between Black English and Standard American English

Black English Grammatical Structure	SAE Grammatical Structure
Possessive -'s	
Nonobligatory where word position expresses possession.	Obligatory regardless of position.
Get *mother* coat.	Get mother's coat.
It be mother's.	It's mother's.
Plural -s	
Nonobligatory with numerical quantifier.	Obligatory regardless of numerical quantifier.
He got ten *dollar*.	He has ten dollars.
Look at the *cat*.	Look at the cats.
Regular past -*ed*	
Nonobligatory; reduced as consonant cluster.	Obligatory.
Yesterday, I *walk* to school.	Yesterday, I *walked* to school.
Irregular past	
Case by case, some verbs inflected, others not.	All irregular verbs inflected.
I *see* him last week.	I *saw* him last week.
Regular present tense third person singular -*s*	
Nonobligatory.	Obligatory.
She *eat* too much.	She *eats* too much.
Irregular present tense third person singular -*s*	
Nonobligatory.	Obligatory.
He *do* my job.	He *does* my job.
Indefinite *an*	
Use of indefinite *a*	Use of *an* before nouns beginning with a vowel.
He ride in *a* airplane.	He rode in *an* airplane.
Pronouns	
Pronominal apposition; pronoun immediately follows noun.	Pronoun used elsewhere in sentence or in other sentence; not in apposition.
Mamma *she* mad. She . . .	Mamma is mad. *She* . . .
Future tense	
More frequent use of *be going to* (gonna)	More frequent use of *will*.
I *be going to* dance tonight.	I *will* dance tonight.
I *gonna* dance tonight.	I *am going to* dance tonight.
Omit *will* preceding *be*.	Obligatory use of *will*.
I *be* home later.	I *will (I'll)* be home later.
Negation	
Triple negative.	Absence of triple negative.
Nobody don't never like me.	*No* one ever likes me.
Use of *ain't*	*Ain't* is unacceptable form.
I *ain't* going.	*I'm not* going.

(continued)

Table A–2. *(continued)*

Black English Grammatical Structure	SAE Grammatical Structure
Modals	
Double models for such forms as *might, could,* and *should.*	Single modal use.
I *might could* go.	I *might* be able to go.
Questions	
Same form for direct and indirect.	Different forms for direct and indirect.
What *it is*?	What *is it*?
Do you know what *it is*?	Do you know what *it is*?
Relative pronouns	
Nonobligatory in most cases.	Nonobligatory with *that* only.
He the one stole it	He's the one *who* stole it
It the one you like.	It's the one (that) you like.
Conditional *if*	
Use of *do* for conditional *if.*	Use of *if.*
I ask *did* she go.	I asked *if* she went.
Perfect construction	
Been used for action in the distant past.	*Been* not used.
He *been* gone.	He left a long time ago.
Copula	
Nonobligatory when contractible.	Obligatory in contractible and uncontractible forms.
He sick.	He's sick.
Habitual or general state	
Marked with uninflected *be.*	Nonuse of *be*; verb inflected.
She *be* workin'.	She's *working* now.

[*Sources*: Data drawn from Baratz (1969), Fasold & Wolfram, and Williams & Wolfram (1977)]

Table A–3. Pragmatic and Nonlinguistic Contrasts Between Black English and Standard American English

Black English	Standard American English
Touching of one's hair by another person is often considered offensive.	Touching of one's hair by another person is a sign of affection.
Preference for indirect eye contact during listening, direct eye contact during speaking as signs of attentiveness and respect.	Preference for direct eye contact during listening and indirect eye contact during speaking as signs of attention and respect.
Public behavior may be emotionally intense, dynamic, and demonstrative.	Public behavior expected to be modest and emotionally restrained. Emotional displays are seen as irresponsible or in bad taste.
Clear distinction between "argument" and "fight." Verbal abuse is not necessarily a precursor to violence.	Heated arguments are viewed as suggesting that violence is imminent.
Asking "personal questions" of someone one has met for the first time is seen as improper and intrusive.	Inquiring about jobs, family, and so forth of someone one has met for the first time is seen as friendly.
Use of direct questions is sometimes seen as harrassment, e.g., asking when something will be finished is seen as rushing that person to finish.	Use of direct questions for personal information is permissible.
Interruption during conversation is usually tolerated. Access to the floor is granted to the person who is most assertive.	Rules of turn-taking in conversation dictate that one person has the floor at a time until all his points are made.
Conversations are regarded as private between recognized participants. "Butting in" is seen as eavesdropping and is not tolerated.	Adding points of information or insight to a conversation in which one is not engaged is seen as being helpful.
Use of expression "you people" is seen as pejorative and racist.	Use of expression "you people" tolerated.
Accusations or allegations are general rather than categorical, and are not intended to be all-inclusive. Refutation is the responsibility of the accused.	Stereotypical accusations or allegations are all-inclusive. Refutations or making exception is the responsibility of the person making the accusation.
Silence denotes refutation of accusation. To state that you feel accused is regarded as an admission of guilt.	Silence denotes acceptance of an accusation. Guilt is verbally denied.

[*Source*: Taylor (in press), Clinical practice as a social occasion. In L. Cole & V. Deal (Eds.), *Communication disorders in multicultural populations*. Rockville, MD: American Speech-Language-Hearing Association.]

Source: From *Language Disorders: A Functional Approach to Assessment and Intervention* by Robert E. Owens, Jr. Copyright © 1991 by Macmillan Publishing Company. (p. 333). Reprinted with permission.

Table A–4. Phonemic Contrasts Between Hispanic English and Standard American English

| SAE Phoneme | Position in Word | | |
	Initial	Medial	Final[†]
/p/	Unaspirated /p/		Omitted or weakened
/m/			Omitted
/w/	/hu/		Omitted
/b/			Omitted, distorted, or /p/
/g/			Omitted, distorted, or /k/
/k/	Unaspirated or /g/		Omitted, distorted, or/g/
/f/			Omitted
/d/		Dentalized	Omitted, distorted, or /t/
/ŋ/	/n/	/d/	/n/ (*sing-sin*)
/j/	/dʒ/		
/t/			Omitted
/ʃ/	/tʃ/	/s/, /tʃ/	/tʃ/ (*wish-which*)
/tʃ/	/ʃ/ (*chair-share*)	/ʃ/	/ʃ/ (*watch-wash*)
/r/	Distorted	Distorted	Distorted
/dʒ/	/d/	/j/	/ʃ/
/θ/	/t/, /s/ (*thin-tin, sin*)	Omitted	/ʃ/, /t/, /s/
/v/	/b/ (*vat-bat*)	/b/	Distorted
/z/	/s/ (*zip-sip*)	/s/ (*razor-racer*)	/s/
/ð/	/d/ (*then-den*)	/d/, /θ/,S /v/ (*lather-ladder*)	/d/

Blends

/skw/ becomes /eskw/[†]
/sl/ becomes /esl/[†]
/st/ becomes /est/[†]

Vowels

/ɪ/ becomes /i/ (*bit-beet*)

[†]Separates clusters of 2 syllables

[*Sources:* Data drawn from Sawyer (1973), Weiner & Lewnau (1979), and Williams, Cairns, & Cairns (1971)].

Table A–5. Grammatical Contrasts Between Hispanic English and Standard American English

Spanish English Grammatical Structure	SAE Grammatical Structure
Possessive -'s	
Use postnoun modifier.	Postnoun modifier used only rarely.
This is the homework *of my brother.*	This is my brother's homework.
Article used with body parts.	Possessive pronoun used with body parts.
I cut *the* finger.	I cut *my* finger.
Plural -s	
Nonobligatory.	Obligatory excluding exceptions.
The *girl* are playing.	The *girls* are playing.
The *sheep* are playing.	The *sheep* are playing.
Regular past -*ed*	
Nonobligatory, especially when understood.	Obligatory.
I *talk* to her yesterday.	I *talked* to her yesterday.
Regular third person present tense -*s*	
Nonobligatory.	Obligatory.
She *eat* too much.	She *eats* too much.
Articles	
Often omitted.	Usually obligatory.
I am going to store.	I am going to *the* store.
I am going to school.	I am going to school.
Subject pronouns	
Omitted when subject has been identified in the previous sentence.	Obligatory.
Father is happy. Bought a new car.	Father is happy. *He* bought a new car.
Future tense	
Use *go + to.*	Use *be + going to.*
I *go to* dance.	I *am going* to the dance.
Negation	
Use *no* before the verb.	Use *not* (preceded by auxiliary verb where appropriate).
She *no* eat candy.	She does *not* eat candy.
Question	
Intonation; no noun-verb inversion.	Noun-verb inversion usually.
Maria is going?	*Is Maria* going?
Copula	
Occasional use of *have.*	Use of *be.*
I *have* ten years.	I *am* ten years old.
Negative imperatives	
No used for *don't.*	*Don't* used.
No throw stones.	*Don't* throw stones.

(continued)

Table A–5 *(continued)*

Spanish English Grammatical Structure	SAE Grammatical Structure
Do insertion	
Nonobligatory in questions. You like ice cream?	Obligatory when no auxiliary verb. *Do* you like ice cream?
Comparatives	
More frequent use of longer form (more). He is *more* tall.	More frequent use of shorter *-er*. He is tall*er*.

[*Sources*: Data drawn from Davis (1972) and Taylor (1986).]

Table A–6. Pragmatic and Nonlinguistic Contrasts Between Black English and Standard American English

Black English	Standard American English
Hissing to gain attention is acceptable.	Hissing is considered impolite and indicates contempt.
Touching is often observed between two people in conversation.	Touching is usually unacceptable and usually carries sexual overtone.
Avoidance of direct eye contact is sometimes a sign of attentiveness and respect; sustained eye contact may be interpreted as a challenge to authority.	Direct eye contact is a sign of attentiveness and respect.
Relative distance between two speakers in conversation is close.	Relative distance between two speakers in conversation is farther apart.
Official or business conversations are preceded by lengthy greeting, pleasantries, and other talk unrelated to the point of business.	Getting to the point quickly is valid.

[*Source*: Taylor (in press), Clinical practice as a social occasion. In L. Cole and V. Deal (Eds.), *Communication disorders in multicultural populations*. Rockville, MD: American Speech-Language-Hearing Association.]

Table A–7. Phonemic Contrasts Between Asian English and Standard American English

SAE Phoneme	Position in Word		
	Initial	**Medial**	**Final**[†]
/p/	/b/[††††]	/b/[††††]	Omission
/s/	Distortion[†]	Distortion[†]	Omission
/z/	/s/[††]	/s/[††]	Omission
/t/	Distortion[†]	Distortion[†]	Omission
/tʃ/	/ʃ/[††††]	/ʃ/[††††]	Omission
/ʃ/	/s/[††]	/s/[††]	Omission
/r/, /l/	Confusion[†††]	Confusion[†††]	Omission
/θ/	/s/	/s/	Omission
/dʒ/	/d/ or /z/[††††]	/d/ or /z/[††††]	Omission
/v/	/f/[†††]	/f/[†††]	Omission
	/w/[††]	/w/[††]	Omission
/ð/	/z/[†]	/z/[†]	Omission
	/d/[††††]	/d/[††††]	Omission

Blends

Addition of /ə/ between consonants[†††]
Omission of final consonant clusters[††††]

Vowels

Shortening or lengthening of vowels (seat-sit, it-eat[†])
Difficulty with /ɪ/, /ɔ/, and /æ/, and substitution of /e/ for /æ/[††]
Difficulty with /ɪ/, /æ/, /ʊ/ and /ə/[†††]

[†] Mandarin dialect of Chinese only
[††] Cantonese dialect of Chinese only
[†††] Mandarin, Cantonese, and Japanese
[††††] Vietnamese only

[*Source*: Adapted from Cheng (1987, June), Cross-cultural and linguistic considerations in working with Asian population. *Asha, 29*, 33–38.]

Source: From *Language Disorders: A Functional Approach to Assessment and Intervention* by Robert E. Owens, Jr. Copyright © 1991 by Macmillan Publishing Company. (p. 337). Reprinted with permission.

Table A–8. Grammatical Contrasts Between Asian English and Standard American English

Asian English Grammatical Structure	SAE Grammatical Structure
Plural -s	
Not used with numerical adjective.	Used regardless of numerical adjective.
three cat	*three cats*
Used with irregular plural.	Not used with irregular plural.
three sheeps	*three sheep*
Auxiliaries *to be* and *to do*	
Omission.	Obligatory and inflected in the present progressive form.
I going home.	I *am* going home.
She not want eat.	She *does* not want to eat.
Uninflected.	
I *is* going.	I *am* going
She *do* not want eat.	She *does* not want to eat.
Verb *have*	
Omission.	Obligatory and inflected.
You been here.	You *have* been here.
Uninflected.	
He *have* one.	He *has* one.
Past tense -ed	
Omission.	Obligatory, nonovergeneralization, and single marking.
He talk yesterday.	He *talked* yesterday.
Overgeneralization.	
I *eated* yesterday.	I *ate* yesterday.
Double-marking	
She *didn't ate*.	She *didn't* eat.
Interrogative	
Nonreversal.	Reversal and obligatory.
You *are* late?	*Are* you late?
Omitted auxiliary.	
You like ice cream?	*Do* you like ice cream?
Perfect marker	
Omission.	Obligatory.
I have write letter.	I have writt*en* a letter.
Verb-noun agreement	
Nonagreement.	Agreement.
He go to school.	*He goes* to school.
You goes to school.	*You go* to school.
Article	
Omission.	Obligatory with certain nouns.
Please give gift.	Please give *the* gift.
Overgeneralization.	
She go *the* school.	She went to school.

Asian English Grammatical Structure	SAE Grammatical Structure
Preposition	
Misuse.	Obligatory specific use.
I am *in* home.	I am *at* home.
Omission.	
He go bus.	He goes *by* bus.
Pronoun	
Subjective/objective confusion.	Subjective/objective distinction.
Him go quickly.	*He* gave it to *her*.
Possessive confusion.	Possessive distinction.
It *him* book.	It's *his* book.
Demonstrative	
Confusion	Singular/plural distinction.
I like *those* horse.	I like *that* horse.
Conjunction	
Omission.	Obligatory use between last two items in a series.
You I go together.	You *and* I are going together.
Mary, John, Carol went.	Mary, John, *and* Carol went.
Negative	
Double-marking	Single obligatory marking.
I didn't see *nobody*.	I *didn't see anybody*.
Simplified form.	
He *no* come.	He *didn't* come.
Word order	
Adjective following noun (Vietnamese).	Most noun modifiers precede noun.
clothes new	*new clothes*
Possessive following noun (Vietnamese).	Possessive precedes noun.
dress her	*her dress*
Omission of object with transitive verb.	Use of direct object with most transitive verbs.
I want.	I want *it*.

[*Source*: Adapted from Cheng (1987, June), Cross-cultural and linguistic considerations in working with Asian populations, *Asha, 29*, 33–38.]

Table A–9. Pragmatic and Nonlinguistic Contrasts Between Asian English and Standard American English

Asian English	Standard American English
Considered impolite, especially for children, to interrupt a conversation.	Appropriate to interrupt in certain circumstances.
Addressing others may be controlled by several hierarchies that govern social interactions. May be many forms of address.	Forms of address less rigid, more informal. Limited number of forms.
Social distance is a factor of age, sex, status, and marital status. Therefore, questions relative to these factors are considered appropriate.	Standards of social distance are less rigid. Questions about age and status may be considered inappropriate.
Kinship terms are very important in determining the relationship between two speakers and extend beyond the immediate and extended family to include nonfamily members.	Kinship terms, such as aunt or uncle, occasionally extended beyond family. Have less rigid effect on speakers in a conversation.
May keep composed when very emotional. May withhold facial expression.	More emotive, expressive.
Do not express public affection.	Kiss and hug in public.
May not maintain eye contact with a superior.	Usually stare at a superior in conversation.
Humility respected and may respond with embarrassment to praise.	Acceptable, within bounds, to be personally boastful.
Giggle when embarrassed or shy.	Giggle when mocking or "making fun" of someone.
Touching or hand-holding between members of the same sex is acceptable.	Touching or hand-holding between members of the same sex is considered a sign of homosexuality.
Hand-holding/hugging/kissing between men and women in public looks ridiculous.	Hand-holding/hugging/kissing between men and women in public is acceptable.
A slap on the back is insulting.	A slap on the back denotes friendliness.
It is not customary to shake hands with persons of the opposite sex.	It is customary to shake hands with persons of the opposite sex.
Finger beckoning is only used by adults to call little children and not vice-versa.	Finger beckoning is often used to call people.

[*Source*: Taylor (in press), Clinical practice as a social occasion. In L. Cole & V. Deal (Eds.), *Communication disorders in multicultural populations*. Rockville, MD: American Speech-Language-Hearing Association. Adapted from Cheng (1987, June), Crosscultural and linguistic considerations in working with Asian populations. *Asha, 29*, 33–38.]

Source: From *Language Disorders: A Functional Approach to Assessment and Intervention* by Robert E. Owens, Jr. Copyright © 1991 by Macmillan Publishing Company. (p. 340). Reprinted with permission.

SOURCES OF ADDITIONAL INFORMATION

Adler, S. (1990). Multicultural clients: Implication for the SLP. *Language, Speech, and Hearing Services in Schools, 21*, 135–139.

American Speech-Language-Hearing Association. (1985, June). Clinical management of communicatively handicapped minority language populations. *Asha, 27*(6), 29–32.

Cheng, L. L. (1991). *Assessing Asian language performance* (2nd ed.). Oceanside, CA: Academic Communication Associates.

Cole, L., & Snope, T. (1981, September). Resource guide to multicultural tests and materials. *Asha, 23*, 639–649.

Deal, V. R, & Yen, M. A. (1985, June). Resource guide to multicultural tests and materials. *Asha, 27*(6), 43–49.

Erickson, J. G., & Omark, D. R (Eds.). (1981). *Communication assessment of the bilingual bicultural child*. Baltimore: University Park Press.

Hamayan, E. V., & Damico, J. S. (Eds.). (1991). *Limiting bias in the assessment of bilingual students*. Austin, TX: PRO-ED.

Kayser, H. (1989). Speech and language assessment of Spanish-English speaking children. *Language, Speech, and Hearing Services in Schools, 20*, 226–241.

Labov, W. (1972). *Language in the inner city*. Philadelphia: University of Pennsylvania Press.

Langdon, H., & Cheng, L. L. (1992). *Hispanic children and adults with communicative disorders: Assessment and intervention*. Gaithersburg, MD: Aspen.

Mattes, L. J., & Omark, D. R. (1991). *Speech and language assessment for the bilingual handicapped* (2nd ed.). Oceanside, CA: Academic Communication Associates.

Owens, R. E. (1995). *Language disorders: A functional approach to assessment and intervention* (2nd ed.). Needham Heights, MA: Allyn & Bacon.

Owens, R. E. (1996). *Language development: An introduction* (4th ed.). Needham Heights, MA: Allyn & Bacon.

Taylor, O. L. (1986a). Language and communication differences. In G. H. Shames & E. H. Wiig (Eds.), *Human communication disorders* (2nd ed., pp. 126–158). Columbus, OH: Merrill.

Taylor, O. L. (Ed.). (1986b). *Nature of communication disorders in culturally and linguistically diverse populations*. San Diego: College-Hill Press.

Taylor, O. L. (1986c). *Treatment of communication disorders in culturally and linguistically diverse populations*. San Diego: College-Hill Press.

Taylor, O. L., & Payne, K. T. (1994). Language and communication differences. In G. H. Shames, E. H. Wiig, & W. A. Sailor (Eds.), *Human communication disorders: An introduction* (4th ed., pp 136–173). Needham Heights, MA: Allyn & Bacon.

Taylor, O. L. (in press). Clinical practice as a social occasion. In L. Cole & V. Deal, *Communication disorders in multicultural populations*. Rockville, MD: American Speech-Language-Hearing Association.

Wolfram, W., & Fasold, R. W. (1974). *The study of social dialects in American English*. Englewood Cliffs, NJ: Prentice-Hall.

Internet Sources

American Speech-Language-Hearing Association
http://www.asha.org

APPENDIX B

Evaluating Formal Tests
Used for Assessment Purposes

This appendix includes two items: excerpts from the *Code of Fair Testing Practices in Education* (1988) and a form for evaluating tests. The *Code of Fair Testing Practices* was developed by the Joint Committee on Testing Practices, which is sponsored by professional associations such as the American Psychological Association, the National Counsel on Measurement in Education, the American Association for Counseling and Development, and the American Speech-Language-Hearing Association.

The guidelines in the *Code* were developed primarily for use with professionally developed tests such as those available commercially from test publishers, and those used in formal testing situations. There are actually two parts to the *Code*: one focuses on test developers and publishers, the other on those who administer and use the tests. Only the sections dealing with the test users are presented here. The second inclusion, the "Test Evaluation Form," is adapted from Mattes and Omark (1991). The form provides a checklist format to use when reviewing information in a test manual. The form can be adapted for your particular needs and purposes.

CODE OF FAIR TESTING PRACTICES IN EDUCATION[1]

A. *Developing/SelectingAppropriate Tests*. Test users should select tests that meet the purpose for which they are to be used and that are appropriate for the intended test-taking populations. Test users should:

1. First define the purpose for testing and the population to be tested. Then, select a test for that purpose and that population based on a thorough review of the available information.
2. Investigate potentially useful sources of information in addition to test scores to corroborate the information provided by the test.
3. Read the materials provided by the test developers and avoid using tests for which unclear or incomplete information is provided.
4. Become familiar with how and when the test was developed and tried out.
5. Read independent evaluations of a test and of possible alternative measures. Look for evidence required to support the claims of test developers.
6. Examine specimen sets, disclosed tests or samples of questions, directions, answer sheets, manuals, and score reports before selecting a test.
7. Ascertain whether the test content and norm group(s) or comparison group(s) are appropriate for the intended test takers.
8. Select and use only those tests for which the skills needed to administer the test and interpret scores correctly are available.

B. *Interpreting Scores*. Test users should interpret scores correctly. Test users should:

9. Obtain information about the scale used for reporting scores, the characteristics of any norms or comparison group(s), and the limitations of the scores.

---

[1]*Source*: From Testing Practices. (Mailing address: Joint Committee on Testing Practices, American Psychological Association, 1200 17th Street, NW, Washington, D.C. 20036). This is not copyrighted material. Reproduction and dissemination are encouraged by the Joint Committee on Testing Practices.

10. Interpret scores taking into account any major differences between the norms or comparison groups and the actual test takers. Also take into account any differences in test administration practices or familiarity with the specific questions in the test.

11. Avoid using tests for purposes not specifically recommended by the test developer unless evidence is obtained to support the intended use.

12. Explain how any passing scores were set and gather evidence to support the appropriateness of the scores.

13. Obtain evidence to help show that the test is meeting its intended purpose(s).

C. *Striving for Fairness.* Test users should select tests that have been developed in ways that attempt to make them as fair as possible for the test takers of different races, gender, ethnic backgrounds, or handicapping conditions. Test users should:

14. Evaluate the procedures used by the test developers to avoid potentially insensitive content or language.

15. Review the performance of the test takers of different races, gender, and ethnic backgrounds when samples of sufficient size are available. Evaluate the extent to which performance differences may have been caused by inappropriate characteristics of the test.

16. When necessary and feasible, use appropriately modified forms of tests or administration procedures for test takers with handicapping conditions. Interpret standard norms with care in the light of modifications that were made.

D. *Informing Test Takers.* Under some circumstances, test developers have direct communication with test takers. Under other circumstances, test users communicate directly with test takers. Whichever group communicates directly with test takers should provide the information described below. Test users should:

17. When a test is optional, provide test takers or their parent/guardians with information to help them judge whether the test should be taken, or if an available alternative to the test should be used.

18. Provide test takers with the information they need to be familiar with the coverage of the test, the types of question formats, the directions, and appropriate test-taking strategies. Strive to make such information equally available to all test takers.

E. Under some circumstances, test developers have direct control of tests and test scores. Under other circumstances, test users have such control. Whichever group has direct control of tests and test scores should take the steps described below. Test developers or test users should:

19. Provide test takers or their parents/guardians with information about rights test takers may have to obtain copies of tests and completed answer sheets, retake tests, have tests rescored, or cancel scores.

20. Tell test takers or their parents/guardians how long scores will be kept on file and indicate to whom and under what circumstances test scores will or will not be released.

21. Describe the procedures that test takers or their parents/guardians may use to register complaints and have problems resolved.

Form B–1 Test Evaluation Form[1]

Title of Test:

Author:

Publisher:

Date of Publication:

Cost:

Directions for Completing This Form: Evaluate the test in each of the areas below using the following scoring system:

    G = Good
    F = Fair
    P = Poor
  NI = No Information
NA = Not Applicable

I. PURPOSES OF THE TEST

_____A. The purposes of the test are described adequately in the test manual.

_____B. The purposes of the test are appropriate for the intended local uses of the instrument.

    Comments

(continued)

Form B–1 *(continued)*

II. CONSTRUCTION OF THE TEST

_____A. Test was developed based on a contemporary theoretical model of speech-language development and reflects findings of recent research.

_____B. Procedures used in developing test content (e.g., selection and field-testing of test items) were adequate.

Comments

III. PROCEDURES

A. Procedures for test administration:

_____ 1. Described adequately in the test manual.

_____ 2. Appropriate for the local population.

B. Procedures for scoring the test:

_____ 1. Described adequately in the test manual.

_____ 2. Appropriate for the local population.

C. Procedures for test interpretation:

_____ 1. Described adequately in the test manual.

_____ 2. Appropriate for the local population.

Comments

IV. ADEQUACY OF NORMS

_____A. Procedures for selection of the standardization sample are described in detail.

_____B. Sample size is adequate.

_____C. Type of subjects studied is adequate.

Comments

V. ADEQUACY OF TEST RELIABILITY DATA

_____A. Intratester reliability

_____B. Intertester reliability

_____C. Test-retest reliability

_____D. Alternate form reliability

_____E. Split-half or internal consistency

Comments

VI. ADEQUACY OF TEST VALIDITY DATA

_____A. Face validity

_____B. Content validity

_____C. Construct validity

_____D. Concurrent validity

_____E. Predictive validity

Comments

VII. LINGUISTIC, CULTURAL, AND NORMATIVE APPROPRIATENESS OF THE TEST WITH DIVERSE POPULATIONS

_____A. Directions presented to the child are written in the dialect used by the local population.

_____B. Test items are written in the dialect used by the local population.

_____C. Types of tasks that the child is asked to perform are culturally appropriate for the local population.

_____D. Content of test items is culturally appropriate for the local population.

_____E. Visual stimuli (e.g., stimulus pictures used with the test) are culturally appropriate for the local population.

Comments

(continued)

Form B–1 *(continued)*

F. Standardization sample is an appropriate comparison group for the local population in terms of:

_____ 1. Age

_____ 2. Ethnic background

_____ 3. Place of birth

_____ 4. Community of current residence

_____ 5. Length of residence in the United States

_____ 6. Socioeconomic level

_____ 7. Language classification (e.g., limited English proficient)

_____ 8. Language most often used by child at home

_____ 9. Language most often used by child at school

_____10. Type of language program provided in school setting

Comments

□ GLOSSARY □

Acoustic reflex: An involuntary movement to sound which stiffens the ossicular chain and decreases the compliance of the tympanic membrane.

Adenoidectomy: Surgical removal of the adenoidal tissue.

Adjective: A word that modifies a noun or pronoun. It adds description or definition of kind (*red* car), which one (*that* man), or how many (*three* children).

Adverb: A word that modifies a verb, adjective, or another adverb. It adds description or definition of how (ran *quickly*), when (went *immediately*), where (walked *here*), or extent (ran *far*).

Agrammaticism: A problem with grammatical accuracy commonly associated with aphasia.

Alternate form reliability: See *Reliability*.

Ambulatory: Capable of walking.

Anterior: See *Distinctive feature*.

Anomia: Inability to identify or to recall names of people, places, or things. Seen with some aphasias.

Aphasia: Loss of language abilities and function as a result of brain damage. It may affect comprehension and/or expression of verbal language, as well as reading, writing, and mathematics.

Apraxia: A neurologically based motor speech disorder that adversely affects the abilities to execute purposeful speech movements. Muscle weakness is not associated with apraxia.

Ataxia: Disturbance of gait and balance associated with damage to the cerebellum. It is a type of dysarthria characterized by errors in articulation, uneven stress patterns, monopitch, and reduced loudness.

Article: A noun modifier that denotes specificity, that is—*a, an,* or *the.*

Articulation: Use of articulators (lips, tongue, etc.) to produce speech sounds. It also describes a person's ability to make sounds, as in "her *articulation* contained several errors."

Aspiration: The action of a foreign material (e.g., food) penetrating and entering the airway below the true vocal folds.

Asymmetry: Lack of similarity of parts of a structure; unevenness or lack of proportion. For example, drooping on one side of the face makes it *asymmetrical* with the other side.

Atresia: Congenital absence, pathological closure, or severe underdevelopment of a normal orifice or cavity. As used in audiology, it often refers to an abnormally small or malformed pinna (the visible outside part of the ear).

Atrophy: The wasting away of tissues or an organ due to disease or lack of use.

Audiogram: A graphic illustration of hearing sensitivity. An audiogram depicts hearing levels (in dB) at different frequencies (Hz) of sound.

Auricle: The outside visible part of the ear. Also called the *pinna.*

Autism: A serious condition typically accompanied by severe deficiencies of speech and language development, as well as nonverbal communication. Difficulties interacting with other people are common.

Automatic speech: Speech that is produced with little conscious effort or thought, such as counting from 1 to 10 or reciting the alphabet. Examples of automatic speech include saying "excuse me" after bumping against something, or responding to a greeting with "fine, how are you?" without thinking about it.

Auxiliary verb: A verb used with a main verb to convey condition, voice, or mood; a "helping verb" *be, do,* or *have,* such as *is* going, *did* go, or *have* gone.

Back: See *Distinctive feature.*

Ballism: Violent or jerky movements observed in chorea (a group of disorders characterized by rapid and usually brief involuntary movements of the limbs, face, trunk, or head).

Bifid uvula: The complete or incomplete separation of the uvula into two parts. Associated with cleft palate.

Bilateral: Pertaining to both sides, such as a *bilateral* hearing loss that involves both ears.

Blue-dye test: A dysphagia test often used with tracheostomized clients. Blue dye is placed in the oral cavity, either directly applied to a client's tongue or mixed in with food or liquid, and then monitored for its progression through the body. If blue dye appears in the lungs or at the site of the stoma, it is an indication of aspiration. Blue dye is used because there are no natural body secretions that are blue.

Bolus: Food in the mouth that is chewed and ready to be swallowed.

Brachydactyly: Shortness of the fingers.

Carhart notch: A dip in bone conduction hearing (seen on an audiogram) of 5 dB at 500 and 4000 Hz, 10 dB at 1000 Hz, and 15 dB at 2000 Hz. It is often observed with otosclerosis because of the inability of fluids to move freely when the footplate of the stapes is fixed firmly to the oval window.

Catenative: A specific type of verb such as *wanna* (want to), *gonna* (going to), and *hafta* (have to).

Central nervous system: Part of the nervous system that includes the brain and spinal cord.

Cerebellar ataxia: See *Ataxia*.

Cerebral vascular accident (CVA): Also called a stroke. Damage to part of the brain due to a disturbance in the blood supply.

Charting: Ongoing recording of client's actions or responses. For example, recording each instance of a correct or incorrect sound production.

Childhood apraxia: See *Developmental apraxia*.

Circumlocution: A round-about way of speaking; or nonuse of a particular sound, word or phrase. In aphasia, the client may be unable to recall the desired word and, therefore, defines or uses a related word. In stuttering, the client may fear stuttering on a particular word and use an alternative word or description.

Cluttering: A speech disorder characterized by rapid and sometimes unintelligible speech; sound, part-word, or whole-word repetitions; and often a language deficit.

Coloboma: A clefting defect of the eye which may involve the iris, choroid (the heavily pigmented tissue in the eye), or retinal structures.

Compliance: The ease with which the tympanic membrane and middle ear mechanism function; mobility of tympanic membrane.

Concurrent validity: See *Validity*.

Conductive hearing loss: Reduced hearing acuity from diminished ability to conduct sound through the outer or middle ear; often due to abnormalities of the external ear canal, eardrum, or ossicular chain.

Congenital: Describes a disease, deformity, or deficiency that is present at birth. The abnormality may be hereditary or acquired prior to birth.

Conjoining: Joined together.

Conjunction: A word that joins two or more grammatical units. Examples include you *and* me, wanted to *but* couldn't, he went *because* he wanted to, I would *if* I could, etc.

Consonantal: See *Distinctive feature*.

Construct validity: See *Validity*.

Content validity: See *Validity*.

Copula: A form of the verb "to be" which links a subject noun with a predicate noun or adjective. For example, the puppy *is* young, or they *were* late.

Coronal: See *Distinctive feature*.

Covert cleft: A cleft of the lip and/or palate which is not overtly visible.

Craniosynostosis: Premature fusion of the cranial sutures that can adversely affect the shape and structure of the head.

Cuff: A part of a tracheostomy tube that can be inflated and deflated to close off the airway.

Cul-de-sac resonance: A hollow sounding, somewhat hyponasal voice quality often associated with cleft palate speech.

CVA: See *Cerebral vascular accident*.

Dementia: Mental deterioration characterized by confusion, poor judgment, impaired memory, disorientation, and impaired intellect.

Denasality: See *Hyponasality*.

Developmental apraxia: A disorder of articulation characterized by difficulty acquiring speech, inconsistent sound errors, and groping or struggle behaviors during speech. Symptoms resemble speech behaviors of apraxia in adults.

Diadochokinesis: Abilities to make rapid, repetitive movements of the articulators to produce speech. Often tested by using preselected syllables such as /pʌ/, /tʌ/, and /kʌ/.

Diplegia: Bilateral paralysis affecting parts of both sides of the body.

Disfluency: See *Dysfluency*.

Distinctive feature: The unique articulatory and/or acoustic characteristics of a phoneme (e.g., voiced or unvoiced, consonant or vowel, tense or lax, etc.) that make it unique from all other phonemes; the specific features attributed to each sound.

> **Anterior:** Produced in the front region of the mouth, at the alveolar ridge, or forward. It includes /l/, /p/, /b/, /f/, /v/, /m/, /t/, /d/, /θ/, /ð/, /n/, /s/, and /z/.

> **Back:** Produced in the back of the mouth with the tongue retracted from the neutral position. It includes /k/, /g/, /ŋ/, /w/, /u/, /oʊ/, /ɑɪ/, /ɔɪ/, /ʌ/, /ʊ/, /o/, and /ɔ/.

> **Consonantal:** Produced with narrow constriction. It includes all consonant sounds except /h/.

> **Continuant:** Produced with partial obstruction of air flow. It includes /r/, /l/, /f/, /v/, /θ/, /ð/, /s/, /z/, /ʃ/, /ʒ/, and /h/.

> **Coronal:** Produced by raising the blade of the tongue above the neutral position, it includes /r/, /l/, /t/, /d/, /θ/, /ð/, /n/, /s/, /z/, /tʃ/, /dʒ/, /ʃ/, and /ʒ/.

> **High:** Produced by raising the body of the tongue above the neutral position. It includes /tʃ/, /dʒ/, /ʃ/, /ʒ/, /k/, /g/, /w/, /j/, /i/, /u/, and /ɪ/.

> **Low:** Produced by lowering the body of the tongue below the neutral position. It includes /h/, /ɑɪ/, /əɪ/, /æ/, and /ɔ/.

> **Nasal:** Produced by lowering the velum to allow air to pass through the oral cavity. It includes /m/, /n/, and /ŋ/.

> **Round:** Produced by narrowing the lips. It includes /u/, /ɔɪ/, /ʊ/, /o/, /ɔ/, and /w/.

> **Strident:** Produced with rapid airflow pressing against the teeth. It includes /f/, /v/, /s/, /z/, /tʃ/, /dʒ/, /ʃ/, and /ʒ/.

> **Tense:** Produced by maintaining muscular effort of the articulators for an extended period of time. It includes /i/, /u/, /e/, /ɑɪ/, and /ɔɪ/.

> **Vocalic:** Produced without significant constriction and with voicing. It includes all vowel sounds and the consonant sound /h/.

> **Voiced:** Produced with vocal fold vibration. It includes /r/, /l/, /b/, /v/, /m/, /d/, /ð/, /n/, /z/, /dʒ/, /ʒ/, /g/, /j/, and all vowel sounds.

Distortion: A speech error whereby the intended sound is recognizable, but is not produced correctly. Examples include "slurred" or imprecise sound productions.

Dysarthria: A group of motor speech disorders associated with muscle paralysis, weakness, or incoordination. It is associated with central or peripheral nervous system damage.

Dysfluency: An interruption that interferes with or prevents the smooth, easy flow of speech. Examples include repetitions, prolongations, interjections, and silent pauses.

Dysphagia: A disturbance in the normal act of swallowing.

Earmold: A fitting designed to conduct amplified sound from the receiver of a hearing aid into the ear.

Echolalia: An involuntary, parrot-like imitation or repeating back of what is heard. It is frequently seen with some autisms and schizophrenias.

Ectrodactyly: Absence of one or more fingers or toes.

Ellipsis: The omission of known or shared information in a subsequent utterance when it would be redundant; construction may be incomplete, but missing parts are understood. In cluttering, it may refer to omission of sounds, syllables, or entire words.

Encephalitis: Inflammation of the brain usually caused by a viral infection.

Eustachian tube: A tube that connects the nasopharynx and the middle ear. It equalizes pressure in the middle ear with atmospheric pressure.

Expressive abilities: The abilities to express oneself. This usually refers to language expression through speech, but it also includes gestures, sign language, use of a communication board, and other forms of expression.

Face validity: See *Validity*.

Failure to thrive: Inability to maintain life functions. People in this condition are bedridden and "just barely alive."

Fasciculations: Tremor-like movements of a band of muscle or nerve fibers.

Fenestrated: A tracheostomy tube that has small holes in it to allow passage of air through the airway.

Fistula: An abnormal channel, often a hole, connecting two spaces. For example, a palatal fistula may connect the oral and nasal cavities.

Fluency: The smooth, uninterrupted, effortless flow of speech; speech that is not hindered by excessive dysfluencies.

Gerund: A verb form that ends in *-ing* and is used as a noun. For example, *stealing* is bad, or *swinging* is fun.

Glossoptosis: A downward displacement of the tongue, typically associated with neurological weakness.

Grammar: Systems, rules, or underlying principles that describe the aspects (phonology, semantics, syntax, pragmatics, morphology) of language.

Hematoma: A collection of blood in an organ, space, or tissue. It is caused by a break in the wall of a blood vessel.

Hemifacial microsomia: A condition in which portions or all of the head are abnormally small.

Hemiparesis: Paralysis or weakness on one side of the body. Commonly associated with stroke.

Hemorrhage: Excessive bleeding typically from a ruptured blood vessel.

Heterochromia irides: More than one color of the iris of one eye (e.g., a brown patch in a blue eye), or differences in color between the two eyes (e.g., one blue eye and one brown eye).

High: See *Distinctive feature*.

Hydrocephaly: Enlargement of the head caused by excessive accumulation of cerebrospinal fluid in the cranial spaces.

Hypernasality: Excessive, undesirable nasal resonance during phonation; nasal resonance on a sound other than /m/, /n/, and /ŋ/.

Hyperplexia: Underdevelopment. For example, a *hyperplexic* mandible is underdeveloped.

Hypertelorism: Increased distance between the eyes.

Hypertonia: Excessive muscle tone or tension.

Hypogonadism: Decreased gonadal function and/or size, often the result of deficient hormone production.

Hyponasality: Lack of normal nasal resonance on the nasal consonants /m/, /n/, and /ŋ/, often a result of obstruction in the nasal tract.

Hypoplasia: Incomplete or underdevelopment of a tissue or organ. For example, lingual *hypoplasia* is an underdeveloped tongue.

Hypotonia: Reduced or absent muscle tone or tension.

Idiom: Short, figurative language expression such as *hit the roof*, *in the ballpark*, or *blew their cool*.

Imitation: Repetition of a behavior. In speech treatment, the client repeats a verbal stimulus. Clinicians use imitation as one technique to teach newly desired behaviors.

Impedance: Resistance to a vibratory source of energy. Resistance may be acoustic, mechanical, or electric. In impedance audiometry, impedance of air pressure and air volume differences are measured to detect conductive hearing loss and middle ear pathology.

Intelligibility: The degree or level to which speech is understood by others.

Interjection: The addition of a sound or word that does not relate grammatically to other words in the utterance. For example, "I want, *you know*, to go," or "He was *uh* going."

Intermittency: Episodic or variable. In voice, it is the inappropriate cessation of phonation during speech. In reference to a hearing aid, it is the inappropriate interruption of the transmission of a signal through the hearing aid.

Intertester reliability: See *Reliability*.

Intonation: Changes in pitch, stress, and prosodic features that affect speech. The lack of intonation makes the speech sound monotone and "colorless."

Intratester reliability: See *Reliability*.

Jargon: (1) Verbal behavior of children (approximately 9–18 months) containing a variety of inflected syllables that resemble meaningful, connected speech. (2) Fluent, well-articulated speech that makes little sense; illogical speech consisting of nonsense words or words used in an inappropriate context. For example, *Get this a splash of arbuckle*.

Klunking: An undesirable, audible sound that occurs when air is injected into the esophagus too quickly during the production of esophageal speech.

Labial pit: A small hole in the lip sometimes seen with cleft lip and/or palate.

Labyrinthitis: An inflammation of the inner ear. Symptoms are vertigo, balance problems, and/or vomiting.

Lesion: A specific site of injury or disease.

Literal paraphasia: See *Paraphasia*.

Low: See *Distinctive feature*.

Malocclusion: Misalignment of the upper and lower teeth. A normal occlusion is the correct alignment of the upper and lower molars; deviations of this are malocclusions.

> **Class I (neutroclusion):** Normal anterior-posterior relationship of the upper and lower molars; individual teeth may be misaligned.

> **Class II (distoclusion):** The lower molars (dental arch) are posterior to the alignment of the upper molars.

> **Class III (mesioclusion):** The lower molars (dental arch) are anterior to the alignment of the upper molars.

Mandible: The lower jaw.

Mandibular hypoplasia: Underdevelopment of the lower jaw.

Mastoiditis: An inflammation of the mastoid process.

Mastoid process: The bony protuberance (bulge) behind and below the outer ear.

Maxilla: The upper jaw.

Mean length of utterance (MLU): The average length of each utterance taken from multiple utterances. It is usually the average number of morphemes per utterance, but it can also be used to describe the average number of words per utterance.

Ménière's disease: A disease of the inner ear characterized by progressive sensorineural hearing loss in the affected ear, recurrent dizziness, tinnitus, nausea, and/or vomiting.

Meningitis: An inflammation of the tissues that surround the brain and spinal cord. It is usually caused by a bacterial infection but can also result from a viral or fungal infection.

Metaphor: A figure of speech with an implied comparison between two entities. For example, *big as a house* or *meaner than a junkyard dog*.

Metathetic errors: Speech errors involving the transposition of sounds or syllables in a word or phrase. For example, *puck* for *cup*, or *warday* for *doorway*.

Microcephaly: Abnormal smallness of the head; imperfect, small development of the cranium.

Micrognathia: Unusually small lower jaw, often associated with a recessed chin.

Microtia: Congenital underdevelopment of the external ear.

Microstoma: Abnormally small mouth.

Mixed hearing loss: A hearing loss with conductive and sensorineural components.

Morpheme: The smallest unit of language that has meaning. Free morphemes (cat, dog, me, etc.) can stand alone to convey meaning and cannot be reduced any further without losing meaning. Bound morphemes (*-ing*, *-s*, *-er*, etc.) cannot stand alone; they must be attached to a free morpheme to convey meaning.

Morphology: The study of how sounds and words are put together to form meaning.

Myopia: Short sightedness; inability to see distances.

Nares: Nostrils.

Nasal: See *Distinctive feature*.

Nasal emission: Escapage of airflow through the nasal cavity. Often seen in the presence of an inadequate velopharyngeal seal between the oral and nasal cavities. It is most frequently heard during the production of voiceless sounds, especially voiceless plosives or fricatives.

Nasality: Sounds made with air moving through the nasal cavities. It is appropriate during productions of /m/, /n/, and /ŋ/; it is inappropriate with all other English sounds.

Nasogastric tube: A tube that leads from the nose to the stomach. It is used to provide liquid nutrients and medications to clients who cannot eat orally.

Nasopharynx: The section of the pharynx located above the level of the soft palate that opens into the nasal cavity.

Neologistic paraphasia: See *Paraphasia*.

Nominal: A word or phrase that acts as a noun.

Nubbin: A small piece on the receiver of a body-level hearing aid that snaps into the snapring of the earmold to attach the receiver to the earmold.

Occult cleft: See *Submucosal cleft*.

Omission: The absence or deletion of a needed sound. For example, articulating *so* instead of *soap*.

Ossicles: The three small bones of the middle ear (incus, malleus, and stapes). Also referred to as the ossicular chain.

Otitis media: An infection of the middle ear frequently acquired by children and often associated with upper respiratory infection. There are three varieties:

   Acute otitis media: A sudden onset of otitis media caused by an infection.

   Chronic otitis media: The permanent condition of a ruptured tympanic membrane. It may or may not be associated with infection.

   Serous otitis media: Inflammation of the middle ear, with the presence of a thick or watery fluid that fills the middle ear space.

Ototoxicity: Damage to the ear caused by a harmful poison. It is usually associated with certain drugs.

Overt cleft: A clearly visible cleft of the lip and/or palate.

Palpebral fissures: The slits of the eyes formed by the upper and lower eyelids.

Paralinguistic cues: Vocal or nonvocal cues which are superimposed (added onto) on a linguistic code to signal the speaker's attitude or emotion or to add or clarify meaning. For example, sarcasm is usually conveyed more through paralinguistic cues than through the actual words or syntax used.

Paralysis: Impairment or loss of muscle power or function due to muscular dysfunction.

Paraphasia: A problem with word or sound substitution commonly associated with aphasia. There are several types:

> **Verbal paraphasia:** Substitution of an entire word for another. There are two types:

>> **Semantic paraphasia:** Substitution of a word that is similar to the intended word. For example, *father* for *mother*.

>> **Random paraphasia:** Substitution of a word that is not similar to the intended word For example, *dog* for *flower*.

> **Neologistic paraphasia:** The use of a nonmeaningful word. For example, "I want *arbuckle*."

> **Phonetic or literal paraphasia:** The substitution of one sound for another or the addition of a sound. For example, *mandwich* for *sandwich* or *skandwich* for *sandwich*.

Paresis: Partial or incomplete paralysis; weakness.

Participle: A verb used as an adjective. For example, the *flowing* water or the *swaying* branch.

Peripheral nervous system: The collection of nerves outside the brain and spinal column that conduct impulses to and from the central nervous system. The peripheral system includes the cranial nerves, spinal nerves, and some portions of the autonomic nerves.

Peristalsis: Alternate contraction and relaxation of the walls of a tube-like structure, which helps its contents move forward (e.g., within the intestinal tract).

Perseveration: Inappropriate continuation or repetition of the same word, thought, or behavior, commonly associated with aphasia and other neurologic impairments.

Phonation: The physiological process by which air moving through the vocal tract becomes acoustic energy in the larynx; production of voiced (versus voiceless) sounds.

Phonetic paraphasia: See *Paraphasia.*

Phonology: The study of the sound system of language, including speech sounds, speech patterns, and rules that apply to those sounds.

Pinna: The outside, visible part of the ear. Also called the *auricle.*

Polydactyly: Extra fingers or toes.

Polyneuritis: The inflammation of multiple nerves.

Pragmatics: The study of the rules that govern and describe how language is used situationally, in light of its context and environment.

Predictive validity: See *Validity.*

Preposition: A word used to relate a noun or pronoun to another word in a sentence. It can be used to modify a noun, adjective, or adverb. For example, *in* there, *on* the bed, *between* them.

Presbycusis: Progressive loss of hearing as a result of the aging process.

Presupposition: Taking the other person into consideration or perspective when communicating. It is the process of understanding what information the other person has or may need.

Prognathic: A marked projection of the jaw.

Prognosis: A prediction or judgment about the course, duration, and prospects for the improvement of a disorder. It may include judgments about future changes with or without professional intervention.

Prolongation: The inappropriate lengthening of a sound production. For example, prolonging the vowel in the word *gooood*.

Pronoun: A word that takes the place of a noun. Examples are *I*, *mine*, *we*, *myself*, *whose*, *which*, and *that*.

Prosody: Variations in rate, loudness, stress, intonation, and rhythm producing the melodic components of speech.

Proverb: A figure of speech that often contains advice or conventional wisdom. For example, *Don't put all your eggs in one basket* or *Nothing ventured—nothing gained*.

Psychosis: A severe mental or behavioral disorder characterized by a disordered personality or inability to deal with reality. It may include disorientation, delusion, and hallucination.

Ptosis: Drooping of the eyelids, usually affecting the upper eyelids.

Puree diet: A diet that consists of foods that are blended to a soft texture, like that of pudding or applesauce. It may be recommended for clients who have dysphagia.

Random paraphasia: See *Paraphasia*.

Receptive abilities: The ability to understand or comprehend language. It usually refers to the ability to understand verbal expression, but it also includes the ability to understand sign language, writing, Braille, and other forms of language.

Reflux: Backward flow of food or liquids that have already entered the stomach.

Regurgitate: Vomiting of food or liquids that have already entered the stomach.

Reliability: The consistency and subsequent dependability of obtained results. For example, a test administered on two occasions produced the same or similar results.

    Alternate form reliability: Consistency of results obtained when using different forms of the test. For example, obtaining similar results after administering Form L and Form M of the *Peabody Picture Vocabulary Test*.

    Intratester reliability: Consistency of results obtained when the same test is administered by the same examiner on two or more occasions.

    Intertester reliability: Consistency of results obtained when the same test is administered by two or more examiners.

    Split-half or internal reliability: Consistency of difficulty throughout a test that is not intended to be progressively more difficult. For example, the first half of a test is equally difficult to the second half.

    Test-retest reliability: Consistency of results of a test administered on two occasions. Administration by one examiner on different occasions is intratester and test-retest reliability. Administration by more than one examiner on different occasions is intertester and test-retest reliability.

Repetition: In dysfluent speech, the abnormal additional productions of a sound, syllable, word, or phrase. For example, *I-I-I-I-I* want to go.

Resonance: Vibration of one or more structures related to the source of the sound; vibration above or below the sound source (the larynx for speech). In voice, resonance relates to the quality of the voice produced.

Respiration: The act of breathing, including drawing air into the body (inspiration) and expulsion of the air from the body (expiration).

Retinitis pigmentosa: A hereditary, deteriorating condition involving inflammation and pigmentary infiltration of the retina.

Revisions: Verbalizations in which a targeted word or phrase is changed and a different word or phrase is substituted.

Round: See *Distinctive feature.*

Schizophrenia: A group of severe mental or behavioral disorders characterized by marked disturbances of reality. It may include severe interpersonal difficulties dealing with other people or marked affective, intellectual, or behavioral disturbances. Bizarre language patterns, including pragmatic deficiencies, are often seen.

Semantic paraphasia: See *Paraphasia.*

Semantics: The study of the meaning of language, including meaning at the word, sentence, and conversational levels.

Sensorineural hearing loss: Reduced hearing acuity due to a pathological condition in the inner ear or along the nerve pathway from the inner ear to the brainstem.

Splay: Spread or turn outward. For example, a hand with the fingers spread apart and turned outward from the palm is called *splayed.*

Split-half reliability: See *Reliability.*

Spoonerism: The transposition of sounds in a word, phrase, or sentence. For example, *half-warmed fish* for *half-formed wish.*

Stoma: A surgically placed opening in the body. Following laryngectomy, the stoma is in the anterior portion of the neck.

Strabismus: A visual disorder in which both eyes do not focus on the same thing at the same time.

Strident: See *Distinctive feature.*

Stridor: An abnormal breathing noise characterized by a tense, nonmusical laryngeal sound.

Submucosal cleft: A cleft of the palate whereby the surface tissues of the hard and soft palate are joined but the underlying bone or muscle tissues are not. Also called an occult cleft.

Substitution: One sound is substituted in place of the target sound. For example *wabbit* for *rabbit.*

Synchondrosis: A joining of two bones by cartilaginous tissue.

Syndactyly: Persistent soft tissue between the fingers or toes; webbing.

Syntax: The order of language, especially the way words are put together in phrases or sentences to produce meaning.

Telecoil switch: A hearing aid switch that allows the induction coil in the hearing aid to pick up signals from a telephone. It is also used in loop induction auditory training units.

Telegraphic speech: Short utterances consisting primarily or exclusively of content words (nouns, verbs, adjectives, adverbs). Grammatical words such as *the*, *to*, or *and* are typically omitted. For example, *I want to go* may be reduced to *want go*.

Tense: See *Distinctive feature*.

Test-retest reliability: See *Reliability*.

Tonsillitis: An inflammation of the tonsils usually caused by a bacterial infection.

Tracheotomy: The operation of cutting into the trachea.

Tracheostomy: The construction of an artificial opening through the neck into the trachea.

Transposition: See *Metathetic errors*.

Traumatic brain injury: An acute assault on the brain that causes mild to severe injury. The two types of traumatic brain injury are penetrating injuries and closed head injuries. The damage is localized or generalized depending on the type and extent of the injury.

Tympanogram: A graph depicting eardrum and middle ear compliance measured during air pressure changes in the external auditory canal.

Unilateral: Pertaining to one side of the body, such as a *unilateral* hearing loss involving only one ear.

Validity: Estimate of the degree to which a test actually measures or evaluates what it is intended to measure or evaluate.

> **Concurrent validity:** The relationship between what a given test measures and the results of a separate test. For example, the relationship between results obtained from two language tests.
>
> **Construct validity:** The relationship between what the test measures and a known construct such as age, sex, or IQ.
>
> **Content validity:** Whether the items contained on the test are appropriate for measuring what it intends to measure.
>
> **Face validity:** Whether a test appears, at face value, to measure what it intends to measure.
>
> **Predictive validity:** The ability of a test to predict future performance or abilities.

Velopharyngeal: Pertaining to the velum (soft palate) and the posterior nasopharyngeal wall.

Ventilation: Movement of air from one place to another.

Ventilation tube: A small tube placed in the tympanic membrane, creating a hole in the ear drum. It is used for the treatment and prevention of chronic otitis media.

Verb: A word expressing action or making a statement about the subject or noun phrase of a sentence.

Verbal paraphasia: See *Paraphasia*.

Vestibular system: The inner-ear structure containing three semicircular canals. The system is important for body position, balance, and movement.

Vitiligo: Unpigmented, pale patches of skin due to loss of pigmentation.

Vocalic: See *Distinctive feature*.

Voiced: See *Distinctive feature*.

□ REFERENCES □

Adams, M. (1980). The young stutterer: Diagnosis, treatment, and assessment of prognosis. *Seminars in Speech, Language, and Hearing, 1*, 289–299.

Adamovich, B. B., Henderson, J. A., & Auerbach, S. (1985). *Cognitive rehabilitation of closed head injured patients: A dynamic approach.* Boston: Little, Brown and Co.

Adamovich, B., & Henderson, J. (1991). *Scales of cognitive ability for traumatic brain injury.* San Antonio, TX: Riverside Publishing.

Adler, S. (1990). Multicultural clients: Implication for the SLP. *Language, Speech, and Hearing Services in Schools, 21*, 135–139.

Albert, M. L. (1973). A simple test of visual neglect. *Neurology, 23*, 658–664.

American Speech-Language-Hearing Association. (1983). *How does your child hear and talk?* Rockville, MD: National Association for Hearing and Speech Action.

American Speech-Language-Hearing Association. (1985, June). Clinical management of communicatively handicapped minority language populations. *Asha, 27*(6), 29–32.

American Speech-Language-Hearing Association. (1989). Competencies for speech-language pathologists providing services in augmentative communication. *Asha, 31*, 107–110.

Andrews, G., & Cutler, J. (1974). Stuttering therapy: The relation between changes in symptom level and attitudes. *Journal of Speech and Hearing Disorders, 39*, 312–319.

Andrews, M. L. (1995). *Manual of voice treatment: Pediatrics through geriatrics.* San Diego, CA: Singular.

Aronson, A. E. (1985). *Clinical voice disorders: An interdisciplinary approach* (3rd ed.). New York: Thieme.

Arwood, E. L. (1991). *Semantic and pragmatic language disorders* (2nd ed.). Gaithersburg, MD: Aspen.

Bailey, D. B., & Wolery, M. (Eds.). (1989). *Assessing infants and preschoolers with handicaps.* Columbus, OH: Merrill.

Baker, H. J., & Leland, B. (1967). *Detroit tests of learning aptitude.* Indianapolis: Bobbs-Merrill.

Bangs, T. E., & Dodson, S. (1979). *Birth to three developmental scales.* Hingham, MA: Teaching Resources.

Bankson, N. W. (1990). *Bankson language test* (2nd ed.). Austin, TX: PRO-ED.

Bankson, N. W., & Bernthal, J. E. (1990). *Bankson-Bernthal phonological process survey test.* Tucson, AZ: Communication Skill Builders.

Baratz, J. C. (1969, March). Language and cognitive assessment of Negro children: Assumptions and research needs. *Asha, 11*(3), 87–91.

Baumgart, D., Johnson, J., & Helmstetter, E. (1990). *Augmentative and alternative communication systems for persons with moderate and severe disabilities.* Baltimore: Paul H. Brookes.

Bayles, K., & Tomoeda, C. (1993). *Arizona battery for communication disorders of dementia* (QBCD). Tucson, AZ: Canyonlands.

Berger, K. W., & Millin, J. P. (1989). Amplification/assistive devices for the hearing impaired. In R. L. Schow & M. A. Nerbonne (Eds.), *Introduction to aural rehabilitation* (2nd ed., pp. 31–80). Austin, TX: PRO-ED.

Berlin, C. I. (1963). Clinical measurement of esophageal speech: I. Methodology and curves of skill acquisition. *Journal of Speech and Hearing Disorders, 28*(1), 42–51.

Bernstein, D. K. (1993). The nature of language and its disorders. In Bernstein, D. K., & Tiegerman, E. (Eds.), *Language and communication disorders in children* (3rd ed., pp. 2–23). New York: Macmillan.

Bernstein, D. K., & Tiegerman, E. (Eds.). (1993). *Language and communication disorders in children* (3rd ed.). New York: Macmillan.

Bernthal, J. E., & Bankson, N. W. (1993). *Articulation and phonological disorders* (3rd ed.). Englewood Cliffs, NJ: Prentice-Hall.

Bess, F. H. (Ed.). (1988). *Hearing impairment in children.* Parkton, MD: York Press.

Bess, F. H., & Hall III, J. W. (1992). *Screening children for auditory function.* Nashville, TN: Bill Wilkerson Center.

Bess, F. H., & Humes, L. E. (1995). *Audiology: The fundamentals* (2nd ed.). Baltimore: Williams & Wilkins.

Beukelman, D. R., & Mirenda, P. (1992). *Augmentative and alternative communication: Management of severe communication disorders in children and adults.* Baltimore: Paul H. Brookes.

Beukelman, D. R., & Yorkston, K. M. (Eds.). (1991). *Communication disorders following traumatic brain injury.* Austin, TX: PRO-ED.

Beukelman, D. R., Yorkston, K. M., & Dowden, P. A. (1985). *Communication augmentation: A casebook of clinical management.* San Diego: CA: College-Hill Press.

Bigler, E. D. (Ed.). (1990). *Traumatic brain injury.* Austin, TX: PRO-ED.

Blakeley, R. W. (1980). *Screening test for developmental apraxia of speech.* Austin, TX: PRO-ED.

Blockcolsky, V. (1990). *Book of words: 17,000 words selected by vowels and diphthongs.* Tucson, AZ: Communication Skill Builders.

Blockcolsky, V. D., Frazer, J. M., & Frazer, D. H. (1987). *40,000 selected words organized by letter, sound, and syllable.* Tucson, AZ: Communication Skill Builders.

Bloodstein, O. (1995). *A handbook on stuttering* (5th ed.). San Diego: Singular Publishing Group.

Bloom, L., & Lahey, M. (1978). *Language development and language disorders.* New York: John Wiley & Sons.

Boehm, A. E. (1986). *Boehm test of basic concepts.* New York: Psychological Corporation.

Bollinger, R., & Hardiman, C. (1990). *Rating scale of communication in cognitive decline.* Buffalo, NY: United Educational Services.

Bolton, S. O., & Dashiell, S. E. (1991). *Interaction checklist for augmentative communication: An observational tool to assess interactive behavior (INCH) (Revised).* Bisbee, AZ: Imaginart.

Boone, D. R. (1986). *The Boone voice program for children: Screening, evaluation, and referral.* Austin, TX: PRO-ED.

Boone, D. R., & McFarlane, S. C. (1994). *The voice and voice therapy* (4th ed.). Englewood Cliffs, NJ: Prentice-Hall.

Boone, D. R., & Plante, E. (1993). *Human communication and its disorders* (2nd ed.). Englewood Cliffs, NJ: Prentice-Hall.

Bosley, E. C. (1981). *Techniques for articulatory disorders*. Springfield, IL: Charles C. Thomas.

Brace, E. R., & Pacanowski, J. P. (1985). *Childhood symptoms*. New York: Harper & Row.

Brookshire, R. H. (1992). *An introduction to neurogenic communication disorders* (4th ed.). St. Louis: Mosby-Year Book.

Brookshire, R. H., & Nicholas, L. E. (1993). *Discourse comprehension test*. Tucson, AZ: Communication Skill Builders.

Brown, R. (1973). *A first language*. Cambridge, MA: Harvard University.

Bryan, K. L. (1989). *The right hemisphere language battery*. Kibworth, England: Far Communications.

Burns, M. S. (1985). Language without communication: The pragmatics of right hemisphere damage. In M. S. Burns, A. S. Halper, & S. I. Mogil (Eds.), *Clinical management of right hemisphere dysfunction* (pp. 17–28). Rockville, MD: Aspen.

Burns, M. S., Halper, A. S., & Mogil, S. I. (1985*). Clinical management of right hemisphere dysfunction*. Rockville, MD: Aspen.

Bzoch, K. R. (Ed.). (1989). *Communicative disorders related to cleft lip and palate*. Austin, TX: PRO-ED.

Bzoch, K. R, & League, R. (1991). *Receptive-expressive emergent language scale* (2nd ed.). Austin, TX: PRO-ED.

Calvert, D. R., & Silverman, S. R. (1983). *Speech and deafness* (rev. ed.). Washington DC: Alexander Graham Bell Association for the Deaf.

Carrow, E. (1973). *Screening test for auditory comprehension of language*. Austin, TX: Urban Research Group.

Carrow, E. (1974). *Carrow elicited language inventory*. Allen, TX: DLM/Teaching Resources.

Carrow-Woolfolk, E. (1985). *Test for auditory comprehension of language—Revised*. Allen, TX: DLM/Teaching Resources.

Case, J. L. (1991). *Clinical management of voice disorders* (2nd ed.). Austin, TX: PRO-ED.

Casper, J. K., & Colton, R. H. (1993). *Clinical manual for laryngectomy and head/neck cancer rehabilitation*. San Diego, CA: Singular Publishing Group.

Cheng, L. L. (1987, June). Cross-cultural and linguistic considerations in working with Asian populations. *Asha, 29*(6), 33–38.

Cheng, L. L. (l991). *Assessing Asian language performance* (2nd ed.). Oceanside, CA: Academic Communication Associates.

Cherney, L. R., Cantieri, C. A., & Pannell, J. J. (1986). *Clinical evaluation of dysphagia*. Rockville, MD: Aspen.

Cherney, L. R., Pannell, J. J., & Cantieri, C. A. (1994). Clinical evaluation of dysphagia in adults. In L. R. Cherney (Ed.)., *Clinical management of dysphagia in adults and children* (2nd ed., pp. 49–92). Gaithersburg, MD: Aspen.

Chomsky, N., & Halle, M. (1968). *The sound pattern of English*. New York: Harper & Row.

Church, G., & Glennen, S. (1991). *The handbook of assistive technology*. San Diego: Singular Publishing Group.

Clark, J. G. (1981, July). Uses and abuses of hearing loss classification. *Asha, 23*(7), 493–500.

Code of Fair Testing Practices in Education. (1988). Washington, DC: Joint Committee on Testing Practices. (Mailing address: Joint Committee on Testing Practices, American Psychological Association, 1200 17th Street, NW, Washington, DC 20036.)

Code, C., & Muller, D. J. (1991). *Aphasia therapy* (2nd ed.). San Diego: Singular Publishing Group.

Cole, L., & Snope, T. (1981, September). Resource guide to multicultural tests and materials. *Asha, 23*(9), 639–649.

Collins, M. (1991). *Diagnosis and treatment of global aphasia*. San Diego: Singular Publishing Group.

Colton, R. H., & Casper, J. K. (1996). *Understanding voice problems: A physiological perspective for diagnosis and treatment* (2nd ed.). Baltimore: Williams & Wilkins.

Compton, A. J. (1978). *Compton speech and language screening evaluation.* San Francisco: Carousel House.

Compton, A. J., & Hutton, S. (1978). *Compton-Hutton phonological assessment.* San Francisco: Carousel House.

Conture, E. G. (1990). *Stuttering* (2nd ed.). Englewood Cliffs, NJ: Prentice-Hall.

Cooper, H. (Ed.). (1991). *A practical guide to cochlear implants.* London: Whurr.

Coplan, J. (1987). *Early language milestone scale.* Austin, TX: PRO-ED.

Creaghead, N. A., Newman, P. W., & Secord, W. (1989). *Assessment and remediation of articulatory and phonological disorders* (2nd ed.). Columbus, OH: Merrill.

Crystal, D. (Ed.). (1979). *Working with the LARSP.* New York: Elsevier.

Crystal, D., Fletcher, P., & Garman, M. (1989). *The grammatical analysis of language disability* (2nd ed.). San Diego: Singular Publishing Group.

Cullum, C. M., Kuck, J., & Ruff, R. M. (1990). Neuropsychological assessment of traumatic brain injury in adults. In E. D. Bigler (Ed.), *Traumatic brain injury* (pp. 129–163). Austin, TX: PRO-ED.

Curlee, R. F. (1984). A case selection strategy for young disfluent children. In W. H. Perkins (Ed.), *Stuttering disorders* (pp. 3–20). New York: Thieme-Stratton.

Curlee, R. F., & Perkins, W. H. (Eds.). (1984). *Nature and treatment of stuttering: New directions.* San Diego: College-Hill Press.

Dabul, B. (1986). *Apraxia battery for adults.* Austin, TX: PRO-ED.

Daly, D. A. (1986). The clutterer. In K. O. St. Louis (Ed.), *The atypical stutterer: Principles and practices of rehabilitation* (pp. 152–192). New York: Academic Press.

D'Antonio, L. L., & Scherer, N. J. (1995). The evaluation of speech disorders associated with clefting. In R. J. Shprintzen & J. Bardach (Eds.), *Cleft palate speech management: A multidisciplinary approach* (pp. 176–220). St. Louis: Mosby.

Darley, F. L. (1982). *Aphasia.* New York: Saunders.

Darley, F. L., Aronson, A. E., & Brown, J. R. (1975). *Motor speech disorders.* Philadelphia: W. B. Saunders Co.

Darley, F. L., & Spriestersbach, D. C. (Eds.). (1978). *Diagnostic methods in speech pathology* (2nd ed.). New York: Harper & Row.

Davis, A. (1972). *English problems of Spanish speakers.* Urbana, IL: National Council of Teachers of English.

Davis, G. A. (1993). *A survey of adult aphasia* (2nd ed.). Englewood Cliffs, NJ: Prentice-Hall.

Deal, V. R., & Yen, M. A. (1985, June). Resource guide to multicultural tests and materials. *Asha, 27*(6), 43–49.

Decker, T. N. (1990). *Instrumentation: An introduction for students in the speech and hearing sciences.* New York: Longman.

Dever, R. B. (1978). *Teaching the American language to kids* (TALK). Columbus, OH: Merrill.

Diedrich, W. M. (1984). Cluttering: Its diagnosis. In H. Winitz (Ed.), *Treating articulation disorders* (pp. 307–323). Baltimore: University Park Press.

Dikeman, K. J., & Kazandjian, M. S. (1995). *Communication and swallowing management of tracheostomized and ventilator-dependent adults.* San Diego, CA: Singular.

DiSimoni, F. G. (1989). *Comprehensive apraxia test.* Dalton, PA: Praxis House.

Drumwright, A. F. (1971). *Denver articulation screening examination.* Denver: University of Colorado Medical Center.

Duffy, J. R. (1995). *Motor speech disorders: Substrates, differential diagnosis, and management.* St. Louis: Mosby.

Duguay, M. J., & Fuedo, P. (1988). The process of postlaryngectomy rehabilitation. In M. P. Fried (Ed.), *The larynx: A multidisciplinary approach* (pp. 603–613). Boston: Little, Brown and Company.

Dunn, L. M., & Dunn, L. M. (1981). *Peabody picture vocabulary test—Revised*. Circle Pines, MN: American Guidance Service.

Dworkin, J. P. (1991). *Motor speech disorders: A treatment guide*. St. Louis: Mosby-Year Book.

Dworkin, J., & Culatta, R. (1980). *Dworkin-Culatta oral mechanism examination*. Nicholasville, KY: Edgewood Press.

Eckel, F. C., & Boone, D. R. (1981). The s/z ratio as an indicator of vocal pathology. *Journal of Speech and Hearing Disorders, 46*, 147–150.

Elbert, M., & Gierut, J. (1986). *Handbook of clinical phonology: Approaches to assessment and treatment*. San Diego: College-Hill Press.

Emerick, L. (1969). *The parent interview*. Danville, IL: Interstate Press.

Emerick, L. L., & Haynes, W. O. (1986). *Diagnosis and evaluation in speech pathology* (3rd ed.). Englewood Cliffs, NJ: Prentice-Hall.

Enderby, P. M. (1983). *Frenchay dysarthria assessment*. Austin, TX: PRO-ED.

Erickson, J. G., & Omark, D. R. (Eds.). (1981). *Communication assessment of the bilingual bicultural child*. Baltimore: University Park Press.

Erickson, R. L. (1969). Assessing communicative attitudes among stutterers. *Journal of Speech and Hearing Research, 12*, 711–724.

Fasold, R., & Wolfram, M. (1970). Some linguistic features of Negro dialect. In R. Fasold & R. Shuy (Eds.), *Teaching standard English in the inner city* (pp. 41--86). Washington, DC: Center for Applied Linguistics.

Feldman, A. S. (1975). Acoustic impedance-admittance measurements. In L. J. Bradford (Ed.), *Physiologic measures of the audio-vestibular system* (pp. 87–145). New York: Academic Press.

Feldman, A. S. (1976). Tympanometry—procedures, interpretations and variables. In A. S. Feldman & L. A. Wilber (Eds.), *Acoustic impedence and admittance: The measurement of middle ear function* (pp. 103–155). Baltimore: Williams & Wilkins.

Fell, A., Lynn, E., & Morrison, K. (1984). *Non-oral communication assessment*. Ann Arbor, MI: Alternatives to Speech.

Fisher, H. B., & Logemann, J. A. (1971). *The Fisher-Logemann test of articulation competence*. Boston: Houghton Mifflin.

Fletcher, S. G. (1972). Time-by-count measurement of diadochokinetic syllable rate. *Journal of Speech and Hearing Research, 15*, 763–770.

Fletcher, S. G. (1978). *Time-by-count test measurement of diadochokinetic syllable rate*. Austin, TX: PRO-ED.

Fluharty, N. B. (1978). *Flaharty preschool speech and language screening test*. Boston: Teaching Resources Corporation.

Folstein, M. F., Folstein, S. E., & McHugh, P. R. (1975). Mini-mental state: A practical method for grading the mental state of patients for the clinician. *Journal of Psychiatric Research, 12*, 189–198.

Foster, R., Giddan, J. J., & Stark, J. (1983). *Assessment of children's language comprehension* (3rd ed.). Palo Alto, CA: Consulting Psychologists Press.

Fox, D. R., & Johns, D. (1970). Predicting velopharyngeal closure with a modified tongue-anchor technique. *Journal of Speech and Hearing Disorders, 35*, 248–251.

Fudala, J. B., & Reynolds, W. M. (1986). *Arizona articulation proficiency scale* (2nd ed.). Los Angeles: Western Psychological Services.

Gard, A., Gilman, L., & Gorman, J. (1980). *Speech and language development chart*. Salt Lake City: Word Making Productions.

Gardner, M. F. (1979). *Expressive one-word picture vocabulary test*. Novato, CA: Academic Therapy Publications.

Gardner, M. F. (1983). *Expressive one-word picture vocabulary test—Upper extension*. Novato, CA: Academic Therapy Publications.

Gardner, M. F. (1985). *Receptive one-word picture vocabulary test*. Novato, CA: Academic Therapy Publications.

Gauthier, S. V., & Madison, C. L (1983). *Kindergarten language screening test*. Austin, TX: PRO-ED.

Gerber, S. E. (1990). *Prevention: The etiology of communicative disorders in children*. Englewood Cliffs, NJ: Prentice-Hall.

Gleason, J. Berko. (Ed.). (1993). The development of language (3rd ed.). New York: Macmillan.

Glennen, S. L., & DeCoste, D. C. (1997). *Handbook of augmentative and alternative communication*. San Diego, CA: Singular.

Golden, C. J., Hammeke, T. A., & Purisch, A. D. (1980). *The Luria-Nebraska neuropsychological battery: Manual*. Los Angeles: Western Psychological Services.

Goldman, R., & Fristoe, M. (1986). *Goldman-Fristoe test of articulation*. Circle Pines, MN: American Guidance Service.

Goodglass, H., & Kaplan, E. (1983a). *Boston diagnostic aphasia examination*. Malvern, PA: Lea & Febinger.

Goodglass, H., & Kaplan, E. (1983b). *Boston naming test*. Malvern, PA: Lea & Febinger.

Groher, M. E. (Ed.). (1992). *Dysphagia: Diagnosis and management* (2nd ed.). Stoneham, MA: Butterworth-Heinemann.

Guitar, B. (1979). A response to Ingham's critique. *Journal of Speech and Hearing Disorders, 44*, 393–405.

Guitar, B., & Bass, C. (1978). Stuttering therapy: The relation between attitude change and long-term outcome. *Journal of Speech and Hearing Disorders, 43*, 393 400.

Hall, P. K. (1994). The oral mechanism. In J. B. Tomblin, H. L. Morris, & D. C. Spriestersbach (Eds.), *Diagnosis in speech-language pathology* (pp. 67–98). San Diego: Singular Publishing Group.

Halper, A. S., Burns, M. S., Cherney, L. R., & Mogil, S. I. (1985). *Rehabilitation Institute of Chicago (RIC) evaluation of communication problems in right hemisphere dysfunction—2 (RICE-2)*. Rockville, MD: Aspen.

Ham, R. (1986). *Techniques of stuttering therapy*. Englewood Cliffs, NJ: Prentice-Hall.

Hamann, B. (1994). *Disease identification, prevention , and control*. St. Louis: Mosby.

Hamayan, E. V., & Damico, J. S. (Eds.). (1991). *Limiting bias in the assessment of bilingual students*. Austin, TX: PRO-ED.

Hamlin, M. A. (1987, October). Problems of mild brain injury victims now more recognized in workplace. *Occupational Health and Safety, 56*(11), 59–64.

Hammill, D. (1985). *Detroit tests of learning aptitude 2*. Austin, TX: PRO-ED.

Hammill, D. D., Brown, V. L., Larsen, S. C., & Wiederholt, J. L. (1987). *Test of adolescent language (TOAL-2)*. Austin, TX: PRO-ED.

Hannah, E. P. (1977). *Applied linguistic analysis II: Synthesis and analysis of language*. Pacific Palisades, CA: SenCom.

Hannley, M. (1986). *Basic principles of audiologic assessment*. Boston: Little, Brown and Co.

Haynes, S. (1985). Developmental apraxia of speech: Symptoms and treatment. In D. L. Johns (Ed.), *Clinical management of neurogenic communicative disorders* (2nd ed., pp. 259–266). Boston: Little, Brown and Co.

Haynes, W. O., & Hartmann, D. E. (1975). The agony of report writing: A new look at an old problem. *Journal of the National Student Speech and Hearing Association, 3*(1), 7–15.

Haynes, W. O., Pindzola, R. H., & Emerick, L. L. (1992). *Diagnosis and evaluation in speech pathology* (4th ed.). Englewood Cliffs, NJ: Prentice-Hall.

Hegde, M. N. (1993). *Treatment procedures in communicative disorders* (2nd ed.). Austin, TX: PRO-ED.

Hegde, M. N. (1994). *A coursebook on scientific and professional writing in speech-language pathology*. San Diego: Singular Publishing Group.

Hegde, M. N. (1995a). *A coursebook on aphasia and other neurogenic language disorders*. San Diego, CA: Singular Publishing Group.

Hegde, M. N. (1995b). *Introduction to communicative disorders* (2nd ed.). Austin, TX: PRO-ED.

Hegde, M. N. (1996). *PocketGuide to assessment in speech-language pathology*. San Diego, CA: Singular Publishing Group.

Hegde, M. N. & Davis, D. (1992). *Clinical methods and practicum in speech-language pathology*. San Diego: Singular Publishing Group.

Helm-Estabrooks, N., & Albert, M. L. (1991). *Manual of aphasia therapy*. Austin, TX: PRO-ED.

Helm-Estabrooks, N., & Hotz, G. (1991). *Brief test of head injury*. Chicago, IL: Applied Symbolix.

Helm-Estabrooks, N., Ramsberger, G., Morgan, A. R., & Nicholas, M. (1989). *Boston assessment of severe aphasia*. Austin, TX: PRO-ED.

Hodson, B. W. (1986). *Assessment of phonological processes* (rev. ed.). Danville, IL: Interstate Printers & Publishers.

Hodson, B. W., & Paden, E. P. (1991). *Targeting intelligible speech: A phonological approach to remediation* (2nd ed.). Austin, TX: PRO-ED.

Holland, A. (1980). *Communicative abilities in daily living (CADL)*. Baltimore: University Park Press.

Holland, A. L. (Ed.). (1984). *Language disorders in children*. San Diego: College-Hill Press.

Hubbell, R. D. (1988). *A handbook of English grammar and language sampling*. Englewood Cliffs, NJ: Prentice-Hall.

Huer, M. B. (1983). *The nonspeech test for receptive/expressive language*. Wauconda, IL: Don Johnston Developmental Equipment, Inc.

Hughes, C. P. (1982). A new clinical scale for the staging of dementia. *British Journal of Psychiatry, 140*, 566–572.

Hutchinson, B. B. (1979). Oral-peripheral and motor examination for speech. In B. B. Hutchinson, M. L. Hanson, & M. J. Mecham (Eds.), *Diagnostic handbook of speech pathology* (pp. 109–178). Baltimore: Williams & Wilkins.

Hutchinson, B. B., Hanson, M. L., & Mecham, M. J. (Eds.). (1979). *Diagnostic handbook of speech pathology*. Baltimore: Williams & Wilkins.

Hutchinson, J. M. (1983). Diagnosis of fluency disorders. In I. J. Meitus & B. Weinberg (Eds.), *Diagnosis in speech-language pathology* (pp. 183–222). Baltimore: University Park Press.

Ingham, R. J. (1979). Comment on "Stuttering therapy: The relation between attitude change and longterm outcome." *Journal of Speech and Hearing Disorders, 44*, 397–403.

Ingram, D. (1981). *Procedures for the phonological analysis of children's language*. Baltimore: University Park Press.

James, S. (1993). Assessing children with language disorders. In D. K. Bernstein & E. Tiegerman (Eds.), *Language and communication disorders in children* (3rd ed., pp. 185–228). New York: Macmillan.

James, S. (1990). *Normal language acquisition*. Boston: Little, Brown and Co.

Jerger, S., & Jerger, J. (1981). *Auditory disorders: A manual for clinical evaluation*. Boston: Little, Brown and Co.

Johns, D. F. (Ed.). (1985). *Clinical management of neurogenic communicative disorders* (2nd ed.). Boston: Little, Brown and Co.

Johnson, T. S. (1985). *Vocal abuse reduction program*. Austin, TX: PRO-ED.

Johnson, W., & Associates. (1959). *The onset of stuttering*. Minneapolis: University of Minnesota Press.

Johnson, W., & Knott, J. R. (1937). The distribution of moments of stuttering in successive readings of the same material. *Journal of Speech Disorders, 2*, 17–19.

Jorgenson, C., Barrett, M., Huisingh, R., & Zachman, L. (1981). *The word test*. East Moline, IL: LinguiSystems.

Jung, J. H. (1989). *Genetic syndromes in communicative disorders*. Boston: Little, Brown and Co.

Kaplan, E., Goodglass, H., & Weintraub, S. (1983). *Boston naming test.* Philadelphia: Lea & Febiger.

Karnell, M. P. (1992). Adductor and abductor spasmodic dysphonia: Related until proven otherwise. *American Journal of Speech-Language Pathology, 1,* 17–18.

Kayser, H. (1989). Speech and language assessment of Spanish-English speaking children. *Language, Speech, and Hearing Services in Schools, 20,* 226–241.

Kempler, D. (1995). Language changes in dementia of the Alzheimer type. In R. Lubinski (Ed.), *Dementia and communication* (pp. 98–111). San Diego, CA: Singular.

Kertesz, A. (1982). *Western aphasia battery.* Orlando, FL: Grune & Stratton.

Kinzler, M., & Johnson, C. (1983). *Joliet 3-minute speech and language screening test.* Tuscon, AZ: Communication Skills Builders.

Kirk, S., McCarthy, J., & Kirk, W. (1968). *Illinois test of psycholinguistic abilities* (rev.). Urbana, IL: University of Illinois Press.

Knepfler, K. (1976). *Report writing.* Danville, IL: Interstate Printers & Publishers.

Kunz, J. R. M., & Finkel, A. J. (Eds.). (1987). *The American Medical Association family medical guide.* New York: Random House.

Labov, W. (1972). *Language in the inner city.* Philadelphia: University of Pennsylvania Press.

Lahey, M. (1988). *Language disorders and language development.* New York: Macmillan.

Lane, V. W., & Molyneaux, D. (1992). *The dynamics of communicative development.* Englewood Cliffs, NJ: Prentice-Hall.

Langdon, H., & Cheng, L. L. (1992). *Hispanic children and adults with communicative disorders: Assessment and intervention.* Gaithersburg, MD: Aspen.

Lanyon, R. (1967). The measurement of stuttering therapy. *Journal of Speech and Hearing Research, 10,* 836–843.

LaPointe, L. L. (1977). Base-10 programmed stimulation: Task specification, scoring and plotting performance in aphasia therapy. *Journal of Speech and Hearing Disorders, 42,* 90–105.

LaPointe, L. L. (1990). *Aphasia and related neurogenic language disorders.* New York: Thieme Medical Publishers.

LaPointe, L. L., & Wertz, R. T. (1974). Oral-movement abilities and articulatory characteristics of braininjured adults. *Perceptual and Motor Skills, 39,* 39–46.

Larson, D. E. (Ed.). (1990). *Mayo Clinic family health book.* New York: William Morrow.

Lee, L. (1974). *Developmental sentence analysis.* Evanston, IL: Northwestern University Press.

Lenneberg, E. (1969). On explaining language. *Science, 164,* 636.

Leonard, L. (1990). Language disorders in preschool children. In G.H. Shames & E.H. Wiig (Eds.), *Human communication disorders* (3rd ed., pp. 159–192). Columbus, OH: Merrill.

Logemann, J. A. (1983). *Evaluation and treatment of swallowing disorders.* San Diego: College-Hill Press.

Logemann, J. A. (1984). Evaluation and treatment of swallowing disorders. *Journal of the National Student Speech-Language-Hearing Association, 12*(1), 38–50.

Logemann, J. A. (1985). The relationship of speech and swallowing. *Seminars in Speech and Language, 6,* 351–359.

Logemann, J. A. (1990). Dysphagia. *Seminars in Speech and Language, 2,* 157–164.

Love, R. J. (1992). *Childhood motor speech disability.* Columbus, OH: Merrill/Macmillan.

Love, R. J., & Webb, W. G. (1992). *Neurology for the speech-language pathologist* (2nd ed.). Boston: Butterworth-Heinemann.

Lowe, R. J. (1986). *Assessment link between phonology and articulation (ALPHA).* East Moline, IL: LinguiSystems.

Lowe, R. J. (1989). *Workbook for the identification of phonological processes.* Danville, IL: Interstate Printers & Publishers.

Lucas, E. V. (1980). *Semantic and pragmatic language disorders: Assessment and remediation.* Rockville, MD: Aspen.

Lund, N. J., & Duchan, J. F. (1988). *Assessing children's language in naturalistic contexts* (2nd ed.). Englewood Cliffs, NJ: Prentice-Hall.

Lund, N. J., & Duchan, J. F. (1993). *Assessing children's language in naturalistic contexts* (3rd ed.). Englewood Cliffs, NJ: Prentice-Hall.

MacNeil, M. R. (1988). Aphasia in the adult. In N. J. Lass, L. V. McReynolds, J. L. Northern, & D. E. Yoder (Eds.), *Handbook of speech-language pathology and audiology* (pp. 738–786). Toronto: B. C. Decker.

Malkus, D., Booth, B., & Kodimer, C. (1980). *Rehabilitation of the head-injured adult: Comprehensive cognitive management.* Downey, CA: Professional Staff Association of Rancho Los Amigos Hospital, Inc.

Markwardt, F. C., (1989). *Peabody individual acheivement test—Revised.* Circle Pines, MN: AGS.

Marquardt, T. P., Stoll, J., & Sussman, H. (1990). Disorders of communication in traumatic brain injury. In E. D. Bigler (Ed.), *Traumatic brain injury* (pp.181–205). Austin, TX: PRO-ED.

Martin, D. E., (1994). Evaluating esophageal speech development and proficiency. In R. L. Keith & F. L. Darley (Eds.), *Laryngectomy rehabilitation* (3rd ed., pp. 331–349). Austin, TX: PRO-ED.

Martin, F. N. (1990). Hearing and hearing disorders. In G. H. Shames & E. H. Wiig (Eds.), *Human communication and its disorders* (3rd ed., pp. 350–392). Columbus, OH: Merrill.

Martin, F. N. (1994). *Introduction to audiology* (5th ed.). Englewood Cliffs, NJ: Prentice-Hall.

Martin, F. N., & Noble, B. (1994). Hearing and hearing disorders. In G. H. Shames, E. H. Wiig, & W. A. Secord (Eds.), *Human communication disorders: An introduction* (4th ed., pp. 388–436). New York: Macmillan.

Mason, R., & Simon, C. (1977). The orofacial examination checklist. *Language, Speech, and Hearing Services in Schools, 8,* 155–163.

Mattes, L. J., & Omark, D. R. (1991). *Speech and language assessment for the bilingual handicapped* (2nd ed.). Oceanside, CA: Academic Communication Associates.

McCormick, L., & Schiefelbusch, R. L. (1984). *Early language intervention.* Columbus, OH: Merrill.

McCormick, L., & Schiefelbusch, R. L. (1990). *Early language intervention* (2nd ed.). Columbus, OH: Merrill.

McDonald, E. T. (1976a). *A screening deep test of articulation with longitudinal norms.* Tucson, AZ: Communication Skill Builders.

McDonald, E. T. (1976b). *A deep test of articulation.* Tucson, AZ: Communication Skill Builders.

McNeil, M. R., & Prescott, T. E. (1978). *Token test—Revised.* Baltimore, MD: University Park Press.

McReynolds, L. V. (1990). Articulation and phonological disorders. In G. H. Shames & E. H. Wiig (Eds.), *Human communication disorders* (3rd ed., pp. 222–265). Columbus, OH: Merrill.

McWilliams, B. J., Morris, H. L., & Shelton, R. L. (1990). *Cleft palate speech* (2nd ed.). Philadelphia: B.C. Decker, Inc.

Meitus, I. J. (1983a). Clinical report and letter writing. In I. J. Meitus & B. Weinberg (Eds.), *Diagnosis in speech-language pathology* (pp. 287–309). Austin, TX: PRO-ED.

Meitus, I. J. (1983b). Talking with patients and their families. In I. J. Meitus & B. Weinberg (Eds.), *Diagnosis in speech-language pathology* (pp. 311–337). Austin, TX: PRO-ED.

Meitus, I. J., & Weinberg, B. (1983a). Gathering clinical information. In I. J. Weinberg (Eds.), *Diagnosis in speech-language pathology* (pp. 31–70). Austin, TX: PRO-ED.

Meitus, I. J., & Weinberg, B. (Eds.). (1983b). *Diagnosis in speech-language pathology.* Austin, TX: PRO-ED.

Miller, J. F. (1981). *Assessing language production in children.* Baltimore: University Park Press.

Miller, J. F., & Chapman, R. (1981). The relation between age and mean length of utterance in morphemes. *Journal of Speech and Hearing Research, 24,* 154–161.

Moller, K. T., & Starr, C. D. (1993). *Cleft palate: Interdisciplinary issues and treatment.* Austin, TX: PRO-ED.

Morley, M. E. (1970). *Cleft palate and speech* (7th ed.). Edinburgh: E. & S. Livingstone.

Morris, H. L. (1990). Clinical assessment by the speech pathologist. In J. Bardach & H. L. Morris (Eds.), *Multidisciplinary management of cleft lip and palate* (pp. 757–762). Philadelphia: W. B. Saunders Company.

Morris, H. L., Spriestersbach, D. C., & Darley, F. L. (1961). An articulation test for assessing velopharyngeal closure. *Journal of Speech and Hearing Research, 4*, 48–55.

Morrison, M., Rammage, L., Nichol, H., Pullan, B., May, P., & Salkeld, L. (1994). *The management of voice disorders.* San Diego, CA: Singular Publishing Group.

Mowrer, D. (1988). *Methods of modifying speech behaviors: Learning theory in speech pathology* (2nd ed.). Prospect Heights, IL: Waveland Press.

Mumm, M., Secord, W., & Dykstra, K. (1980). *Merrill language screening test.* Columbus, OH: Merrill.

Musselwhite, C. R., & St. Louis, K. W. (1988). *Communication programming for persons with severe handicaps: Vocal and augmentative strategies* (2nd ed.). Austin, TX: PRO-ED.

Nation, J. E., & Aram, D. M. (1991). *Diagnosis of speech and language disorders* (2nd ed.). San Diego: Singular Publishing Group.

National Center for Health Research. (1989). *The role of speech language pathologists in the management of dysphagia* (Health Tech. Rep., No. 1). Rockville, MD: National Center for Health Services Research.

National Institutes of Health. (1984). *Head injury: Hope through research.* Bethesda, MD: National Institutes of Health.

Naugle, R. I. (1990). Epidemiology of traumatic brain injury in adults. In E. D. Bigler (Ed.), *Traumatic brain injury* (pp. 69–103). Austin, TX: PRO-ED.

Neidecker, E. A. (1987). *School programs in speech-language: Organization and management* (2nd ed.). Englewood Cliffs, NJ: Prentice-Hall.

Nemoy, E. M., & Davis, S. F. (1980). *The correction of defective consonant sounds* (16th printing). Londonberry, NH: Expression Co.

Newcomer, P. L., & Hammill, D. D. (1988a). *Test of language development-2 intermediate.* Austin, TX: PRO-ED.

Newcomer, P. L., & Hammill, D. D. (1988b). *Test of language development-2 primary.* Austin, TX: PRO-ED.

Newman, P. W., Creaghead, N. A., & Secord, W. (1985). *Assessment and remediation of articulatory and phonological disorders.* Columbus, OH: Merrill.

Nicolosi, L., Harryman, E., & Kreshek, J. (1996). *Terminology of communication disorders speech-language-hearing* (4th ed.). Baltimore: Williams & Wilkins.

Northern, J. L. (Ed.). (1996). *Hearing disorders* (3rd ed.). Needham Heights, MA: Allyn & Bacon.

Northern, J. L., & Downs, M. P. (1991). *Hearing in children* (4th ed.). Baltimore: Williams & Wilkins.

Olin, W. H. (1960). *Cleft lip and palate rehabilitation.* Springfield: C. C. Thomas.

Oller, D. K, & Eilers, R. E. (Eds.). (1988). Tactile artificial hearing for the deaf. In F. H. Bess (Ed.), *Hearing impairment in children* (pp. 310–328). Parkton, MD: York Press.

Overman, C. A., & Geoffrey, V. C. (1987). Alzheimer's disease and other dementias. In H. G. Mueller & V. C. Geoffrey (Eds.), *Communication disorders in aging: Assessment and management* (pp. 271–297). Washington, DC: Gallaudet University Press.

Owens, E., & Kessler, D. K. (Eds.). (1989). *Cochlear implants in young deaf children.* Boston: College-Hill Press.

Owens, R. E. (1991). *Language disorders: A functional approach to assessment and intervention.* Columbus, OH: Merrill/Macmillan.

Owens, R. E. (1995). *Language disorders: A functional approach to assessment and intervention.* (3rd ed.). Needham Heights, MA: Allyn & Bacon.

Owens, R. E. (1996). *Language development: An introduction* (4th ed.). Needham Heights, MA: Allyn & Bacon.

Owens, R. E., Haney, M. J., Giesow, V. E., Dooley, L. F., & Kelly, R. J. (1983). Language test content: A comparative study. *Language, Speech, and Hearing Services in Schools, 14*, 7–21.

Palmer, J. M., & Yantis, P. A. (1990). *Survey of communication disorders.* Baltimore: Williams & Wilkins.

Payne, J. C. (1997). *Adult neurogenic language disorders: Assessment and treatment.* San Diego, CA: Singular.

Pendergest, K., Dickey, S., Selmar, J., & Sudar, A. (1984). *Photo articulation test* (2nd ed.). Interstate Printers & Publishers.

Perkins, W. H. (1977). *Speech pathology: An applied behavioral science* (2nd ed.). St. Louis: C. V. Mosby.

Perkins, W. H: (Ed.). (1980). *Strategies in stuttering therapy.* New York: Thieme-Stratton.

Perkins, W. H. (Ed.). (1983). *Dysarthria and apraxia.* New York: Thieme-Stratton.

Perkins, W. H. (Ed.). (1984). *Stuttering disorders.* New York: Thieme-Stratton.

Perkins, W. H., & Kent, R. D. (1986). *Functional anatomy of speech, language and hearing.* San Diego: College-Hill Press.

Perlman, A. L., & Schulze-Delrieu, K. S. (Eds.). (1997). *Deglutition and its disorders.* San Diego, CA: Singular.

Peters, T. J., & Guitar, B. (1991). *Stuttering: An integrated approach to its nature and treatment.* Baltimore: Williams & Wilkins.

Peterson, C. W. (1981). *Conversation starters for speech-language pathology.* Danville, IL: Interstate Printers & Publishers.

Peterson, H. A., & Marquardt, T. P. (1994). *Appraisal and diagnosis of speech and language disorders* (3rd ed.). Englewood Cliffs, NJ: Prentice-Hall.

Pimental, P. A., & Kingsbury, N. A. (1989). *Mini inventory of right brain injury (MIRBI).* Austin, TX: PRO-ED.

Poole, E. (1934). Genetic development of articulation of consonant sounds in speech. *Elementary English Review, 11*, 159–161.

Porch, B. E. (1981). *Porch index of communicative ability* (3rd ed.). Palo Alto, CA: Consulting Psychologists Press.

Prater, R. J., & Swift, R. W. (1984). *Manual of voice therapy.* Boston: Little, Brown and Co.

Prather, E. M., Breecher, S., Stafford, M. L., & Wallace, E. (1980). *Screening test for adolescent language.* Seattle: University of Washington Press.

Prather, E., Hedrick, D., & Kern, C. (1975). Articulation development in children aged two to four years. *Journal of Speech and Hearing Disorders, 40*, 179–191.

Purcell, R. M., & Runyan, C. M. (1980). Normative study of speech rates of children. *Journal of the Speech and Hearing Association of Virginia, 21*, 6–14.

Reed, V. A. (1994). *An introduction to children with language disorders* (2nd ed.). New York: Macmillan.

Reese, R. E., & Douglas, R. G. (Eds.). (1983). *A practical approach to infectious diseases.* Boston: Little, Brown and Co.

Reich, P. A. (1986). *Language development.* Englewood Cliffs, NJ: Prentice-Hall.

Reisberg, B., Feris, S. H., DeLeon, M. S., & Crook, T. (1982). The global deterioration scale for assessment of primary degenerative dementia. *American Journal of Psychiatry, 139*, 1136–1139.

Reitan, R. M., & Davison, L. A. (Eds.). (1974). *Clinical neuropsychology: Current status and applications.* New York: Winston-Wiley.

Retherford, K. (1993). *Guide to analysis of language transcripts* (2nd ed.). Eau Claire, WI: Thinking Publications.

Riley, G. D. (1981). *Stuttering prediction instrument*. Austin, TX: PRO-ED.

Riley, G. D. (1986). *Stuttering severity instrument*. Austin, TX: PRO-ED.

Ripich, D. N. (1991). Language and communication in dementia. In D. Ripich (Ed.), *Handbook of geriatric communication disorders* (pp. 255–283). Austin, TX: PRO-ED.

Ripich, D. N. (1995). Differential diagnosis and assessment. In R. Lubinski (Ed.), *Dementia and communication* (pp. 188–222). San Diego, CA: Singular.

Roeser, R. J. (1986). *Diagnostic audiology: The PRO-ED studies in communicative disorders*. Austin, TX: PRO–ED.

Roeser, R. J., & Downs, M. P. (Eds.). (1995). *Auditory disorders in school children: The law, identification, remediation* (3rd ed.). New York: Thieme Medical.

Rodgers, W. C. (1976). *Articulation and language screening test*. Austin, TX: PRO–ED.

Rosenbek, J. C. (1985). Treating apraxia of speech. In D. F. Johns (Ed.), *Clinical management of neurogenic communicative disorders* (2nd ed., pp. 267–312). Boston: Little, Brown and Co.

Rosenbek, J. C., Kent, R. D., & LaPointe, L. L. (1984). Apraxia of speech: An overview and some perspectives. In J. C. Rosenbek, M. R. McNeil, & A. E. Aronson (Eds.), *Apraxia of speech: Physiology, acoustics, linguistics, management* (pp. 1–72). San Diego: College-Hill Press.

Rosenbek, J. C., & LaPointe, L. L. (1985). The dysarthrias: Description, diagnosis, and treatment. In D. F. Johns (Ed.), *Clinical management of neurogenic communicative disorders* (2nd ed., pp. 97–152). Boston: Little, Brown and Co.

Rosenbek, J. C., LaPointe, L. L., & Wertz, W. T. (1989). *Aphasia: A clinical approach*. Austin, TX: PRO-ED.

Ross-Swain, D. (1996). *Ross information processing assessment* (2nd ed.). Austin, TX: PRO-ED.

Ross-Swain, D., & Fogle, P. (1996). *Ross information processing assessment—Geriatric*. Austin, TX: PRO-ED.

Roth, F., & Spekman, N. (1984a). Assessing the pragmatic abilities of children: Part 1. Organizational and assessment parameters. *Journal of Speech and Hearing Disorders, 49*, 2–11.

Roth, F., & Spekman, N. (1984b). Assessing the pragmatic abilities of children: Part 2. Guide lines, considerations, and specific evaluation procedures. *Journal of Speech and Hearing Disorders, 49*, 12–17.

Rothenberg, M. A., & Chapman, C. F. (1989). *Dictionary of medical terms for the nonmedical person* (2nd ed.). New York: Barron's Educational Series.

Sander, E. (1972). When are speech sounds learned? *Journal of Speech and Hearing Disorders, 37*, 55–63.

Sander, D. A. (1993). *Management of hearing handicap: Infants to elderly* (3rd ed.). Englewood Cliffs, NJ: Prentice-Hall.

Sanders, L. J. (1979). *Procedure guides for evaluation of speech and hearing disorders in children* (4th ed.) Danville, IL: Interstate Printers & Publishers.

Sawyer, J. (1973). Social aspects of bilingualism in San Antonio, Texas. In R. Bailey & J. Robinson (Eds.), *Varieties of present-day English* (pp. 226–235). New York: Macmillan.

Saxton, J., McGonigle, K. L., Swihart, A. A., & Boller, F. (1993). *Severe impairment battery*. Bury St. Edmunds, UK: Thames Valley Test Company.

Schow, R. L., & Nerbonne, M. A. (Eds.). (1989). *Introduction to aural rehabilitation* (2nd ed.). Austin, TX: PRO-ED.

Schuell, H. (1965). *The Minnesota test for differential diagnosis of aphasia*. Minneapolis: University of Minnesota Press.

Schulman, E. D. (1991). *Intervention in human services: A guide to skills and knowledge* (4th ed.). New York: Merrill.

Sell, D., Harding, A., & Grunwell, P. (1994). A screening assessment of cleft palate speech (Great Ormond Street Speech Assessment). *European Journal of Disorders of Communication, 29*, 1–15.

Semel, E., Wiig, E. H., & Secord, W. (1987). *Clinical evaluation of language fundamentals—Revised*. New York: Psychological Corporation.

Semel, E., Wiig, E. H., & Secord, W. (1989). *CELF-R test (Clinical evaluation of language fundamentals—Revised)*. New York: Psychological Corporation.

Semel-Mintz, E., & Wiig, E. H. (1982). *Clinical evaluation of language functions*. New York: Psychological Corporation.

Shames, G. H. (1990). Disorders of fluency. In G. H. Shames & E. H. Wiig (Eds.), *Human communication disorders* (3rd ed., pp. 306–349). Columbus, OH: Merrill.

Shane, H. C., & Sauer, M. (1986). *Augmentative and alternative communication*. Austin, TX: PRO-ED.

Shipley, K. G. (1981). Interpreting results obtained from Carrow's TACL. *Journal of Speech and Hearing Disorders, 46*, 222–223.

Shipley, K. G. (1990). *Systematic assessment of voice*. Oceanside, CA: Academic Communication Associates.

Shipley, K. G. (1992). *Interviewing and counseling in communicative disorders: Principles and procedures*. New York: Merrill/Macmillan.

Shipley, K. G., Recor, D. B., & Nakamura, S. M. (1990). *Sourcebook of apraxia remediation activities*. Oceanside, CA: Academic Communication Associates.

Shipley, K. G., Stone, T. A., & Sue, M. B. (1983). *Test for examining expressive morphology (TEEM)*. Tucson, AZ: Communication Skills Builders.

Shprintzen, R. J., & Bardach, J. (1995). *Cleft palate speech management: A multidisciplinary approach*. St. Louis: Mosby.

Shriberg, L. D., & Kent, R D. (1995). *Clinical phonetics* (2nd ed,). Boston: Allyn & Bacon.

Shriberg, L. D., & Kwiatkowski, J. (1980). *Natural process analysis*. New York: John Wiley & Sons.

Shriberg, L. D., & Kwiatkowski, J. (1983). Computer-assisted natural process analysis (NPA): Recent issues and data. *Seminars in Speech and Language, 4*, 397–406.

Shumak, I. C. (1955). A speech situation rating sheet for stutterers. In W. Johnson & R. R. Leutenegger (Eds.), *Stuttering in children and adults* (pp. 341–347). Minneapolis: University of Minnesota Press.

Silverman, F. H. (1980). Dimensions of improvement in stuttering. *Journal of Speech and Hearing Research, 23*, 137–151.

Silverman, F. H. (1995). *Communication for the speechless* (3rd ed.). Needham Heights, MA: Allyn & Bacon.

Simon, C. S. (1986). *Evaluating communicative competence: A functional pragmatic procedure* (rev. ed.). Tucson, AZ: Communication Skill Builders.

Sohlberg, M. M., & Mateer, C. A. (1989). *Introduction to cognitive rehabilitation: Theory and practice*. New York: The Guilford Press.

Sparks, S. N. (1984). *Birth defects and speech-language disorders*. San Diego: College-Hill Press.

Spriestersbach, D. C., Morris, H. L., & Darley, F. L. (1978). Examination of the speech mechanism. In F. L. Darley & D. C. Spriestersbach (Eds.), *Diagnostic methods in speech pathology* (2nd ed., pp. 322–345). New York: Harper & Row.

Starkweather, C. W. (1987). *Fluency and stuttering*. Englewood Cliffs, NJ: Prentice-Hall.

Starkweather, C. W., Gottwald, S. R., & Halfond, M. H. (1990). *Stuttering prevention: A clinical method*. Englewood Cliffs, NJ: Prentice-Hall.

Stemple, J. C. (1992). *Clinical voice management: Techniques for children*. St. Louis: Mosby Year Book.

Stemple, J. C., Glaze, L. E., & Gerdeman, B. K. (1995). *Clinical voice pathology: Theory and management* (2nd ed.). San Diego, CA: Singular.

Stephens, I. (1977). *The Stephens oral language screening test*. Penninsula, OH: Interim Publishers.

St. Louis, K. O. (Ed.). (1986). *The atypical stutterer: Principles and practices of rehabilitation*. New York: Academic Press.

St. Louis, K. O., Hinzman, A. R., & Hull, F. M. (1985). Studies of cluttering: Disfluency and language measures in young possible clutterers and stutterers. *Journal of Fluency Disorders, 10,* 151–172.

St. Louis, K. O., & Ruscello, D. M. (1987). *Oral speech mechanism screening examination* (rev.). Austin, TX: PRO-ED.

Stewart, C. J., & Cash, W. B. (1991). *Interviewing: Principles and practices* (6th ed.). Dubuque, IA: William C. Brown.

Stoel-Gammon, C., & Dunn, C. (1985). *Normal and disordered phonology in children.* Austin, TX: PRO-ED.

Taylor, J. S. (1992). *Speech-language pathology services in the schools* (2nd ed.). Needham Heights, MA: Allyn & Bacon.

Taylor, O. L. (1986a). Language differences. In G. H. Shames & E. H. Wiig (Eds.), *Human communication disorders* (2nd ed., pp. 385–413). Columbus, OH: Merrill.

Taylor, O. L. (Ed.). (1986b). *Nature of communication disorders in culturally and linguistically diverse populations.* San Diego: College-Hill Press.

Taylor, O. L. (Ed.). (1986c). *Treatment of communication disorders in culturally and linguistically diverse populations.* San Diego: College-Hill Press.

Taylor, O. L. (1990). Language and communication differences. In G. H. Shames & E. H. Wiig (Eds.), *Human communication disorders* (3rd ed., pp. 126–158). Columbus, OH: Merrill.

Taylor, O. L. (in press). Clinical practice as a social occasion. In L. Cole & V. Deal (Eds.), *Communication disorders in multicultural populations.* Rockville, MD: American Speech-Language-Hearing Association.

Templin, M. (1957). *Certain language skills in children: Their development and interrelationships* (Institute of Child Welfare, Monograph, No. 26). Minneapolis: The University of Minnesota Press.

Templin, M. C., & Darley, F. L. (1969). *Templin-Darley tests of articulation* (2nd ed.). Iowa City: University of Iowa.

Thomas, C. L. (Ed.). (1989). *Taber's cyclopedic medical dictionary* (16th ed.). Philadelphia: F. A. Davis Co.

Tompkins, C. A. (1995). *Right hemisphere communication disorders: Theory and management.* San Diego, CA: Singular.

Trost, J. E. (1981). Articulatory additions to the classical description of the speech of persons with cleft palate. *Cleft Palate Journal, 18*(3), 193–203.

Trost-Cardamone, J. E., & Bernthal, J. E. (1993). Articulation assessment procedures and treatment decisions. In K. T. Moller & C. D. Starr (Eds.), *Cleft palate: Interdisciplinary issues and treatment* (pp. 307–336). Austin, TX: PRO-ED.

Tyack, D., & Gottsleben, R. (1974). *Language sampling, analysis, and training: A handbook for teachers and clinicians.* Palo Alto, CA: Consulting Psychologists Press.

Ulliana, L., & Ingham, R. J. (1984). Behavioral and nonbehavioral variables in the measurement of stutterers' communication attitudes. *Journal of Speech and Hearing Disorders, 49,* 83–93.

Van Riper, C. (1971). *The nature of stuttering.* Englewood Cliffs, NJ: Prentice-Hall.

Van Riper, C. (1973). *The treatment of stuttering.* Englewood Cliffs, NJ: Prentice-Hall.

Van Riper, C., & Emerick, L. (1996). *Speech correction: An introduction to speech pathology and audiology* (9th ed.). Needham Heights, MA: Allyn & Bacon.

Van Riper, C., & Erickson, R. L. (1973). *Predictive screening test of articulation* (3rd ed.). Kalamazoo: Western Michigan University.

Watterson, T., & McFarlane, S. C. (1992). Adductor and abductor spasmotic dysphonia: Different disorders. *American Journal of Speech Pathology, 1,* 19–20.

Wechsler, D. (1981). *Wechsler adult intelligence scale—Revised.* New York: Psychological Corporation.

Wechsler, D. (1987). *Wechsler memory scale—Revised.* New York: Psychological Corporation.

Weiner, A. E. (1984). Vocal control therapy for stutterers. In M. Peins (Ed.), *Contemporary approaches in stuttering therapy* (pp. 217–269). Boston: Little, Brown and Co.

Weiner, F., & Lewnau, L. (1979, November). *Nondiscriminatory speech and language testing of minority children: Linguistic interferences*. Paper presented at the Annual Convention of the American Speech-Language-Hearing Association, Atlanta.

Weiner, F. F. (1979). *Phonological process analysis*. Austin, TX: PRO-ED.

Weiss, C. E., Gordon, M. E., & Lillywhite, H. S., (1987). *Clinical management of articulation disorders* (2nd ed.). Baltimore: Williams & Wilkens.

Weiss, D. A. (1964). *Cluttering*. Englewood Cliffs, NJ: Prentice-Hall.

Wellman, B., Case, I., Mengurt, I., & Bradbury, D. (1931). *Speech sounds of young children* (University of Iowa Studies in Child Welfare No. 5). Iowa City: University of Iowa Press.

Wells, G. B. (1987). *Stuttering treatment: A comprehensive clinical guide*. Englewood Cliffs, NJ: Prentice-Hall.

Wertz, R. T., LaPointe, L. L., & Rosenbek, J. C. (1991). *Apraxia of speech in adults: The disorder and its management*. San Diego: Singular Publishing Group.

Wiener, S., & Young, J. (1988). *FullWrite™ Professional Version 1.1* [computer software]. Torrance, CA: Ashton-Tate Corp.

Wiig, E., & Semel, E. (1995). *Clinical evaluations of language functions—3*. San Antonio, TX: The Psychological Corporation.

Wiig, E., Secord, W., & Semel, E. (1992). *Clinical evaluation of language functions—preschool*. San Antonio, TX: The Psychological Corporation.

Wiig, E. H., & Semel, E. (1984). *Language assessment and intervention for the learning disabled* (2nd ed.). Columbus, OH: Merrill.

Williams, D. E. (1978). The problem of stuttering. In F. L. Darley & D. C. Spriestersbach (Eds.), *Diagnostic methods in speech pathology* (2nd ed., pp. 284–321). New York: Harper & Row.

Williams, F., Cairns, H., & Cairns, C. (1971). *An analysis of the variations from standard English pronunciation in the phonetic performance of two nonstandard-English-speaking children*. Dallas: Center for Communication Research, University of Texas.

Williams, R., & Wolfram, W. (1977). *Social dialects: Differences vs. disorders*. Washington, DC: American Speech-Language-Hearing Association.

Williams, W. B., Stemach, G., Wolfe, S., & Stanger, C. (1993). *Lifespace access profile: Assistive technology planning for individuals with severe or multiple disabilities*. Sebastopol, CA: Lifespace Access.

Wilson, D. K. (1987). *Voice problems of children* (3rd ed.). Baltimore: Williams & Wilkins.

Wilson, F. B., & Rice, M. (1977). *A programmed approach to voice therapy*. Allen, TX: DLM/Teaching Resources.

Wingate, M. (1976). *Stuttering theory and treatment*. New York: Irvington Publishers.

Witzel, M. A., & Stringer, D. A. (1990). Methods of assessing velopharyngeal function. In J. Bardach & H. L. Morris (Eds.), *Multidisciplinary management of cleft lip and palate* (pp. 763–775). Philadelphia: W. B. Saunders Company.

Wolery, M. (1989). Using direct observation in assessment. In D. B. Bailey & M. Wolery (Eds.), *Assessing infants and preschoolers with handicaps* (pp. 64–96). Columbus, OH: Merrill.

Wolfram, W., & Fasold, R. W. (1974). *The study of social dialects in American English*. Englewood Cliffs, NJ: Prentice-Hall.

Woodcock, R. W., & Johnson, M. B. (1977). *Woodcock-Johnson psychoeducational battery, part one: Tests of cognitive ability*. Hingham, MA: Teaching Resources.

Ylvisaker, M. S., & Holland, A. L. (1985). Coaching, self-coaching, and rehabilitation of head injury. In D. F. Johns (Ed.), *Clinical management of neurogenic communicative disorders* (pp. 243–257). Boston: Little, Brown and Co.

Yorkston, K. M., Beukelman, D., & Bell, K. R. (1988). *Clinical management of dysarthric speakers*. Austin, TX: PRO-ED.

Yorkston, K. M., Beukelman, D. P., & Traynor, C. (1984). *Assessment of intelligibility of dysarthric speech*. Austin, TX: PRO-ED.

Yoss, K. A., & Darley, F. L. (1974). Therapy in developmental apraxia of speech. *Language, Speech, and Hearing Services in Schools, 5*, 23–31.

Zimmerman, I., Steiner, V., & Evatt-Pond, R. (1991). *The preschool language scale III*. San Antonio, TX: The Psychological Corporation.

□ INDEX □